NURSING CARE OF THE BURN-INJURED PATIENT

Rita Bolek Trofino, R.N., M.N.Ed.
Assistant Professor
Department of Nursing
Saint Francis College
Loretto, Pennsylvania

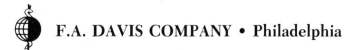

F.A. DAVIS COMPANY • Philadelphia

Printed in the United States of America

Last digit indicates print number: 10 9 8 7 6 5 4 3 2 1

NOTE: As new scientific information becomes available through basic and clinical research, recommended treatments and drug therapies undergo changes. The author(s)
and publisher have done everything possible to make this book accurate, up-to-date, and
in accord with accepted standards at the time of publication. The authors, editors and
publisher are not responsible for errors or omissions or for consequences from application of the book, and make no warranty, expressed or implied, in regard to the contents
of the book. Any practice described in this book should be applied by the reader in
accordance with professional standards of care used in regard to the unique circumstances that may apply in each situation. The reader is advised always to check product
information (package inserts) for changes and new information regarding dose and
contraindications before administering any drug. Caution is especially urged when using
new or infrequently ordered drugs.

Library of Congress Cataloging-in-Publication Data

Nursing care of the burn-injured patient / [editor] Rita Bolek
    Trofino.
        p.   cm.
    Includes bibliographical references and index.
    ISBN 0-8036-8658-7 (hardcover : alk. paper)
        1. Burns and scalds — Nursing.   I. Trofino, Rita Bolek, 1954–
    [DNLM: 1. Burns — nursing.   WY 161 N9737]
    RD96.4.N87   1991
    610.73′677 — dc20
    DNLM/DLC
    for Library of Congress   90-15722
                                                                    CIP

PREFACE

Nursing care of the patient with burns is a specialized area of nursing that requires a unique body of knowledge. It encompasses a wide variety of nursing roles and responsibilities. New developments in this area of nursing, and especially in the care of the patient with a major burn, make this nursing specialty a difficult but rewarding challenge.

The purpose of this book is to provide a reference for the nurse, in different settings, in caring for patients of all ages with various types of burn injuries. Selected contributors with exceptional expertise provide comprehensive information. Key features of this book are the care plans which utilize approved nursing diagnoses, as proposed by the North American Nursing Diagnosis Association. Additionally, care plans are prioritized and differentiated into independent and collaborative areas.

Rita Bolek Trofino

ACKNOWLEDGMENTS

This book is dedicated to my loved ones, my patient and supportive husband Ralph, and my loving children, Joseph, Thomas, and Maria. I would also like to thank my father, Walter Bolek and late mother, Irene, for their constant encouragement and support throughout my nursing career.

To the F. A. Davis Company, I am truly grateful, especially to the following people for their time and effort in this project, as well as their encouragement and support: Linda Nold, former Nursing Editor, Robert G. Martone, Senior Editor, Ruth De George, Alan Sorkowitz, who helped bring this project to fruition; Herb Powell, Gail Chaiken and finally, to Judy Ilov who brought this project to the attention of the nursing department.

I would also like to acknowledge and thank all of the contributing authors who shared their educational and clinical expertise in writing the chapters. Without their contributions, this book would not exist.

This book is further enriched by the color graphics. I would like to especially thank Dr. Harvey Slater from the Burn Trauma Unit at The Western Pennsylvania Hospital, Pittsburgh, PA, for the many color slides that he so graciously provided to enhance this book.

Finally, I dedicate this book to all nurses who care for patients with burns. And especially the burn patients who daily face the challenge of recovery.

Rita Bolek Trofino

FOREWORD

Nursing care of the burn-injured patient has changed dramatically over the past two decades. These changes have paralleled the advances in medical therapy, technological innovations, and the profession of nursing itself. Changes in medical therapy and advances in medical technology have led to decreased morbidity (as evidenced by decreased hospital stays), improved survival and improved functional and cosmetic results. These changes have been accomplished by the dedication of nurses, physicians, therapists, and a myriad of other health care workers, working together as a team. Although there may be innovations that are closely associated with a specific nurse's name, there are those associated with physicians' names such as the Evan's or Baxter's Resuscitation Formulas, Burke's Artificial Skin or the Swan Ganz Catheter; nurses have been instrumental in these and other innovations.

Likewise, the advances in nursing towards professional status has had its impact on the nursing care of burn patients. The movement toward clinical specialization at the graduate level and the development, in the early 1970's, of the first clinical nurse specialist program in burn nursing was a major factor in advancing the role of nurses and nursing in the care of these complex patients. In addition, the development of Guidelines for Burn Nursing Practice developed jointly by the American Burn Association and the American Nurses Association in the late 1970's provided the recognition of burn nursing as a clinical subspecialty in nursing.

Burn nursing encompasses many of the fields of nursing whether one uses the more conventional titles such as medical-surgical, pediatrics, obstetrical, psychiatric, and public health nursing or whether one prefers to view nursing by its many subspecialties such as parent-child nursing, oncological, gerontological, neurological, cardiac, critical care, etc. or whether one takes a broader approach and considers the fields of nursing to be individual or group adaptation to physical, psychological, or environmental derangements. Thus, the nurse involved in burn care must possess the knowledge and skills related to many of the fields of nursing. It is not enough to be an expert critical care nurse and deal with the physiologic derangements caused by the patient's response to the burn injury; but one must possess the skills, knowledge, and patience to deal with the psychological and rehabilitation problems as they affect the patients with burn injury across the life-span. To this end a nursing text which emphasizes nursing process and focuses on all aspects of burn care from emergency treatment through rehabilitation and across all age groups should make a significant contribution to the care of these complex patients.

Janet A. Marvin, R.N., M.N.

CONTRIBUTORS

Elizabeth W. Bayley, Ph.D., R.N.
Associate Professor
Burn, Emergency and Trauma Nursing
Widener University
Chester, Pennsylvania

Lisa Marie Bernardo, R.N., M.S.N., CCRN
Instructor of Nursing
Parent Child Graduate Program
University of Pittsburgh
Trauma Clinical Nurse Specialist
Children's Hospital of Pittsburgh
Pittsburgh, Pennsylvania

Anne E. Braun, R.N.C., M.S.N., CCRN, C.E.N.
Instructor
Critical Care Nursing
Crozer-Chester Medical Center
Chester, Pennsylvania

Elizabeth I. Helvig, R.N., M.S.
Director of Nursing Education
Shriners Burns Institute
Galveston, Texas

Doreen J. Konop, R.N., B.S.N.
Nurse Manager
Burn Trauma Center
The Western Pennsylvania Hospital
Pittsburgh, Pennsylvania

Melva Kravitz, R.N., PH.S.
Director of Nursing
Shriners Burns Institute
    and
Associate Professor
University of Texas
Medical Branch
School of Nursing
Galveston, Texas

Madeleine T. Martin, R.N., M.S.N., Ed.D.
Professor
University of Cincinnati
College of Nursing and Health
Cincinnati, Ohio

Janet A. Marvin, R.N., M.N.
Associate Professor
Department of Surgery
University of Washington
School of Medicine
    and
Department of Physiological Nursing
University of Washington
School of Nursing
    and
Associate Director
University of Washington
Burn Center at Harborview Medical Center
Seattle, Washington

Patricia M. Orr, R.N., M.B.A., CCRN, C.N.A.
Director — Critical Care
Saint Agnes Medical Center
Philadelphia, Pennsylvania

Denise A. Sadowski, R.N., M.S.N.
Burn Clinical Specialist
Shriners Burns Institute
Cincinnati, Ohio

Lorna L. Schumann, Ph.D., R.N., C.S., CCRN, A.R.N.P.
Assistant Professor of Nursing
Intercollegiate Center for Nursing Education
Spokane, Washington

Roslyn Seligman, M.D.
Associate Professor
Department of Psychiatry
University of Cincinnati
Medical Sciences Building
Cincinnati, Ohio

Patricia Smith-Regojo, R.N., B.S.N.
Head Nurse
Burn Treatment Center
Saint Agnes Medical Center
Philadelphia, Pennsylvania

Kathleen Sullivan, Ph.D., R.N.
Director of Nursing for Patient Care and Research
Children's Hospital of Pittsburgh
Pittsburgh, Pennsylvania

Yvonne Troiani Sweeney, M.S.N., R.N.
Burn Nurse Consultant
Burn Foundation Nurse Advisory Council
Philadelphia, Pennsylvania

Patricia Vaccaro, R.N., CCRN
Clinical Instructor
Burn Center/Plastics Unit
The Allentown and Lehigh Valley Hospital Center
Allentown, Pennsylvania

Mary M. Wagner, M.S., R.N., C.S.
Clinical Assistant Professor
University of South Carolina
College of Nursing
Columbia, South Carolina

CONSULTANTS

Barbara J. Bunker, R.N., M.S.N.
Associate Professor
University of North Carolina
School of Nursing
Chapel Hill, North Carolina

Suzanne S. Cooke, R.N., C.S., M.S.N.
Associate Professor of Clinical Nursing
Texas Tech University
Health Sciences Center
School of Nursing
Lubbock, Texas

Deanna Epley, M.Ed., M.S.N.
Assistant Professor
School of Nursing
Barry University
Miami, Florida

Janice M. Fitzgerald, M.S.N., R.N.
Doctoral Candidate and Research Assistant
University of Maryland
School of Nursing
Baltimore, Maryland

Mary D. Gordon, R.N., M.S.
Associate Editor
Journal of Burn Care and Rehabilitation
Dallas, Texas

Cynthia A. Horvath, B.S., M.S.
University of Alabama at Birmingham
School of Nursing
Assistant Professor of Nursing
Birmingham, Alabama

Deborah Goldenberg Klein, M.S.N., CCRN, C.S.
Clinical Nurse Specialist
Trauma/Critical Care Nursing
Metro Health Medical Center
Cleveland, Ohio
and
Clinical Instructor
Medical-Surgical Nursing
Frances Payne Bolton School of Nursing
Case Western Research University
Cleveland, Ohio

Jane M. Kurz, B.S.N., M.S.N., R.N.
Instructor in Nursing
Holy Family College
Philadelphia, Pennsylvania

Arlene C. Miller, R.N., M.S.N.
Burn Clinical Nurse Specialist
University Hospital
University of Cincinnati, Medical Center
Cincinnati, Ohio

M.K. Gaedeke Norris, R.N., B.S.N.
Instructor, School of Nursing
Good Samaritan Hospital
Cincinnati, Ohio

Gwendolyn A. Smith, B.S.N., M.B.A.
Clinical Coordinator of Burn Treatment Center
Crozer-Chester Medical Center
Chester, Pennsylvania

Mary L. Stoeckel, R.N., M.S.N., CCRN
Clinical Nurse Specialist
Our Lady of Mercy Hospital
Cincinnati, Ohio

CONTENTS

NURSING CARE PLANS

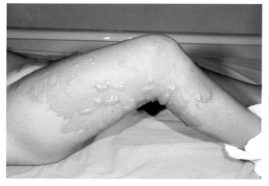

Color Plate 1.

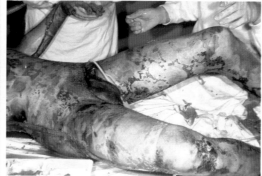

Color Plate 2.

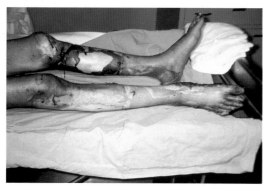

Color Plate 3.

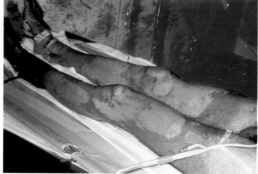

Color Plate 4.

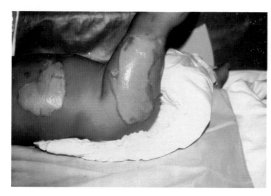

Color Plate 5.

Color Plate 6.

Color Plate 1. Superficial partial-thickness burn. (Courtesy of The Western Pennsylvania Hospital Burn Trauma Center, Pittsburgh, PA.)

Color Plate 2. Deep partial-thickness burn. (Courtesy of The Western Pennsylvania Hospital Burn Trauma Center, Pittsburgh, PA.)

Color Plate 3. Full-thickness burn. (Courtesy of The Western Pennsylvania Hospital Burn Trauma Center, Pittsburgh, PA.)

Color Plate 4. Flame burn. (Courtesy of The Western Pennsylvania Hospital Burn Trauma Center, Pittsburgh, PA.)

Color Plate 5. Scald burn (leg and chest). (Courtesy of The Western Pennsylvania Hospital Burn Trauma Center, Pittsburgh, PA.)

Color Plate 6. Chemical burn (legs). (Courtesy of The Western Pennsylvania Hospital Burn Trauma Center, Pittsburgh, PA.)

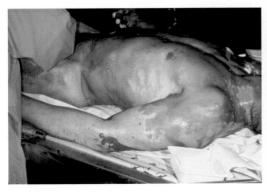

Color Plate 7.

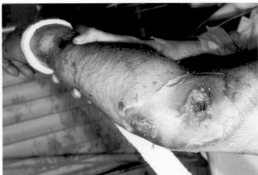

Color Plate 8.

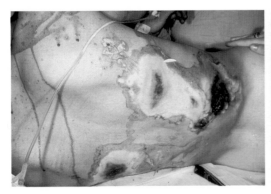

Color Plate 9.

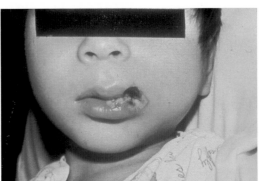

Color Plate 10.

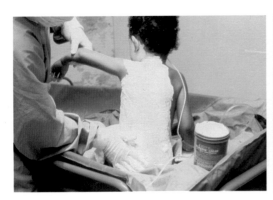

Color Plate 11.

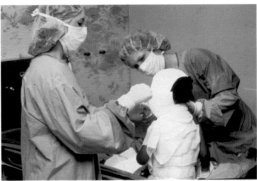

Color Plate 12.

Color Plate 7.   Chemical burn. (Courtesy of The Western Pennsylvania Hospital Burn Trauma Center, Pittsburgh, PA.)

Color Plate 8.   Electrical burn (elbow). (Courtesy of The Western Pennsylvania Hospital Burn Trauma Center, Pittsburgh, PA.)

Color Plate 9.   Electrical burn (back.) (Courtesy of The Western Pennsylvania Hospital Burn Trauma Center, Pittsburgh, PA.)

Color Plate 10.   Electrical burn sustained from biting an electrical cord. (Courtesy of The Western Pennsylvania Hospital Burn Trauma Center, Pittsburgh, PA.)

Color Plate 11.   Application of silver sulfadiazine. (Courtesy of The Western Pennsylvania Hospital Burn Trauma Center, Pittsburgh, PA.)

Color Plate 12.   Application of dressings (closed technique). (Courtesy of The Western Pennsylvania Hospital Burn Trauma Center, Pittsburgh, PA.)

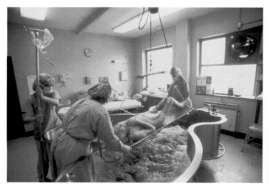

Color Plate 13.

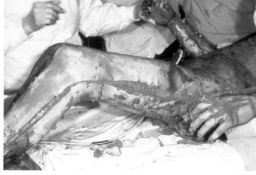

Color Plate 14.

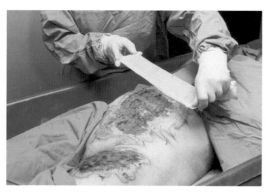

Color Plate 15.

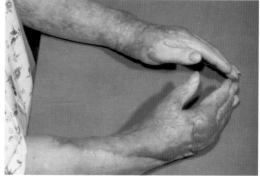

Color Plate 16.

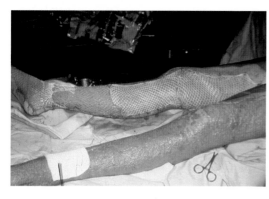

Color Plate 17.

Color Plate 18.

Color Plate 13. Hubbard tank and hydrotherapy. (Courtesy of The Western Pennsylvania Hospital Burn Trauma Center, Pittsburgh, PA.)

Color Plate 14. Portable shower trolley and routine washing of wounds. (Courtesy of The Western Pennsylvania Hospital Burn Trauma Center, Pittsburgh, PA.)

Color Plate 15. Mechanical debridement using coarse mesh gauze (wet to moist). (Courtesy of The Western Pennsylvania Hospital Burn Trauma Center, Pittsburgh, PA.)

Color Plate 16. Escharotomy. (Courtesy of The Western Pennsylvania Hospital Burn Trauma Center, Pittsburgh, PA.)

Color Plate 17. Meshed and expanded split thickness skin grafts. (Courtesy of The Western Pennsylvania Hospital Burn Trauma Center, Pittsburgh, PA.)

Color Plate 18. Hypertrophic scarring of hand. (Courtesy of The Western Pennsylvania Hospital Burn Trauma Center, Pittsburgh, PA.)

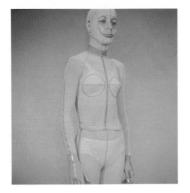

Color Plate 19.

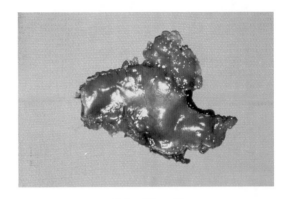

Color Plate 20.

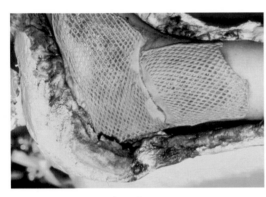

Color Plate 21.

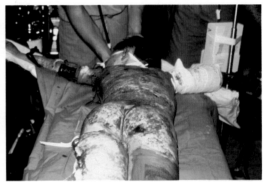

Color Plate 22.

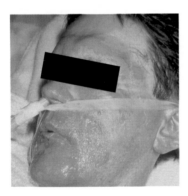

Color Plate 23.

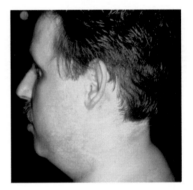

Color Plate 24.

Color Plate 19. Pressure garment. (Courtesy of The Western Pennsylvania Hospital Burn Trauma Center, Pittsburgh, PA.)

Color Plate 20. Gastric ulcer in an electrical burn patient.

Color Plate 21. Wound care in a patient with a cast.

Color Plate 22. Surgical excision and grafting in a patient with a fractured arm and leg.

Color Plate 23. Chemical burn to face. (Courtesy of The Western Pennsylvania Hospital Burn Trauma Center, Pittsburgh, PA.)

Color Plate 24. Chemical burn to eyes and face. (Courtesy of The Western Pennsylvania Hospital Burn Trauma Center, Pittsburgh, PA.)

Unit ONE

BASICS OF BURN CARE

Chapter 1

LORNA L. SCHUMANN

INTRODUCTION

HISTORY OF BURN CARE

Ancient Times to 1940

Early man's use of fire inevitably led to accidental burn injury. Evidence points to the use of herbs as the earliest burn wound therapy.[1] Early attempts at burn care are documented in the writings of ancient Egypt, Greece, and Europe. Such care involved removal of foreign bodies, suturing, and protecting wounds with clean materials. Recorded history reveals that the early Egyptians (approximately 1600 B.C.) used incantations, magic, and a special sequence of topical agents, such as goat's milk, mother's milk, beeswax, gum mixtures, cow's fat, papyrus, and bean paste. The application of such agents varied with the specific day of therapy and the appearance of the wound. It appears that some of the early agents used may in fact have had medicinal value.[2] Figure 1–1 depicts an artist's rendition of typical burn care in ancient times.

Hippocrates (circa 400 B.C.), a Greek physician, recommended using bandages soaked in a mixture of swine's fat, resin, and bitumin.[3-5] The Hippocratic corpus, possibly written by Hippocrates, emphasizes that burn treatment should include the use of diagnostic evaluations, surgical intervention, drug therapies, and the consideration of the anatomic area burned.[6-8] Other areas emphasized in his early works are as follows:

1. Maintain a clean wound by irrigation with clean water or wine
2. Avoid the formation of pus in the wound
3. Keep the wound dry
4. Apply clean, warm dressings of swine's fat, pine resin, and bitumen[9-11]

The Roman Empire (1st century A.D.) brought about a resurgence in medical writings. Cornelius Celsus in his book *DeMedicina* emphasized the use of herbs for wound therapy and surgical excision of contracted burn scars. Early "researchers" of the day were using trial-and-error methods of burn wound therapy with new kinds of herbs.[12]

Onions and leeks found favor in burn therapy both as a topical covering and as a dietary supplement from the 7th century until the late 1800s. Animal dung was also a

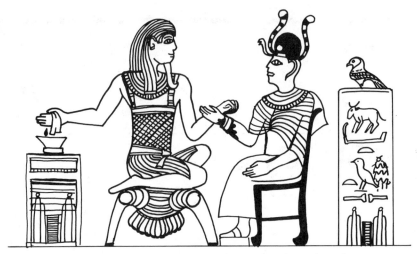

FIGURE 1-1. Artist's conception of burn care in ancient times.

highly recommended topical agent during this period. Other major historic develop-ments between 1600 and 1850 include:

1. The first description of three degrees of burn by Hilanus in 1607
2. The first use of ice and ice water to alleviate burn pain and prevent local edema by Earle in 1799
3. The first description of six depths of burn injury by Dupuytren in the early 1800s.[13]

In the 1800s, when Lister and Semmelweis recognized the influence of bacteria on wound sepsis and the infectious process, the use of vegetables and animal dung was greatly lessened. At that time, and even today in some areas, maggots were used for debridement of eschar. Sheepskin and other animal skins were used as burn wound coverings. It was also during the 1800s that bloodletting for cholera and burn victims fell into disfavor with the discovery that both groups were volume-depleted.

In 1897, the first saline solution infusions were given by Tommasoli in Sicily for fluid replacement in major burns.[14] In 1905, an article appeared in the *Journal of the American Medical Association* emphasizing the importance of using parenteral saline and early skin grafting in the treatment of burn victims. This same year Wiedenfeld and Zumbush performed early excision (first 3 days) of the burn wound. This treatment built on the successful excision and wound grafting done by Wilms 3 years earlier.[15]

A research study by Underhill and associates in 1921 demonstrated that burn shock was primarily a result of fluid loss during the initial burn period. The researchers measured serum hematocrit, hemoglobin, and chloride on a population of 20 burn victims. This fluid loss was secondary to translocation of fluids and electrolytes into interstitial spaces. This finding opposed the current theory of the day, which stated that burn shock was due to the release of toxins. This research laid the foundation for modern fluid and electrolyte therapy and served as the basis for further study in the pathophysi-ology of burns.[16]

During the 19th century, substances such as dry cotton, wool, oils, picric acid, aluminum acetate, and tannic acid were advocated to improve wound care. Initially, tannic acid was used as a wound coagulant and later (1925) as a method of decreasing fluid loss and relieving pain.[17]

Burn wound management in the early 20th century involved the use of dressings soaked with sodium bicarbonate, normal saline, or zinc oxide. Dressings were often not changed for 5 days, thus allowing for enhanced bacterial growth. Silver nitrate became a mainstay in burn wound therapy in 1934 and has continued as a therapeutic agent to the present.

The advent of modern skin grafting began with the techniques of the Swiss surgeon, Reverdin, who performed the first epithelial graft in 1869.[18] This laid the foundation for modern split-thickness skin grafting. Prior to his work minimal success was made with skin grafting techniques. Tissue for transplantation was procured with scalpels. In 1939, the dermatome was developed for procuring thin layers of skin for skin grafting.[19] This aided the move toward early wound closure and enhanced patient survival. Table 1–1 summarizes these historic developments in burn management.

1940 to Present

Historically, the Coconut Grove Night Club fire of 1942, where 492 lives were lost and hundreds were treated for minor to major burn injuries, created a public movement for changes in building codes, building designs, and standards of fire protection and prevention. This disaster also provided the impetus for gathering further information on fluid shifting. Researchers again emphasized the need for large volume fluid resuscitation.[20] The use of special formulas for fluid resuscitation had its beginnings with Evans in 1952. The Evans formula using normal saline at 1 ml/kg per percent burn plus colloids

TABLE 1–1. Treatment of Burns Throughout Time

Year	Treatment
1600 B.C.	Magic, beeswax, gum mixtures, bean paste
400 B.C.	Keep wound dry. Irrigate wound. Apply dressings.
1st century A.D.	Herbs. Surgical incision
600 A.D.	Onions, leeks, animal dung
1850 A.D.	Description of 3 degrees of burns. Use of ice and ice water. Use of maggots.
Late 1800s	First epithelial graft. Use of saline for fluid replacement.
1900	Use of soaked dressings. Use of skin grafts. Early excision of wounds.
1920	Use of tannic acid. Etiology of burn shock from translocation.
1930s	Silver nitrate
1940s	First burn unit established. Coconut Grove fire. Large volume fluid replacement.
1950s	Invention of Brown dermatome. Septicemia as cause of death recognized.
1960s	0.5% silver nitrate. Mafenide. Silver sulfadiazine.
1970s–1980s	138 burn units. Burn Nurse Clinical Specialists

TABLE 1-2. History of the Major Fluid Resuscitation Formulas

Name	Year	Crystalloid	Amount of Fluid (ml/kg per percent burn)	Colloid	Other Elements
Tommasoli	1897	Saline	Not specified	0	0
Cope and Moore	1942	Saline	"Large volumes"	0	0
Evans	1952	Saline	1.0	+	2 L D_5W
Brooke	1954	Ringer's lactate	1.5	+	0
Baxter's Parkland Formula	1970	Ringer's lactate	4.0	0	0

(whole blood, plasma, or plasma expanders) of 1 ml/kg per percent burn was later modified by Brooke Army Medical Center to use Ringer's lactate at 1.5 ml/kg per percent burn plus colloids at 0.5 ml/kg per percent burn. A more recent development of the Baxter's Parkland formula utilizes only Ringer's lactate during the first 24 hours.[21] The history of fluid resuscitation formulas development is presented in Table 1-2.

Burn wound care advances accelerated during World War II, the Korean War, and the Vietnam War. As often is the case with wars, the great numbers of burned victims, and the extensiveness of the burns, provided a vast clinical trial for new and developing therapies. The development of the Brown dermatome is one example of this trend. Brown was a prisoner of war in the Philippines during World War II when he developed the idea for an electrical dermatome which would increase the speed and accuracy of procuring skin. It remains in wide use today.[22,23]

Leidberg, Reiss, and Artz in 1954[24] emphasized that septicemia was a common cause of death in burn victims. Further study into septicemia and burn wound sepsis led to intensive research for more powerful topical antimicrobial agents that has continued to the present.

The historic aspects of burn care cannot be complete without mentioning the amazing advancements that have been made in topical antimicrobial therapy. The 20th century has seen the advancement from tannic acid spray and gentian violet to the use of 0.5 percent silver nitrate in 1965. This was soon followed by the development of mafenide. Both of these topical agents could be used to control gram-positive and gram-negative organisms. In 1969, silver sulfadiazine was introduced as a broad-spectrum topical agent. Although septicemia continues to be a severe threat to major burns, the use of topical antimicrobials and parenteral agents has greatly increased survival rates and controlled infection.

Since 1940, advances in burn therapy have escalated, leading to improved survival, improved cosmetic results, and improved quality of life. Patients who would not have survived 10 years ago are now making remarkable recoveries. These advances in burn therapies include:

1. Early excision and autologous grafting of the wound surface
2. Development of specialized units for burn care which contain proper equipment, a well-trained burn team, and specialized medical supplies
3. Skin cultures and tissue biopsies to monitor bacterial growth
4. The use of pressure garments to minimize hypertrophic scarring and improve circulation
5. The use of synthetic skin as a temporary wound covering
6. Improved fluid resuscitation therapy

Fluid resuscitation has advanced far from the hit-and-miss therapy of giving large volumes of normal saline orally. Developments include various intravenous formulas based on kilograms of body weight and percent calculation of the burn with variations in the amount of fluid for the first 24 hours as compared with the second and third 24-hour periods. Chapter 9 presents a more in-depth discussion of advancements in fluid resuscitating.

HISTORY OF BURN UNITS

The impetus for burn unit development came from the studies of Dr. Frank Underhill. His study of the 20 patients who were burned in a fire at the Rialto Theater in New Haven, Connecticut, in 1921, led to more intense studies on pathophysiology of burns and therapy intended to promote survival rates.[25-27]

World War II produced many burns and wounds requiring the development of burn-trauma units to handle the casualties. This prompted the Office of Scientific Research and Development to appoint a committee to study war casualties. This committee awarded 23 contracts to 10 trauma units for the purpose of studying wound contamination. It was not until 1947 that the first official Burn Unit was established at Brooke Army Medical Center.[28]

Currently 138 units are designated as units specifically designed for the care of burn patients.[29] Approximately 1700 beds are available for burn patients in these units, although many units have the capability of expanding their burn beds when the need occurs.

BURN UNIT NURSING

The development of the burn nursing specialty evolved from a need for specially trained nurses who provide extensive wound care in addition to the basic intensive care. The burn nurse must be competent in critical care, infection control, wound care, rehabilitation, psychotherapy, and coordination of the functions of the multidisciplinary burn team. The burn nurse must be flexible and knowledgeable enough to perform nursing care across the age continuum, from the newborn to the elderly. It is an area of nursing in which creativity in care planning and care giving is of the essence.

The University of Rochester Burn Nursing Education Project was developed under a federal grant for the purpose of developing a core curriculum on burn nursing. It is packaged in outline and modular form so that the user can select specific modules or specific areas of burn care to teach.[30]

Traineeship Programs

The American Burn Association offers traveling fellowship grants for nurses who seek training in burn care. These grants pay a stipend plus air fare for the nurse to go to a burn center of choice. The National Institute for Burn Care in Ann Arbor, Michigan, also has a special burn care training program.

Clinical Specialists

The burn clinical specialist represents a means of improving the quality of patient care and nursing practice. Ideally, the specialist is a master's-prepared nurse who has specialized in burn care. Various master's programs for burn nursing have developed in the United States. The first program developed was at Texas Women's University in 1972. This was followed by the development of programs at the University of Cincinnati in 1975, University of Washington in 1976, and Widener University in 1978. The University of Washington Burn program was broadened to include critical care nursing in 1987.[31]

The role of the clinical specialist is multifocal, encompassing the components of a practitioner, researcher, teacher, consultant, and change agent. The specialty role of the clinical nurse specialist is covered in detail in Chapter 24.

THE BURN TEAM

Monitoring the progress of the burn patient is an important team function. The burn team includes members from each of the following supporting departments: dietary, respiratory therapy, physical therapy, occupational therapy, play therapy, nursing, psychiatry, social work, physicians, infection control, pharmacy, utilization review, and others who may be peripherally involved. The team approach to burn care has proven very effective in dealing with even the most complex patient situations and in individualizing patient care. Patients and their families should be made aware that they have access to a wide variety of team members to help them in all aspects of burn management.

The philosophic foundation of the team approach is improved patient care. The nurse provides bedside nursing care, coordinates team efforts, and promotes the return to activities of daily living. The physician provides comprehensive medical-surgical care that promotes wound healing. Physical therapists and occupational therapists assist the patient to regain and achieve optimal physical function. Play therapists are essential to pediatric burn cases. They help children deal with their environment and the emotional stress they are undergoing. The psychiatry department and social workers coordinate activities to improve the patient's psychosocial well-being. Emotional adjustments for victims of major burns require the coordinated efforts of the burn team, the patient, and the patient's family. The respiratory therapy department and the dietary department are each responsible for their respective functions and coordinate their activities with members of the team. Although each member of the team has specific functions, no member is an island. Many of the functions overlap and require a blending of activities to promote high-quality patient care and successful patient outcomes.

Interdisciplinary Conferences

The means by which team efforts for quality burn care are promoted and coordinated are the institution of burn rounds, or interdisciplinary conferences. Burn rounds consist of weekly or biweekly team meetings that include at least one member from each of the supporting departments. The purpose of these meetings is to review the chart and progress of each patient as well as to discuss and plan the individual short- and long-term goals for each patient. As with other patient care management, discharge planning is initiated at admission.

At times family members and patients attend the meetings to provide essential information and discuss long-term goals that promote the effectiveness of patient care.

The culmination of the conference establishes an individualized plan for patient care for the following week(s).

ASSOCIATIONS FOR BURN CARE

American Burn Association

The American Burn Association (ABA) was formed in 1958, under the direction of Curtis Artz, Irving Feller, Bruce MacMillan, Boyd Haynes, and John Boswick. Prior to that time there were fewer than 10 U.S. hospitals that had specialty burn units. The purpose of the organization was to promote burn care, teaching, and research. In 1972, prevention of burns was added to the purpose of the organization. This purpose has led to the dissemination of educational material to the public.[32-35] The ABA granted full membership with voting privileges to nurses and other nonphysician members in 1982, thus acknowledging the interdisciplinary nature of burn care.

Nurses influence the ABA by serving on various committees of the association, presenting papers, serving as group moderators, and presenting sessions. Because burn care requires an integrated approach, nurses serve on a variety of committees. Examples of these committees are the Education Committee, Federal Issues Committee, Research Committee, Program Committee, Membership Committee, Burn Prevention, Organization and Delivery of Burn Care, Rehabilitation Committee, the Standards of Care Committee, and two Advisory Committees to the Board. Another example of nurse members' impact on burn nursing is the joint effort of the American Nurses Association and the ABA to develop "Guidelines for Burn Nursing Practice."

A nurse special interest group (NSIG) meets every year at the annual ABA meeting to share information and ideas for improvement in burn care. The NSIG of the ABA was initiated by Florence Jacoby and Elizabeth Bayley and was officially established in 1980. The official journal of the ABA is *The Journal of Burn Care and Rehabilitation.*

Nurse members of the ABA also influence the association and burn nursing by becoming involved in regional nursing activities such as:

1. Prevention of fires and burns via mass media and public burn conferences
2. Education of emergency care providers
3. Education of nursing students
4. Preparation of burn educational materials
5. Development of burn educational exchange programs
6. Development of family support groups
7. Development of family re-entry programs
8. Development of work re-entry programs

International Societies

The impetus for the international movement in burn medicine was World War II. During the 1950s, burn centers were developed worldwide for the purpose of providing specialized care. The 1960s saw the development of many burn units in the United States. Shriners of North America advanced the care of children with burns by establishing units specific to their needs.

In 1960, the First International Congress on Research in Burns was held in Washington, DC. It was followed by a Second International Burn Congress in 1965 in Edinburgh, Scotland.[36] At this meeting the International Society for Burn Injuries was formed. The International Burn Congress has continued to meet every 4 to 5 years for the purpose of disseminating information about new research and new techniques in burn therapy. Other goals of the organization are education in the treatment of burn wounds, improvement in morbidity and mortality statistics, and international dissemination of information among physicians and nurses. The official journal of the organization is *Burns*.

LEGAL AND ETHICAL ISSUES

Legal Issues

Legal issues involving burn injuries can be divided into two major categories: those involving the cause of the burn and those involving the burn patients' care. Both categories of legal cases may bring the burn nurse into the courtroom.

Legal issues involving the cause of burns include accidental injury issues such as vehicles that explode in flames when rear-ended, other types of explosive fires, malfunction of equipment in industrial settings, and fires involving areas where large numbers of people are housed or entertained: hotels, convalescent homes, hospitals, supper clubs, and the like.

Special types of burns within this category are attempted murder; attempted suicide; victims of arson; and elderly, child, or spouse abuse. These burns require careful documentation of the injury itself and the history of the burn injury.

Approximately 25 percent of all burns occur in children under age 10. Of these, approximately 10 percent involve child abuse.[37] Burns occurring in children are suspected as abuse when the history and the type of burn injury do not match. Health personnel should be alert to the possibility of child abuse and report such to appropriate authorities. Certain types of burns are more prevalent in child abuse (e.g., cigarette burns and scalding injuries of the back, buttocks, perineum, and feet). These burns may require the nurse to testify to the type and extent of burn injury and the ability of the burn victim to give testimony in court. The nurse may be required to go with the patient to give physical and emotional care. In some cases, the courtroom setting may be in the burn unit itself.

The second major category of legal issues involves patient care delivery. Patients and their families may challenge medical authority with the right-to-die issue. This issue has come to the forefront in all areas of medical treatment and requires individual treatment and decision making. State laws vary in regard to the refusal of medical care and the right to die.

Malpractice is a separate issue that is best treated by prevention. Nursing practice that exemplifies the standard of care that a prudent nurse would follow in the delivery of patient care and produces well-documented nursing notes and flow sheets are the best defense against malpractice suits. The nurse's actions must fall within the scope of practice established by the State Nurse Practice Act in the state where he or she is working and meet established standards. The burn nurse must assume the responsibility of keeping up with nursing standards by attending continuing education courses and maintaining competency.

Another preventative measure, in addition to excellence in patient care, is demonstration of a sincere, positive, caring attitude that shows patients and their families that nurses are truly concerned about their welfare.

Ethical Issues

The ethical issues seen in burn nursing are similar in some respects to those in other areas of nursing, but different in the aspects of severe disfiguring disability requiring major emotional adjustment. On a daily basis in the burn unit, the nurse is faced with issues of impending death, severe disfiguring burns, and physical and emotional dysfunction that impairs activities of daily living and the quality of life. As with other ethical issues, the answers are not clear-cut. To work so hard to keep someone alive for 3 months and then to participate in the decision to remove ventilatory support and let the patient die is not an easy decision. Being faced daily with a patient's screaming "Let me die, let me die" may make nurses question their own purpose in care giving. When faced with major disfiguring burns, the nurse may in fact question the intense push to keep that patient alive.

Working with such challenging and difficult situations is both rewarding and draining. To see a severely burned individual discharged to the home setting is a touching, rewarding accomplishment. Yet accomplishing the goal of discharge loses its rewards when one sees that some of these individuals have severe emotional scars and have not been able to adjust to their disfigurement and impaired mobility. Some of these burn patients not only have to face their own disabilities but have to reflect on those of significant others involved in the same fire.

More than 2 million persons with burn injuries seek medical care each year in the United States. Mortality figures show that death due to burns averages about 12,000 per year.[38] The evolution of burn centers utilizing the team approach to burn care has met the challenge of treating the multifocal problems of major burns. The burn nurse plays an important role in coordinating the multidisciplinary care necessary to return the patient to society as a productive member.

REFERENCES

1. Solecki, RS and Shanidar, N: A Neanderthal flower burial in Northern Iraq. Sci 190:880, 1975.
2. Bryan, CP: Ancient Egyptian medicine: The Papyrus Ebers. Ares, London, 1930.
3. Archambeault-Jones, CA and Feller, I: Burn care. In Kinney, MR. et al: AACN's Clinical Reference for Critical-Care Nursing. McGraw-Hill, New York, 1981, p 741.
4. Haynes, BW: The history of burn care. In Boswick, JA: The Art and Science of Burn Care. Aspen Publishers, Rockville, MD, 1987, p 3.
5. Artz, CP: History of burns. In Artz, CP, Moncrief, JA, and Pruitt, BA (eds): Burns: A Team Approach. WB Saunders, Philadelphia, 1977, p 3.
6. Lloyd, GE: The Hippocratic question. Classical Quarterly 25:171, 1975.
7. Archambeault-Jones, CA, p 741.
8. Haynes, BW, p 3.
9. Lloyd, GE, p 171.
10. Archambeault-Jones, CA, p 741.
11. Haynes, BW, p 3.
12. Ibid.
13. Bayley, B: Personal communication, May, 1988.
14. Tommasoli, E: Le iniezioni di sieri artificiali come metodo per iscongiurare in morte nelle scottature. Riforma Medica 13:39, 1897.
15. Haynes, BW, p 6.
16. Underhill, EP, et al: Blood concentration changes in extensive superficial burns, and their significance for systemic treatment. Arch Intern Med 32:31, 1923.
17. Artz, CP and Yarbrough, DR: Burns: Including cold, chemical and electrical injuries. In Sabiston, DC (ed): Davis-Christopher Textbook of Surgery: The Biological Basis of Modern Surgical Practice. WB Saunders, Philadelphia, 1977, p 295.
18. Haynes, BW, p 6.
19. Archambeault-Jones, CA, p 742.
20. Haynes, BW, p. 5.
21. Ibid, p 6.
22. Archambeault-Jones, CA, p 742.
23. Haynes, BW, p 7.
24. Leidberg, NC, Reiss, E, and Artz, CP: Infection in burns, III. Septicemia, a common cause of death. Surg Gynecol Obstet 99:151, 1954.

25. Haynes, BW, p 5.
26. Underhill, EP, p. 31.
27. Artz, CP, History of burns, p 6.
28. Macmillan, BG: The development of burn care facilities. In Boswick, JA (ed): The Art and Science of Burn Care. Aspen Publishers, Rockville, MD, 1987, p 19.
29. Ibid.
30. Bayley, B: Personal communication, May, 1988.
31. Marvin, J: Personal communication, May, 1988.
32. Macmillan, BG, p 21.
33. Marvin, JA: Burn nursing as a speciality. Heart Lung 8:913, 1979.
34. Silverstein, P and Lack, B: Fire prevention in the United States: Are the home fires still burning? Surg Clin North Am 67:1, 1987.
35. Feller, I and Jones, CA: The National Burn Information Exchange: The use of a National Burn Registry to evaluate and address the burn problem. Surg Clin North Am 67:167, 1987.
36. Artz, CP, History of burns, p 11.
37. Height, DW, Bakala, HR, and Lloyd, JR: Inflicted burns in children. JAMA 242:517, 1979.
38. Trunkey, DD: Transporting the critically burned patient. Surg Clin North Am 67:11, 1987.

Chapter 2

RITA BOLEK TROFINO
ANNE E. BRAUN

PATHOPHYSIOLOGY OF BURNS

A burn can be a catastrophic injury in terms of the physical and psychologic damage to the patient as well as the psychologic insult to the patient's family and friends. For the nurse to effectively treat the patient and family, an understanding of the pathophysiology of the burn is necessary.

ANATOMY AND PHYSIOLOGY OF THE SKIN

The skin, or integumentary system, is the largest organ of the body. It serves as the first line of defense against infection and trauma. The skin also performs other important functions in temperature regulation and sensation.

Normal Skin Anatomy

Normal skin anatomy consists of two main layers—the epidermis and the dermis. The subcutaneous tissue is under the dermis but is not considered a layer of skin. Muscle and bone lie underneath the subcutaneous tissue (Fig. 2–1).

EPIDERMIS

The epidermis is the outer layer of the skin and, as such, is the first line of defense to the environment. It consists of five cellular layers: stratum corneum, stratum lucidum, stratum granulosum, stratum spinosum, and stratum germinativum. The two layers that are of most significance in burn care are the stratum corneum, or surface layer, and the deepest layer, the stratum germinativum. Composed of dead keratinized cells surrounded by a lipid monolayer, the stratum corneum acts as a vapor barrier to the body and protects the body from microorganisms and chemicals. When this is damaged by burns, body fluids are allowed to escape. The stratum germinativum generates new cells

13

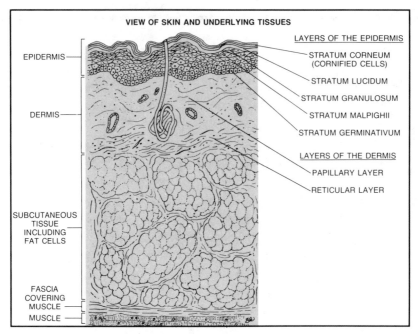

VIEW OF SKIN AND UNDERLYING TISSUES

EPIDERMIS

DERMIS

SUBCUTANEOUS
TISSUE
INCLUDING
FAT CELLS

FASCIA
COVERING
MUSCLE

MUSCLE

LAYERS OF THE EPIDERMIS

STRATUM CORNEUM
(CORNIFIED CELLS)

STRATUM LUCIDUM

STRATUM GRANULOSUM

STRATUM MALPIGHII

STRATUM GERMINATIVUM

LAYERS OF THE DERMIS

PAPILLARY LAYER

RETICULAR LAYER

FIGURE 2-1. Normal skin anatomy: view of skin and underlying structures. (From Thomas, CL: Taber's Cyclopedic Medical Dictionary, 16th ed., FA Davis, Philadelphia, 1989, p. 1987, with permission.)

that regenerate a new epithelial covering. Following burn injury, the epidermis will regenerate if portions of the stratum germinativum remain undamaged.

The epidermis contains no blood vessels, but new epithelial cells produced by the stratum germinativum are nourished by the capillaries in the upper part of the dermis. If the epidermal layer is destroyed in a burn injury but appendages of the dermis remain undamaged, then the epithelial cells of the sheaths of the hair follicles, along with sebaceous and sweat glands, will regenerate a new epithelium.

In general, the entire epidermal layer varies in thickness. For example, it is thickest on the upper back and thinnest on the eyelids. Thus, exposure to the same temperature for the same length of time will result in different degrees of burns on different areas of the body. The thickness of the epidermis and dermis layers varies with age, leaving the very young and the very old with thin skin that will progress to full-thickness burns in a much shorter exposure time than that of people in the prime of life.

DERMIS

The dermis, the second layer of the skin, consists primarily of collagen and fibrous connective tissue. It is also called the corium or true skin since it is not continuously being shed and replaced as is the epidermis. The dermal surface is uneven due to papillae that attach it to the epidermis. The dermis contains arterioles and capillaries from arteries that lie just beneath the dermis. The nerve supply is located throughout the dermis and contains special sensory nerve fibers, discussed later. The dermis also contains the lymph system of the skin.

APPENDAGES

The main appendages of the skin are the sebaceous glands, sweat glands, and hair follicles. Sebaceous glands, the oil-secreting glands of the skin, are found in the dermis with their excretory ducts opening near the top of the hair follicle. Sweat glands also are found in the dermis. Their ducts pass through the epidermis to the surface of the skin where they open in pores. The roots of the hair follicles are located in the deep dermis.

There are also special nerve fibers with specific sensory functions. In the dermis, just beneath the epidermis, are Meissner's corpuscles, which respond to light touch. Deeper in the dermis and in the subcutaneous tissue are the corpuscles of Vater-Pacini, Ruffini, and Krause, which respond to pressure, heat, and cold, respectively.

SUBCUTANEOUS TISSUE

Subcutaneous tissue or superficial fascia lies below the dermis and is firmly attached to the dermis by collagen fibers. These fibers also hold burn slough and eschar securely, making their removal difficult. The subcutaneous tissue is composed of areolar, adipose, and loose connective tissue. Since the amount of adipose tissue varies in individuals, this tissue varies in thickness. The deep fascia lies underneath the superficial fascia, and surrounds muscles and blood vessels. This layer is connected to the periosteum of bones.

Normal Skin Function

The main function of the skin is to protect the body from injury and infection. It also performs other important functions, however (Table 2–1). The skin conserves body fluids to prevent dehydration and assists in the maintenance of fluid balance. Body temperature is regulated by vasoconstriction and vasodilatation of the capillaries and by control of evaporation of water from sweat glands. Vitamin D is produced by the reaction of sunlight with cholesterol compounds in the skin. The skin senses pressure, pain, touch, and temperature, allowing individuals to react to their environment and respond to danger. The skin secretes oil from the sebaceous glands to lubricate the skin, keep it pliable, prevent cracks and fissures, and protect the individual from invasion by microorganisms. When skin is damaged or destroyed, the individual becomes a target for infection and disease.

The skin excretes excess water, small amounts of sodium chloride and cholesterin, and trace amounts of albumin and urea from the sweat glands. Normal fluid loss is 30 to 50 ml per hour.

In addition to these physiologic functions, the skin is also used for psychosocial purposes. The characteristics of the skin are often used to describe or identify people, as by race, distinguishing marks, or fingerprints. Because the skin is a visible organ, there

TABLE 2–1. Normal Skin Functions

Defense against trauma and infection
Retention of body fluids
Regulation of body temperature
Production of vitamin D
Sensation
Secretion
Regeneration of new skin

are also cosmetic factors, and many people are concerned about the texture, condition, and appearance of their skin.

PHYSIOLOGIC RESPONSE TO BURN INJURY

Thermal injury is caused by a transfer from a heat source to the body, heating the tissue enough to cause damage. There are three dimensions to the burn wound. The most superficial is the zone of hyperemia, similar to a sunburn. The middle layer is the zone of stasis. The microcirculation is damaged and capillary permeability allows fluid to leak into the extravascular space. This leads to burn edema and burn shock. There is more constriction of the venous circulation than of the arterial circulation in the zone of stasis. The inside layer is the zone of coagulation or necrosis. Here there is obstruction of the microcirculation that prevents the humoral defenses of the immune response from reaching the burned tissue.

Other types of burn injuries include electrical, chemical, and radioactive burns (refer to Chapter 3). Electrical injury results from exposure to electrical current. The amount of damage depends on the type of circuit, voltage of the circuit, resistance offered by the body, amperage of the current that flows through the tissue, pathway of the current through the body, and duration of the contact. Chemical burns cause coagulation of tissue protein by oxidation, corrosion, protein denaturation, desiccation, and vesication. Absorption of the chemical into the body can cause systemic toxicity. Tissue damage is dependent on the concentration of the agent, the quantity of the agent, the manner and duration of skin contact, the extent of penetration into the tissue, and the mechanism of action. Alkalines cause a liquefaction necrosis, whereas acids cause a coagulation necrosis. Radiation burns occur from the absorption, by the tissue, of different protons of the electromagnetic spectrum.

Integumentary Alterations

As a result of a burn injury, there are alterations in normal skin functioning. Some of the common changes that can occur due to burns are summarized in Table 2–2. These physiologic changes and others depend upon the extent, type, and depth of the burn. For example, major burns (refer to Chapter 9) can cause significant systemic alterations, as summarized in Table 2–3.

TABLE 2–2. Alterations in Normal Skin Functions that can Occur Following Thermal Injury

Loss of protection
Impaired thermoregulation
Impaired defense against infection
Decreased or absent sensory function
Loss of fluids
Decreased vitamin D production
Impaired skin regeneration
Impaired secretory function
Impaired excretory function
Loss of hair growth
Alteration in appearance

**TABLE 2-3. Alterations in Systemic Functions
Associated with Major Burns**

Anemia
Curling's ulcer
Decreased cardiac output
Electrolyte imbalances
Hypoproteinemia
Increased capillary permeability
Increased metabolism
Renal failure

Vascular Alterations

The vasculature supplying the full-thickness injury is completely occluded almost immediately after injury, primarily due to thrombosis. Vasoconstriction occurs as a result of exposure to the heat source and from norepinephrine release during the stress response. The decrease in blood flow causes ischemia which further potentiates the anaerobic metabolism. The decreased blood flow to areas of full-thickness and deep partial-thickness burns occurs secondary to slugging of damaged cells and microemboli formation. Dehydration has been implicated as a primary cause of tissue necrosis in the zone of stasis. In partial-thickness burns, blood flow is normally restored within 24 to 48 hours. However, in full-thickness burns, circulation may not be restored for 3 weeks.

After the initial vasoconstriction, dilatation of adjacent vessels and capillaries occurs, along with increased capillary permeability. This is caused by vasoactive substances, released by the damaged cells, such as bradykinin, serotonin, prostaglandins, complement system by-products, lysosomal components, and histamine. Within 30 seconds of injury arterioles of greater than 12 micrometers undergo immediate vasoconstriction followed by vasodilatation up to 30 percent greater than the preburn diameter, with the vessel recovery occurring about 30 minutes postburn. Arterioles less than 12 μm do not change appreciably. Venules dilate up to 40 percent greater than preburn size.

Endothelial cells swell when heated by the burn. These cells become spherical and pull away from the other cells. Due to this increased capillary permeability, plasma protein along with fluids and electrolytes seep into interstitial tissues, producing blisters and edema. This fluid leaks toward the surface of the wound because of the destruction of lipoproteins that normally would retain the fluid in the interstitial space. This fluid leak varies according to the depth and percentage of the burn but generally continues for 18 to 36 hours postburn, peaking by 12 hours. With a major burn, this fluid leak can continue for several weeks, due to the slow reabsorption of large hydrophilic molecules. In a patient with a major burn this increased capillary permeability may be so widespread as to cause a great deal of edema or fluid shift, referred to as burn shock (refer to Chapter 9).

Pulmonary Alterations

Capillary permeability may increase at the pulmonary level also. Excess fluid and protein can cross the capillary membranes and increase the space between the alveolar and capillary membranes, producing extrinsic pressure on bronchioles, causing wheezing and decreased dynamic lung compliance. This fluid can compress vessels and impair blood flow, creating a ventilation perfusion mismatch. When the pressure rises too much, the fluid and protein move into the alveolar space, with frothy pulmonary edema and marked hypoxia. The inflammatory process immediately postburn causes an increase in tissue oxygen requirements. The increased carbon dioxide component from hypermetabolism can potentiate underlying pulmonary injury because of the strong demands on the lung for increased minute ventilation. The patient with impaired lung function is unable to provide the needed oxygen or to remove the increased carbon dioxide.

Fluid and Electrolyte Alterations

The sodium pump slows down due to hypoxia leading to an increase of sodium chloride inside the cell and potassium outside the cell. Initially, the patient has hyperkalemia from the release of potassium from the cells and fluid shifts from the intravascular space. Under the influence of aldosterone, potassium is lost in the urine, leading ultimately to hypokalemia.

The fluids that leak into the extravascular, extracellular space create edema. This edema causes pain, and puts pressure on the tissues and on the vascular system, slowing the blood flow, which also leads to ischemia.

Insensible water loss also contributes to a deficit in the extracellular fluid volume. Fluid loss from burned skin is 5 to 10 times greater than that from undamaged skin. If a patient has burns on 50 percent of his or her body, water loss can amount to 4000 to 5000 ml per day.

In addition to this loss of water, a heat loss may also result in hypothermia. Approximately 2000 to 4000 calories are expended in the evaporation process resulting in hypothermia. These water and heat losses contribute to a hypermetabolic state.

METABOLIC ACIDOSIS

Metabolic acidosis develops in response to the inability to maintain the proper acid-base balance. The buffering action of the body is disrupted by the fluid shift from the vascular to the extracellular tissue space. In addition, there is an accumulation of acids released into the extracellular fluid from the injured and ischemic tissues. The altered concentrations of sodium, potassium, bicarbonate, and chloride ions also contribute to the development of acidosis.

Hematologic Alterations

Major thermal burns cause a variety of hematologic changes. There is a destruction of red blood cells in the burned area and reduced red cell half-life secondary to increased fragility. Anemia results from red cell damage and reduced half-life. There is engorgement of red blood cells in the area. Some of these cells hemolyze, causing hemoglobinemia; eventually they are eliminated via the urinary tract, which becomes manifested as hemoglobinuria. Red blood cells usually remain inside blood vessels during this fluid shift, which often results in an increase in the hematocrit and hemoglobin initially in the immediate postburn period.

White blood cells and macrophages migrate to the burn area by chemotaxis. This migration is facilitated by the increased capillary permeability. They begin phagocytosis to prepare the injured area for healing. All of this activity, however, is impaired by the burn itself. Chemotaxic activity and serum complement levels are present but decreased. Platelets adhere to the inner walls of the blood vessels. Platelet function and half-life are also diminished.

As fluid leaks into the extravascular space, the cellular components of the blood become more concentrated, resulting in an increased hematocrit and sluggish blood flow. This causes ischemia in the underlying tissues to a depth of perhaps three to seven times the thickness of the directly damaged tissue. Thrombi may develop in the blood vessels, which contributes to ischemia. This ischemia eventually leads to necrosis of unburned tissue, increasing the severity of the burn.

The increased hematocrit, as well as erythrocyte damage and loss, results in stasis and impaired microcirculation contributing to burn shock and possibly disseminated intravascular coagulation (DIC). Large amounts of tissue thromboplastin are released into the circulation following extensive burn injury. The tissue thromboplastin stimulates the intrinsic and/or extrinsic clotting pathways, beginning the cycle of clot formation, followed by rapid use of clotting factors with depletion of these factors, creating a state in which hemostasis cannot be maintained.

Fibrinogen normally comes into an area of injury to line the injured area and decrease bleeding, but albumin and globulin, which normally do not pass through the capillary walls, escape to the interstitial area. The albumin molecules are smaller than globulin; therefore, more albumin molecules leak out. The fluid lost into the interstitial spaces is no longer available for circulation. Instead albumin and globulin increase the concentration of the interstitial fluid and pull more fluid by osmosis from the vascular space. When the walls of the capillaries regain their normal integrity and osmotic pressure is re-established, the fluid is reabsorbed into the bloodstream and excreted; the outward sign of this is a profound diuresis. However, some protein extravasate remains trapped in the extravascular spaces contributing to the slow late phase resolution of tissue edema lasting for 2 to 3 weeks.

Cardiovascular Alterations

Cardiovascular instability occurs because of the microvascular and cell membrane alterations (refer to Vascular Alterations, p 17). Cardiac output is initially depressed, primarily due to hypovolemia. Arterial blood pressure is well maintained even in the presence of severe hypovolemia as massive quantities of catecholamines are released immediately postburn. This maintains pressure but severely impairs tissue perfusion. Blood pressure alone will be very deceptive when trying to calculate fluid volume loss. Central venous pressure and pulmonary artery wedge pressure readings, which reflect volume, are often low due to the large fluid losses.

Children have a very labile cardiovascular system. The pulse, rather than the blood pressure, is a better indicator of change. The child has a poor peripheral compensatory response to volume changes. This labile cardiovascular system leads the child to decompensate quickly in the presence of shock or sepsis. The small diameter of the toes and fingers of a child leads to a greater compromise of the circulation in the presence of circumferential burns.

Endocrine Alterations

All body systems of burn patients are stressed. Due to increased energy expenditures and requirements, the body moves from an anabolic or energy-storage mode to a catabolic or energy-utilizing process. Much of this is due to the hypermetabolic state due to the burn injury, but most is due to the hormonal changes after burn injury. Catecholamines (epinephrine and norepinephrine) are released immediately after the burn injury. Epinephrine stimulates glycogenolysis and promotes hyperglycemia. Norepinephrine causes an initial vasoconstriction after the burn injury. Catecholamines also cause an increase in lipolysis, which releases free fatty acids as an energy source. Glucagon levels are increased, which stimulates production of hepatic glucose. Liver function is decreased by the initial hypoxia, which is caused by the vasoconstriction of catecholamine release and decreased systemic circulation.

The adrenal cortex is stimulated to form cortisol by adrenocorticotropic hormone

(ACTH) release immediately following the burn injury. Cortisol is a factor in the early phases of the catabolic response. Aldosterone secretion is increased in response to the decrease in intravascular sodium and hypovolemia.

Burn patients are not only hypermetabolic with an increased expenditure of resting energy, but also hypercatabolic with loss of tissue with a large excretion of nitrogen products and a negative nitrogen balance. The hypercatabolism leads to depletion of the albumin needed for oncotic activity, the immunoproteins for defense against infections, and the cell synthesis needed for tissue repair.

Immune Response

Thermal injury damages the skin, providing an area for microbial invasion. In terms of nonspecific immunity, an inflammatory reaction occurs. This reaction includes increased capillary permeability and local vasodilatation. Also, the complement system is activated by the abnormal proteins in the damaged tissue. This leads to chemotaxis, opsonization, and surface immune adherence to the cell bacteria; release of kinin, histamine, and lysosomal enzymes; and cytolysis. Defects in the complement system occur in burn patients due to activation of the system and consumption of the factors (Fig. 2−2).

With humoral immunity, there is a decrease of circulating IgA, IgM, and IgG. It has further been correlated that, postburn, depletion of IgG can be correlated with sepsis.[1] IgG is the major antibody involved in the secondary immune responses and antitoxin responses. Thus, a decrease in IgG impedes the formation of specific antibodies. Beyond all of these changes, more extensive alterations in the immune reactivity of patients with major burns are further compromised by general anesthesia, surgical procedures, transfusion, and the administration of antibiotics.[2]

In cellular immunity, all cell types are affected. T-helper cell activity is suppressed and T-suppressor cell activity is enhanced. This leads to a decline in the production of antibodies by B cells and suppression of B-cell activity, respectively. A decline in immune potential results.

Among the possible etiologies of immunosuppression in the burn patient are the following drugs: tetracycline, chloramphenicol, clindamycin, streptomycin, gentamicin, kanamycin, and neomycin. All inhibit cellular immunity. Mafenide (acetate) and silver sulfadiazine can inhibit movement of polymorphonuclear neutrophils into an area of inflammation. The anti-inflammatory action of steroids decreases the number of cells available to participate in the inflammatory response and can lead to a temporary lymphocytopenia.

Stress alters the enzymes in the immunoreactive cells. The immune system of the very young is not fully developed, and the immune system of the elderly is slowing down. The very young and the elderly cannot tolerate the stress of the burn as well as the adult can.

Protein and caloric malnutrition decrease immune responses and resistance to infection. Malnourished patients cannot generate adequate numbers of immunoreactive cells such as white blood cells (WBCs), and this leads to (1) a decreased ability to form antibodies, (2) defects in recognizing and processing antigens, and (3) a decrease in neutrophil function. Defects in the functioning of the reticuloendothelial system occurs because of an overload of particulate matter from the burn wound. Phagocytosis is impaired in the malnourished individual.

The need for repeated surgical procedures and for general anesthesia further compromise immune activity. Halothane, cyclopropane, ether, and nitrous oxide depress humoral and cellular immunity, depress the allergic response, and inhibit phagocytosis.

Postburn immunosuppression can also be caused by immunologic tolerance pro-

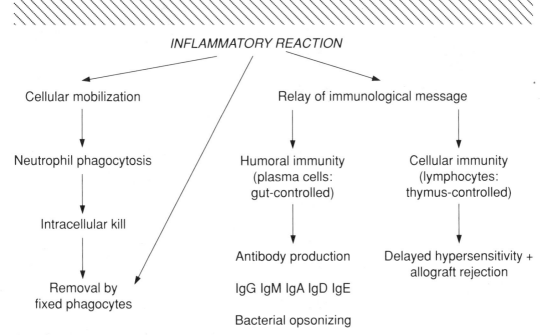

FIGURE 2–2. Immunologic response: factors associated with defense against invasion by various microorganisms. (From Munster, AM: Surgical Clinics of North America, 50:1217, 1970, with permission.)

duced by exposure to vast numbers of new antigens following tissue injury. Also, some patients who are completely recovered and whose wounds are healed can still experience postburn immunosuppression. Suppression of the immune response can lead to an inability to prevent and/or fight infection.

DEPTH OF DESTRUCTION

Classification of a burn injury includes the degree of injury according to the depth of destruction. This classification can include first-, second-, third-, and sometimes fourth-degree burns. More appropriately burns are divided into partial-thickness and full-thickness burns (Fig. 2–3). First- and second-degree burns are classified as partial-thickness burns, and third- and fourth-degree burns as full-thickness.

Partial-Thickness Burns

First-degree burns, or superficial partial-thickness burns (Color Plate 1), involve only the epidermis and are red or pink, dry, and painful without blister formation; a mild sunburn is an example. They heal in 5 to 10 days.

Second-degree burns, or deeper partial-thickness burns, include the epidermis and varying degrees of the dermis. These burns are painful, moist, red, and blistered. Blisters prevent excess water loss, dehydration, and death of superficial dermal cells. If the

CLASSIFICATION OF BURNS

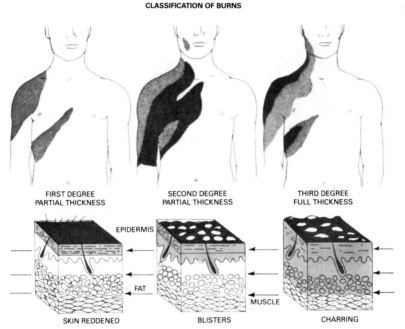

FIGURE 2-3. Classification of burns. (From Thomas, CL: Taber's Cyclopedic Medical Dictionary, 15th ed., FA Davis, Philadelphia, 1985, p. 243, with permission.)

blister were to be torn or removed, the underlying skin would be weeping, bright pink or red, and extremely sensitive to temperature changes, exposure to air, and light touch. They usually heal in approximately 1 to 2 weeks.

The deep second-degree burn, or deep partial-thickness burn, involves the entire epidermal and dermal layers. Sweat glands and hair follicles remain intact. These burns are very painful, and can appear mottled with pink or red to waxy white areas with blisters and edema (Color Plate 2). This burn is still soft and elastic but may be insensitive to light pressure. Deep partial-thickness burns usually heal in about 1 month but with a large amount of scar formation. Spontaneous restoration of skin coverage, or re-epithelialization, occurs with all partial-thickness burns if the wound receives adequate hydration, nutrients, oxygen, and appropriate tissue bases, and if the patient remains free from infection. Further damage caused from infection, mechanical trauma such as occlusive dressings, or obliteration of the blood supply can transform the deep dermal partial-thickness burn into a full-thickness third-degree burn.

Full-Thickness Burns

Third-degree or full-thickness burns extend into the subcutaneous tissue and may involve muscle and bone. They include direct damage to the vasculature underlying the burned skin. Thrombosed vessels can be seen beneath the surface of the wound. These burns vary in color from tan, deep red, black, waxy white, yellow, or brown (Color Plate 3). Full-thickness burns are hard, dry, and leathery. Much edema is usually noted. The wound will leak fluid absorbed from the underlying tissues. Scald injuries, which appear red but dry, are full-thickness burns. The red discoloration is from hemoglobin fixed in the tissues. Normally, third-degree burn injuries are painless, unless surrounded by areas of partial-thickness burns. Full-thickness burns are not capable of self–re-epithelialization.

Fourth-degree burns are also full-thickness injuries but definitely involve muscle, fascia, and bone. The wound appears blackened and depressed. If the bone is involved in the injury the wound appears dull and dry. Bones and ligaments may be exposed. Since nerve fibers in the dermis are destroyed with full-thickness burn injury, these burns are anesthetic. It is important to note that most burns are a combination of partial- and full-thickness injury, so some pain is usually present. All full-thickness burns require skin grafting for closure.

EXTENT OF INJURY

The depth of a burn wound is not the only factor that affects the magnitude of these injuries. An estimation of the extent of the burn injury is also necessary. A common method for determining the extent of the injury is the "Rule of Nines" method.[3] This method divides the body into segments whose areas are either 9 percent or multiples of 9 percent of the total body surface, with the perineum counted as 1 percent (Fig. 2–4).

This formula is simple but is inaccurate in assessing children. A more accurate method, such as that used in the Lund and Browder chart,[4] requires a table with a relative anatomic scale or diagram that estimates total burned area by ages and by smaller anatomic areas of the body (Fig. 2–4). For example, the head of an infant would be counted as twice the percentage of an adult's head. The extent of the burn is expressed as a percentage of the total body surface area. An adaptation of both methods utilizes the palm of the patient's closed hand. This is equal to 1 percent of that patient's body. However, for children, the anatomic scale or diagram is recommended.

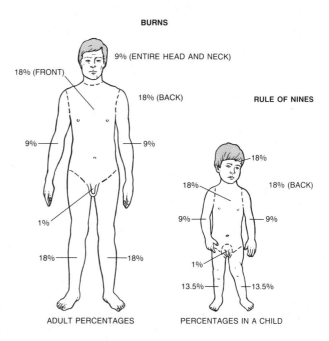

FIGURE 2–4. Estimation of percentage of burns ("rule of nines"). (From Thomas, CL: Taber's Cyclopedic Medical Dictionary, 16th ed., FA Davis, Philadelphia, 1989, p. 260, with permission.)

BURNS

9% (ENTIRE HEAD AND NECK)

18% (FRONT)

18% (BACK)

RULE OF NINES

9%   9%

1%

18%   18%

ADULT PERCENTAGES

18%

18%   18% (BACK)

9%   9%

1%

13.5%   13.5%

PERCENTAGES IN A CHILD

CLASSIFICATION OF BURNS

BURN SEVERITY

The depth of burn injury is determined by the burning agent, the temperature of the burning agent, the duration of exposure, the conductivity of the tissue, and the thickness of the dermal structures involved. The severity of the burn injury — minor, moderate, or major — is determined by the depth of the burn, the extent of the burn, patient's age, past medical history, concomitant injuries, and the location of the wound (refer to Table 8 – 1).

Agent and Circumstance

It is important to note the agent that caused the injury as well as the duration of exposure. In thermal burns, the higher the heat and the longer the duration of exposure, the deeper the wound will be. In chemical burns, the more destructive the agent and the longer the duration of exposure, the deeper the wound will be. In electrical burns, the greater the current, the longer the exposure, and the extent of local tissue resistance, the more internal damage to fascia, muscle, and bone there will be. Electrical burns can also produce cutaneous burns from the ignition of clothing. In radiation injuries, the closer to the source of the radiation the patient is and the longer the exposure, the worse the injuries will be.

Knowledge of the agent can provide valuable information, which assists in the determination of the extent of injury. For example, electrical burns are almost always full-thickness injuries, because the current enters the full thickness of the skin and travels through the body and usually exits elsewhere. Flame burns, particularly if the victim's clothing is involved, can cause full-thickness or third-degree burns. Synthetic materials retain heat longer than natural materials. Burns caused by exposure to extremely hot liquids or prolonged contact with hot metal or melted plastic are usually full-thickness. Immersion burns, in most cases, are also full-thickness as a result of increased exposure time.

The circumstances of the burns can also suggest whether there are any other injuries. One example would be the patient who was in a fire in an enclosed space. Inhalation injury should be highly suspected. Because the duration of exposure is one factor that determines the depth of the burn, it is important to ascertain whether the injury was accidental or intentional. Intentional burns usually result in a much deeper and more serious burn injury because of increased time of exposure to the heat source. These patients cannot remove themselves from the source of the burn.

Location

In determining the severity of a burn injury, the location of the injury is always taken into consideration. For example, burns of the eyes, face, feet, hands, and perineum are rarely considered to be minor or moderate burns, regardless of the estimated percentage. The reasons they are usually considered to be major burns are varied. Determining the depth of injury to burns of the face and neck may be difficult due to early swelling that occurs. A patient with a periorbital burn should be examined by an ophthalmologist. Burns of the ears may result in chondritis leading to loss of cartilage and deformities. Flame burns of the face and neck are highly indicative of inhalation injury (refer to Chapter 18). Burns of the face may interfere with adequate nutrition. Cosmetic and functional deformities may occur if burns of the face and neck are not properly treated. Burns of the hands and feet require special treatment to minimize swelling and preserve optimum mobility. Burns of the hands, while covering only a small body area, may necessitate in-hospital nursing care. Perineal burns are especially prone to infection and maceration in all patients, especially young children who are not toilet trained and incontinent adults. Burns of the head, neck, and chest may lead to increased incidence of pulmonary problems (refer to Chapter 18).

Age

Age is always a major factor in determining the severity of a burn injury. Patients under age 2 or over age 60 have a higher mortality than other age groups for a similar-size injury. The skin in the very young is thin. The skin of the elderly is also thin and has less elasticity. Because of the thinness of their skins, the dermal appendages are shallower and a deeper injury will occur. Both age groups are also more prone to infection due to their lowered immune status. Young children have a larger head surface and smaller extremity surface area. Psychosocial needs vary greatly in these age groups and must be considered in all aspects of nursing care.

The infant has minimal protein stores which are rapidly depleted during the period of capillary permeability. The child also has poor antibody responses to infection, which results in less resistance, leading to a more frequent occurrence of sepsis. Also, the infant has less body mass to provide metabolism, and more body water in proportion to size. The child has immature renal function which negatively affects the ability to retain sodium and water. Reduced mobility may be a factor in the severity of the burn.

The older patient most likely has latent degenerative processes that may prove fatal. Sensory loss and motor paralysis prevent the patient from feeling the burn and escaping the burning process. Anemia, arteriosclerosis, and pre-existing edema have already created some cellular hypoxia.

Concomitant Injuries

Many patients with burns also have other injuries that occurred along with the burn injury (refer to Chapter 19). Many patients in house fires must jump from a window to escape. These jumps can result in fractures and other trauma. The patient with an electrical injury may have associated fractures due to the tetanic contraction of muscle groups. In this way, a jolt from the electrical current can cause a fall or fractures. Inhalation injuries are commonly seen in patients who are injured in house fires. Patients injured in car accidents in which the vehicle caught fire may have related trauma such as spinal cord injuries, chest trauma, head trauma, or abdominal injuries. A patient who suffers a myocardial infarction trying to put out a fire or escape from it will require delicate adjustment of fluids and pain relief. Often, the burn injury has a lower priority due to the more serious concomitant injuries.

Patients who abuse alcohol and drugs or have high blood alcohol or drug levels are difficult to manage in surgery. These patients also tend to have a low tolerance to pain and may resist all efforts to help them. Patients who were burned in suicide attempts will have ongoing psychiatric problems. Many times the patients' desire to die threatens their desire and ability to get well.

Pre-existing Conditions

Pre-existing conditions such as heart disease, diabetes, sickle cell anemia, and lung disease complicate wound management and healing. Conversely, the burn injury can exacerbate pre-existing conditions. Certain medications that the patient has been taking for other illnesses can also alter the body's response to the burn injury. Steroids have an anti-inflammatory effect and alter protein synthesis. They also cause bone degeneration and suppression of the immune response. Aspirin also has an anti-inflammatory effect and influences the clotting activity of platelets. Dipyridamole decreases the adhesiveness of thrombocytes and leukocytes and decreases the vasoconstrictive effects of thromboxane.

Patients who were immobilized prior to the burn, such as quadriplegics or paraplegics, have skin that has atrophied and thinned. They fail to perceive the burning process and are unable to remove themselves from the source, thus prolonging exposure time.

Malnutrition can lead to a thinning of the skin and also to a decrease in the immune response following burn injury. It also leads to a decrease in metabolic reserves needed to appropriately respond to hypovolemia, infection, hypothermia, or operative stress.

The stress caused by a severe burn may activate a latent disease process, worsen an active process, or cause resuscitative efforts to be changed in consideration of the disease process. A patient with diabetes mellitus would be prone to ketoacidosis because of the hormonal changes (relative insulin deficiency and hyperglycemia) brought about by the stress response. A patient with arthritis might be unable to move to get away from the burning process. Patients with heart or lung disease, or both, are prone to pulmonary insufficiency and congestive heart failure. This in turn could lead to acute tubular necrosis. Patients with liver disease would not be able to mobilize glucose in response to glucagon stimulation. There is a very narrow margin of error that can be tolerated in the elderly with underlying heart, lung, renal, or liver dysfunction.

Mental confusion and significant disorientation may be the cause of the burn or be exacerbated by the injury circumstances or the initial treatment process. This will also affect the cooperation of the patient in subsequent treatment modalities.

SUMMARY

When caring for the burn patient, a thorough understanding of the pathophysiology of burns guides the nurse in planning, implementing, and evaluating care. A foundation of knowledge in normal anatomy and physiology of the skin provides the basis for applying the pathologic changes that occur with burn injuries. Not confined to local manifestations, the nurse applies this knowledge to assessing for and treating systemic manifestations as well. Major burn injuries result in changes in most body systems including the cardiovascular, hematologic, pulmonary, and immune systems as well as fluid and electrolyte function.

The depth of destruction, percentage of body surface affected, and the nature of the causative agent also affect the nurse's plan of care. These factors help determine the severity of the burn, helping to classify each injury as a minor, moderate, or major burn. Severity is also defined by other factors such as anatomic location of the burn, age of the patient, pre-existing conditions and any other concomitant injuries.

A thorough understanding of the pathophysiology of burns is imperative in the nurse's care of the burn patient. This foundation serves as the scientific basis for the delivery of professional nursing care.

BIBLIOGRAPHY

Achauer, BM and Martinez, SE: Burn wound pathophysiology and care. Critical Care Clinics 1(1):47, March 1985.

American College of Emergency Physicians: Minor Burns: Evaluation and Treatment. Marion Laboratories, Scientificom, Kansas City, Mo, 1979.

Arturson, MG: The pathophysiology of severe thermal injury. Journal of Burn Care and Rehabilitation 6(2):129, March/April 1985.

Bayley, EW and Smith, GA: The three degrees of burn care. Nursing 17(3):34, March 1987.

Bernstein, N and Robson, M: Comprehensive Approaches to the Burned Person. Medical Examination Publishing, New York, 1983.

Feller, I and Archambeault, C: Nursing the Burned Patient. Institute for Burn Medicine, Ann Arbor, MI, 1973.

Freeman, JW: Nursing care of the patient with a burn injury. Critical Care Nurse 4(6):52, November/December 1984.

Hills, SW and Birmingham, JJ: Burn Care. Fleschner Publishing, Bethany, CT, 1981.

Hurt, R: More than skin deep, guidelines for caring for the burn patient. Nursing 15(6):52, June 1985.

Jacoby, FG: Nursing Care of the Patient with Burns, ed 2. CV Mosby, St. Louis, 1976.

Malkiewicz, J: The integumentary system. RN 44:54, 1981.

Morath, MA, et al: Interpretation of assessment data in burn patients. Bulletin and Clinical Review of Burn Injuries 2:21, 1985.

Ogle, CK, et al: A long term study and correlation of lymphocyte and neutrophil function in the patient with burns. Journal of Burn Care and Rehabilitation, 11(2):105, 1990.

Robertson, KE, et al: Burn care: The crucial first days. AJN 85(1):30, January 1985.

Robson, MC, Krizek, TJ, Wrary, RC: Care of the thermally injured. In Zuimeda, GD, Rutherford, RB, and Ballinger, WF: The Management of Trauma. Saunders, Philadelphia, 1979.

Warden, GD: Outpatient care of thermal injuries. Surg Clin North Am 67(1):147, February 1987.

Wilkenstein, A: What are the immunological alterations induced by burn injury? J Trauma 24(9):572, September 1984.

Zimmerman, TJ and Krizek, TJ: Thermally induced injury: A review of pathophysiological events and therapeutic interventions. Journal of Burn Care and Rehabilitation, 5(33):193, 1984.

REFERENCES

1. Moran, K and Munster AM: Alterations of the host defense mechanism in burned patients. Surg Clin North Am 67(1):51, 1987.
2. Hansbrough, JF, Zapata-Sirvent, RL, and Peterson, VM: Immunomodulation following burn injury. Surg Clin North Am 67(1):70, 1987.
3. Artz, CP, Moncrief, JA, and Pruitt, BA: Burns: A Team Approach. WB Saunders, Philadelphia, 1979, p 153.
4. Lund, CC and Browder, NC: Estimation of areas of burns. Surg Gynecol Obstet 79:352, 1944.

Chapter 3

RITA BOLEK TROFINO
PATRICIA M. ORR

TYPES OF BURNS

Two million burn injuries occur within the United States each year, 70,000 of which are potentially life threatening.[1] The causes of burn injuries include (1) dry heat, (2) contact, (3) moist heat, (4) chemicals, (5) electricity, and (6) radiation (Table 3–1). Identification of the causative agent is of primary importance due to the relationship of the agent to patient prognosis and treatment.

FLAME/FLASH INJURY

Flame injury (Color Plate 4), the second most common cause of burn injury, is the leading cause of mortality and morbidity in burns.[2] This injury usually occurs in the home and is commonly associated with inhalation injury. Inhalation injuries occur when fire is contained in a closed space; the victim is overcome by smoke; the victim runs and fans flames up toward the face. In addition, many synthetics burn or smolder, producing toxic fumes.

House fires can be caused by faulty electrical wiring, gas or wood stoves, unextinguished cigarettes, smoking combined with substance abuse, cooking accidents, and kerosene heaters. Young men are frequently burned by the ignition of gasoline poured into carborators of cars for cleaning purposes. Car fires from exploding gasoline tanks can be catastrophic events. Children playing with matches often hide and start fires in bedrooms or closets, usually involving the whole house. Flame injury can result in a combined partial- and full-thickness injury. The depth of a flame injury is directly proportional to the duration of contact with the flame and the intensity of the heat.

Flash injury results from a sudden ignition or explosion of short duration. This injury is caused by the ignition of explosives such as gasoline fumes or by an electrical flash. Flash injury can often involve inhalation of superheated air causing laryngeal edema.

Nursing Considerations

Of primary importance when a burn victim arrives in an emergency facility is stopping the burning process. If heat is evident on the wound, the nurse cools it with tap water or normal saline solution because the depth of injury increases in relation to the

TABLE 3–1. Causes of Burn Injuries

Dry Heat	Chemicals
Flame injury	Acids
Flash injury	Alkalis
Contact Heat	Vesicants
Hot tar	Desiccants
Industrial metals	Electricity
Hot grease	Direct current
Hot surfaces	Alternating current
Moist Heat	Lightning
Steam	Radiation
Hot water	Ultraviolet rays
	X-rays
	Radioactive substances

length of exposure to the burning agent. The airway, breathing, and circulation (ABCs) of resuscitation are initiated, especially if inhalation injury is suspected. The nurse removes all clothing from the victim—including shoes, boots, or jewelry—as these can retain heat and increase the depth of injury. If the clothing adheres to the skin, it is soaked with cool tap water or normal saline solution and the patient is covered with a clean sheet. After removing clothes, a head-to-toe inspection is done to assess for any other injuries. The burn wound does not bleed. Ice is not applied to the burn victim for cooling. This causes vasoconstriction which damages surrounding tissues and decreases core body temperature. The victim is covered with a clean sheet or blanket to prevent excessive heat loss, decrease pain from exposure to air, and protect the wound from contamination. If other trauma is suspected in the patient this takes priority over the burn wound at this time. Definitive wound care is accomplished only after the patient has been stabilized and burn trauma resuscitation has been instituted.

CONTACT INJURY

Hot tar, hot metals, or hot grease will produce full-thickness burn injury on contact with the skin. Tar or asphalt temperature is usually greater than 400° and the victim will present with a splatter-type injury. Burns from hot metals at temperatures greater than 200° are usually industrial-type injuries. These types of injuries usually occur to the lower legs and feet, even though protective clothing is worn by workers, because the molten metals will go down the tops of boots or penetrate the victim's boots. Burns from hot grease at temperatures greater than 200° constitute a household or job related injury particularly common in fast food restaurants.

Nursing Considerations

Again, critical management of the burn victim on arrival at an emergency facility involves the cooling of the wound. The ABCs of resuscitation are initiated, and burn trauma resuscitation is instituted. Prior to the removal of agents adherent to the skin the patient must be medicated for pain. Hot tar and asphalt are not peeled off of the skin because it can potentially harm the skin and hair that is attached to the agent. Removal of tar or asphalt can be facilitated by the use of Medisol, a citrus and petroleum distillate that contains 70 percent petroleum distillate, 25 to 27 percent limonene, 2 to 3 percent lanolin, and 1 percent surfactant.[3] If the victim is to be admitted to a hospital, tar can be removed with the application of silver sulfadiazine ointment with an occlusive dressing every 4 hours. Other agents used for tar removal are mineral oil, petroleum ointments, and Tween-80. To remove hot grease, the nurse cleanses the area with a mild soap and water or Betadine solution.

SCALD INJURY

Scald injury (Color Plate 5) is the most common burn injury in toddlers and accounts for 17 percent of hospitalized burn-injured children.[4] Populations most at risk are children under age 5 and adults over age 65. This type of burn can be subdivided into two categories: immersion scald and spill scald. With an immersion scald, there are usually no splash marks. The burn is uniform with a linear demarcation between the normal skin and the burned skin. Splash scalds occur when the agent is thrown, poured, or spilled onto the patient. The burn appears nonuniform and may be shallower than an immersion scald. Immersion scald burns usually involve the lower region of the body; spill scald burns usually involve the upper regions. Children, curious, adventurous, and trying to be helpful, may pull hot water off a stove or spill hot coffee or tea on themselves. Unattended children run hot water for a bath and climb in, not realizing the water's temperature. Table 3–2 indicates time-temperature relationships for partial-thickness scald burns.[5]

Elderly individuals are at risk for scald injuries due to decreased sensation from peripheral neuropathies. They frequently get into a tub or shower and are not aware of the temperature of the water. In attempting to get out, these elderly people, often in impaired physical condition, slip and fall into the water and are unable to get out of the tub.

Nursing Considerations

Scald burns caused by spill scalds are usually a clean partial-thickness burn. The skin may appear moist and blisters may be present on or near the wound. Blisters may remain intact, especially on hands, fingers, and soles of the feet, which decreases pain and contamination of the wound. Scald burns in children and the elderly may present as dry, even though the tissue appears red, due to hemoglobin trapped in the tissues. An immersion scald is usually a full-thickness injury.

Much of identified child abuse is often evidenced as thermal injury. Scald burns sustained through abuse occur in children under age 3. Table 3–3 summarizes condi-

TABLE 3–2. Time-Temperature Relationships in Scalds

Temperature (°F)	Time to Produce Partial-Thickness Burn
120	5 min
125	1.5–2 min
130	30 sec
135	10 sec
140	5 sec
145	3 sec
150	1.5 sec
155	1.0 sec

From Moritz and Henriques,[5] with permission.

TABLE 3–3. Assessment Findings Suspicious of Burn Abuse

History of major burn incompatible with physical findings
Burn incompatible with developmental age of child
"Mirror image" burns of the extremities
Localized burns of the perineum, genitalia, and buttocks
Burns assessed as older than the historic account
Unrelated hematomas, lacerations, fingernail marks, or scars

tions that alert the nurse to investigate for burn abuse.[6] If child or adult abuse or neglect is suspected, a complete objective documentation of the circumstances is necessary. A thorough physical and psychosocial assessment along with blood levels and bone series to determine other signs of abuse are also appropriate.

CHEMICAL INJURY

Burns due to chemicals compose less than 10 percent of the burn population in most burn centers. Types of chemical injuries are usually specific to geography, industry, and culture of the population. The population at risk for this work-related injury is male. Fifty-five percent of all burn center admissions from chemical injury ranged from age 21 to 50.[7] Injuries occur most often in laboratory accidents, industrial spills, inexperience in medical applications, and agriculture. Chemical burns are rarely seen in children, although esophageal stricture in children is caused by the ingestion of caustic chemicals from household items. Chemical burns (Color Plates 6 and 7) occur most frequently on upper and lower extremities, followed by injury to the trunk.

Toxic chemical products utilized in industry, agriculture, military science, and the home are capable of producing severe burn injury (Table 3–4). These products produce tissue destruction by precipitation of chemical compounds in the cell, cellular dehydration, protoplasmic poisoning, and the dissolution of tissue proteins. The mechanism of action is coagulation of protein by reduction, oxidation, salt formation, corrosion, protoplasmic poisoning, desiccation, or vesication. In general, acids cause coagulation necrosis and immediate pain, and alkalis cause liquefaction necrosis with deeper penetration and less pain. The extent and depth of the injury is directly proportional to the concentration and quantity of the agent, the activity and penetrability of the agent, as well as the duration of contact and the resistance of the involved tissues. Chemical action will continue to destroy tissue until all toxic properties are neutralized. Chemical burns, as other burns, cause initial vasodilation and hyperemia. Tissue congestion and an inflammatory reaction result from fluid and white blood cell filtration of the injured tissue. In severe chemical injuries, tissue necrosis and dissolution may occur.

Nursing Considerations

Of immediate concern in caring for a victim with a chemical burn is to stop the burning process. Copious water or physiologic saline lavage with simultaneous removal of clothing should be performed immediately at the scene of the injury or in the emergency department. Nurses at this time protect themselves from chemical injury through the use of protective clothing and heavy rubber gloves or thick layers of cloth. All of the patient's garments that were penetrated by the chemical are wrapped in a towel or blanket, placed in a heavy plastic bag, and saved in case an investigation into the incident is warranted. Any dry chemicals are brushed off prior to initiating lavage. It is

TABLE 3-4. Chemicals—Uses and Exposure Effects

Chemicals	Uses	External Effects	Internal Effects
Oxidizing Agent Chromic acid	Metal cleaning	Ulcerates and coagulates tissue	Violent gastroenteritis, peripheral vascular collapse, vertigo, muscle cramps, coma, toxic nephritis with glycosuria
Potassium permanganate	Disinfectants, bleach, medicine for skin disorders	Concentrated solutions and dry crystals create a thick brown-purple eschar of coagulated protein	Edema of the glottis after swallowing; no systemic effects
Sodium hypochlorite	Disinfectants bleaches, deodorants	Released chlorine coagulates cutaneous protein as well as mucous membrane proteins	Esophageal stricture (late complication); vomiting, circulatory collapse, edema of larynx, glottis, and pharynx
Reducing Agents Hydrochloric Acid	Industrial laboratories	Converts protein to respective chloride or nitrate salt; causes erythema with blister formation	Ingestion can cause an esophagitis with stricture; inhalation of the fumes can result in pulmonary injury
Gasoline	Fuel	Causes erythema and blister formation	Produces CNS, pulmonary, cardiovascular, renal, and hepatic injuries; absorption is rapid once skin is broken
Corrosives Phenols	Deodorants, sanitizers, disinfectants	Extensive protein denaturation forms a white or dull grey stain with soft eschar and shallow ulcer formation; causes demyelination of nerve fiber; thus, there is absence of pain or discomfort	Absorbed rapidly percutaneously leading to pulmonary edema, hemolysis, and cardiovascular collapse; can also lead to nephrotoxicity and hepatic failure
Lyes Potassium hydroxide Sodium hydroxide Ammonium hydroxide Lithium hydroxide Barium hydroxide Calcium hydroxide Sodium metal	Industrial cleaning Washing powders Drain cleaners Urine-sugar reagent Tablets Cement Agriculture	Causes liquefaction necrosis—a gelatinous, friable, often brown eschar forms; saponifies tissue cells	Ingestion causes severe pain, spasms, leading to circulatory collapse, asphyxia from glottal or laryngeal edema, pulmonary and gastrointestinal problems
White phosphorus	Incendiaries, insecticides, fertilizers	Painful second- and third-degree burns occur due to	Absorbed and causes systemic toxicity as evidenced by

TABLE 3-4. Chemicals—Uses and Exposure Effects (*Continued*)

Chemicals	Uses	External Effects	Internal Effects
		thermal activity when exposed to air; cellular dehydration due to chemical activity	hepatic and renal failure, and hematemesis
Protoplasmic poisons			
Acids			
Tungstic Sulfosalicylic Tannic Trichloroacetic Cresylic Acetic Formic	Industrial use	Form thin to hard, thick eschars	Hepatic necrosis or nephrotoxicity may result after ingestion or systemic absorption
			Rapidly penetrates causing metabolic acidosis, hemolysis and renal failure
Oxalic acid	Industrial use	Chalky, white, indolent ulcers form	Causes hypolcalcemia
Hydrofluoric acid	Glass etching, plastics production, component of rust removers	Painful, deep ulcerations forms under coagulated eschar; bone decalcifies	Fluoride ion penetrates tissue, causing continued injury over a period of time; chemical pneumonitis can result from inhalation of fumes; corneal loss due to eye exposure; severe hypocalcemia produces refractory cardiac dysrythmias
Desiccants			
Sulfuric acid	Toilet bowl cleaner, industrial use	Forms coagulation necrotic eschar with deep indolent ulcers; extremely painful due to the exothermic reaction	Ingestion causes oral burns, injury to the hypopharynx and epiglottis; esophageal injury is a frequent complication
Muriatic acid	Sheet-metal workers, plumbers	Coagulation necrosis is slow and deep, more severe ulcers are produced	(same as sulfuric acid)
Vessicants			
Cantharides Dimethyl sulfoxide (DMSO) Mustard gas	Veterinary aphrodisiac Linement carrier Military use	Produces blisters and edema, liberates histamine and serotonin at the site, may also cause local tissue anoxia	

extremely important to achieve dilution and removal of chemicals with continuous irrigation for at least 20 to 30 minutes, or until skin pH returns to normal. The water lavage decreases the rate of reaction between the tissue and the chemical. The water should be tepid to avoid further trauma. Neutralizing agents are not recommended for initial use, as many can produce heat by interacting with a chemical. Precious time is lost identifying the chemical and neutralizing agent because the chemical continues to destroy tissue as long as it remains in contact with the skin.

The nurse attempts to identify the offending agent by obtaining a history from either the patient or the rescuers. Chemical pH is assessed for identification as an acid or an alkali. Skin pH can be elevated 5.9 units above normal following an alkali burn and can last 12 hours. Skin pH following an acid burn can be depressed by about 2.5 units and lasts only 2 hours. If skin pH does not return to normal after 30 minutes, lavage can be continued for 12 to 24 hours postinjury. Chemical-specific interventions are necessary following dilution (Table 3–5).

When assessing this injury, it is important to note that chemical burns can be deceptive in the initial estimation of injury. Most chemical burns are more serious than they appear and what may look like a superficial burn may actually be extensive and deep. Also, tissue destruction can occur for up to 72 hours after chemical injury.

As with any other thermal injury, the nurse initiates burn trauma resuscitation as quickly as possible. A thorough assessment is begun for any other concurrent injury. Inhalation of certain chemical fumes can irritate the tracheobronchial tree, leading to retained secretions, atelectasis, and adult respiratory distress syndrome (ARDS). If a chemical injury occurred around or near the face, head, or neck, the nurse must suspect eye injury and lavage the eyes in addition to the skin.

Chemical injury of the eyes requires special consideration. If the eyes are affected, they are lavaged with a minimum of 2 to 3 liters of normal saline solution using a low flow from a standard intravenous line. If blepharospasm occurs during irrigation, an order is obtained for a topical ophthalmic anesthetic agent. Contact lenses, if worn by the patient, may be difficult to remove. Contacts are left in place and eye irrigations continued. An immediate ophthalmology consultation is requested for examination and further treatment. Frequent complications of chemical injury to the eye are corneal ulcerations, eye infections, and loss of sight.

ELECTRICAL INJURY

Electrically injured patients (Color Plates 8 and 9) compose a small portion of the burn population, but true electrical burns cause devasting injuries frequently involving loss of one or more limbs. This injury occurs most frequently in men between the ages of 20 and 34, and is usually job related.[8] Risk-taking behavior of young men combined with substance abuse also leads to critical electrical injury. These accidents are more frequent in the spring and summer months and are usually related to home repairs. Although most electrically injured patients have been in contact with high- or low-voltage current by direct contact, lightning strikes can be an infrequent cause of electrical injury.

Ohm's law states that an electric current (measured in amperes) equals the force (in volts) divided by the resistance of the conductor (in ohms). Joule's law states that the quantity of heat produced is directly proportional to the square of the current strength, the resistance of the conductor, and duration of contact.[9] The effect of electricity on the body is directly related to the factors summarized in Table 3–6.

Electrical current can be of high or low voltage, and either direct or alternating current. Low-voltage direct current is less dangerous than low-voltage alternating cur-

TABLE 3-5. Chemical Injury Management

Chemical	Injury Treatment
Hydrofluoric Acid	Application of magnesium sulfate paste, hyamine 0.2% in ice water (quaternary ammonium compound), soaks bind fluoride ions. Use subcutaneous infiltration of 10% calcium gluconate 0.5 ml/cm² burn surface area if the acid concentrations are 20% or more. If subcutaneous infiltration is used, provide analgesia or anesthetic block. 2.5% calcium gluconate topical gel with dimethyl sulfoxide (DMSO) as a penetrant-carrier to transport calcium across the skin can prevent conversion to full-thickness injury. Topical therapy can be discontinued after pain has decreased to minimal or no analgesia required.
Elemental Phosphorous	Submerge injured area in water to prevent spontaneous ignition of this chemical. Irrigate with a 2% copper sulfate solution, which will stain the phosphorus particles blue-grey to black, facilitating particle identification and removal. Aspirate blister fluid. Three principles to remember are (1) wound must not be allowed to desiccate as the dry chemical ignites, (2) each particle must be mechanically removed, and (3) blisters must be aspirated.
Phenol	Swab the wound with a solvent such as polyethylene glycol, propylene glycol, glycerol, vegetable oil, or detergent soap and water. Keep urine alkaline to decrease precipitation of hemoglobin in the tubules of the kidneys.
Sodium, Lithium, and Magnesium Metals	Remove particles, submerge them in oil, and cover the wound in oil to prevent ignition.

rent due to tetanic muscle contractions produced by alternating current. Conversely, high-voltage direct current is more frequently fatal than high-voltage alternating current. As the electrical current passes through the tissues, it can produce pain and progress to an inability of the individual to let go of the source due to tetanic muscle contractions. Ultimately, the increasing injury can lead to cardiac fibrillation, respiratory failure, convulsions, and burns. A low-voltage current contacting skin with low resistance (wet) can produce an injury similar to high-voltage injury in contact with skin of high resistance (dry). Lightning is high-voltage, high-amperage direct current.

The resistance of the body and the pathway of the electrical current are of extreme importance. Certain areas of the skin, such as the palms of the hands and soles of the

TABLE 3-6. Factors Determining Severity of Electrical Burns

Type and voltage of circuit
Amperage of current
Resistance of the body
Pathway of current
Duration of contact

feet, have a higher resistance due to the thickness of the skin. Resistance of the skin can vary due to the presence or absence of water. Bones offer the greatest resistance of the body to electrical current. Electrical current travels through the body on the path of least resistance—through tissue fluid, blood vessels, and nerves. Electrical current produces a more localized burn if the skin resistance is high at the area of contact, and produces a more systemic injury if skin resistance is low at the area of contact.

In general, there are three types of electrical burn injury. Thermal surface burns are caused by the ignition of clothing from heat or flames produced by electrical sparks or arcing. An arc-type injury is produced by the leaping of electricity to the skin producing severe, deep injuries and is usually associated with a high-tension current. A true electrical injury is caused by direct contact of the body with an electrical source. The current travels through the tissues, creating injuries to deeper areas and produces entrance and exit wounds.

There have also been three types of lightning strikes identified. Ground current produces damaging effects and creates circuits between the ground and legs of victims. Flash discharge injury occurs when lightning "splashes" to a victim from a struck object such as a tree. Direct strikes occur when the victim has a metal object attractant, such as an umbrella, and electricity hits and travels through the body, frequently beginning at the head.

The victim of an electrical injury may present with many different cutaneous injuries. Limbs may be contracted, frozen in position, and charred. Entrance wounds from an electrical injury may present as whiteish-yellow area that is ischemic, charred, and depressed with blister formation on the periphery of the wound. Exit wounds have an explosive appearance with a black depressed center surrounded by grey-white tissue, extensive skin discoloration, edema, charring, and complete tissue loss with exposed bones. Often compared to a crush-type injury, more critical electrical injuries occur from the current passing through vital organs, muscle compartments, nerve, or vascular pathways.

Wounds of lightning injury are frequently superficial with "feathering" or "spidery" patterns which disappear after several days. Cutaneous injuries of the head or leg or cardiopulmonary arrest are predictive of mortality in the lightning-injured patient.

Electrical burns in children frequently occur as children chew on electrical cords (Color Plate 10). An arc injury of the oral commissure is a local injury and can be healed quickly with skin grafts. Called a "kissing" injury, scarring has long-lasting social effects on the child.

Of immediate concern at the scene of an electrical injury is removal of the electrical source from the victim. Institution of cardiopulmonary resuscitation may be necessary as electricity may disrupt cardiac rhythm causing ventricular fibrillation or standstill. Tetanic contractions of muscles or falls can cause fractures or dislocations of long bones or spinal cord injuries.

Nursing Considerations

Electrically injured clients on arrival at emergency facilities are immediately assessed for vital organ function. Cardiopulmonary resuscitation is instituted or continued if necessary. Burn trauma resuscitation is instituted. A quick history is obtained from rescuers, witnesses, or the patient as to the voltage of the current and the duration of contact with electricity. The nurse ascertains whether the victim was thrown or fell any distance at the time of injury.

It is critically important to monitor the cardiac rate and rhythm of this patient, as dysrhythmias occur due to disruption of the cardiac cycle. A 12-lead electrocardiogram (ECG) is obtained as quickly as possible to assess possible cardiac damage from this injury. The nurse monitors vital signs for any changes. Pulses on affected limbs, both proximal and distal to the entrance and exit wounds, are assessed. A Doppler device may be used if necessary. The nurse elevates limbs to help decrease edema. The patient is observed for any disruption in blood flow as electricity degenerates blood vessel walls and thrombi formation causes tissue ischemia.

Damage to muscle compartments initially is due to edema formation and later to progressive loss of blood supply. If the patient complains of numbness, tingling, or increased pain in the extremities and on direct examination has decreased or absent pulses with no capillary refill, muscle compartment pressures are assessed. The patient is prepared for a fasciotomy if muscle compartment pressures are greater than approximately 32 mm Hg. To measure compartment pressure, a saline-filled needle is introduced into the muscle compartment, attached to an air-filled extension and manometer. With the use of a stopcock the intracompartment pressure is read as the air-fluid level stabilizes. A fasciotomy, an incision to split the fascia of the muscle compartment, is performed to allow for muscle expansion, inspection, and debridement if necessary. Daily inspection of this wound is important as muscle tissue will continue to become necrotic due to the thrombosis of the vascular supply to the area. Frequent debridement of this necrotic tissue may occur over 7 to 10 days and eventually may necessitate amputation.

In the electrically injured, there is a higher incidence of hemaglobinuria and hematuria from damaged tissue. Damaged muscles release myoglobin in the urine which can lead to acute tubular necrosis and renal failure. Renal damage can also occur due to the flow of electrical current through the renal arteries or kidneys, or both. Initial fluid therapy in the adult is sufficient to maintain a urine output of 75 to 100 ml per hour to maintain myoglobin clearance and prevention of renal failure. Osmotic diuretics can be used to aid in this clearance and maintain output. The nurse continues to assess the urine for the presence of myoglobin. Continuation of tea-colored or brown urine is indicative of myoglobinuria. Patients with severe muscle injury may continue to excrete myoglobin or hemaglobin in the urine. Additional therapy to aid in clearance may include the use of low-dose dopamine to improve renal perfusion.

All electrically injured patients are treated as spinal cord injured until x-rays are obtained. The cervical spine is immobilized and the patient is log rolled if necessary. Even though the wounds may seem minor, compression fractures of the vertebra or disruption of the blood supply to the spinal cord may lead to transient paresthesia or permanent quadriplegia.

Frequent neurologic assessments are predictive of central nervous system insult. Neurologic deficits may be late findings and can be evidenced as confusion, convulsions, decreased level of consciousness, and respiratory depression and failure. Peripheral neuropathies occur along local nerve roots and usually are transient in nature.

Other late findings from electrical injuries are the incidence of cholelithiasis and cataract formation. In general, these complications are long-term and the patient is encouraged to continue with appropriate medical followup.

RADIATION INJURY

Although radiation injuries are rare, mishaps and injuries will increase due to the increased use of radioisotopes and ionizing radiation in the production of electrical power; diagnosis and treatment of disease; and scientific, industrial, and consumer applications. Five types of injuries from a radioactive incident are summarized in Table 3–7.

TABLE 3–7. Radioactive Injuries

Trauma with no irradiation or radioactive contamination
X-ray or gamma ray irradiation with no radioactive residue to create a hazard
Radioactive contamination within the body with or without trauma
Radioactive contamination within a wound with or without trauma
Radioactive contamination on the skin with or without trauma

Ionizing radiation injuries are rarely life threatening. Injuries that become apparent over a period of time are dependent on the amount of energy deposited. The energy deposited is related to the dose, dose-rate, and volume of tissue irradiated. Ionizing radiation is composed of electromagnetic and/or particulate matter. Alpha particles have extremely poor penetration and are stopped by the outer layer of skin. If ingested, inhaled, or deposited in an open wound, delayed radiation damage can occur. Beta particles penetrate the first few centimeters of soft tissue and are hazardous if improperly handled. High doses may cause thermal burns. Gamma rays and x-rays easily penetrate body tissue, damaging tissue, and are capable of inducing radioactivity in the body.[10]

Burns caused by radiation exposure due to medical therapies can be classified as early, moderate, late, and chronic (Table 3–8). Skin reactions secondary to radiation were once used as a gauge for measuring dosage levels of radiotherapy. Megavoltage doses or fractionated doses of radiation therapy produce relatively minor changes in the skin. It is not a limiting factor and can be circumvented if further therapy is needed.

Of primary importance is the identification of the carcinogenic effect of radiation. Sources of data on the relationships of radiation exposure to malignancies include occupational exposure, atomic bomb exposure, medical exposure, and fallout accidents in the Pacific testing grounds. The most common cancers identified with radiation are leukemias and skin carcinomas. Osteosarcomas and other cancers such as those involving lung and thyroid have a higher incidence in populations exposed to radioactivity.

More recently, exposure to ultraviolet lights in tanning booths or suntanning parlors has lead to the incidence of cutaneous burn injury. Although these tanning agents using high-intensity radiation are advertised as harmless, evidence is beginning to appear that

TABLE 3–8. Classifications of Radiation Exposure Burns

Early	Inflammation, erythema, and dry or moist denudation of skin surface. This reaction appears the same as a deep sunburn; hair falls out and may or may not regrow. Occasionally, patient will experience dry desquamation evidenced by itching and peeling within exposed areas.
Moderate	Blisters may be present with the erythema deeper, a purplish color. Moist desquamation occurs. Sweat glands become atrophied or fibrosed and hair loss may become permanent. Healing occurs in 3 to 4 wk.
Late	Radiation "burn" is usually related to a therapeutic misadventure. It is evidenced by deep dermal blisters and sloughing of an entire skin area. This is very painful and slow healing due to vascular changes.
Chronic	Occurs due to exposure to radiation over a long period of time. These formerly occurred specifically to people who worked around radiation, such as physicians and technicians as well as patients. These changes can occur in individuals who did not experience early changes. Evidence of these changes includes ischemia, decreased or increased pigmentation, atrophy, ulcerations, necrosis, and malignancy.

the effects on the skin can manifest as burn injury, skin cancer, wrinkling, and aging of the skin.[11]

Nursing Considerations

If prewarned of an irradiated or contaminated patient, the hospital must prepare to care for the patient safely. The irradiated person can be cared for in the same manner as any other patient arriving in the emergency department because there is no health hazard to others. A contaminated patient, however, must be treated in an area that can contain the hazardous materials and control the spread of radioactivity. Protocols are similar to "dirty" surgical cases or patients in strict isolation. Beta and gamma radiation survey instruments (Geiger counter) and personal dosimeters are available.

Rarely are radiation injuries life-threatening to the victim or treating staff. ABCs of trauma resuscitation are initiated if acute trauma is evident. Staff prevents the spread of radioactive contamination to themselves, to other persons, or to the environment and limits exposure to as low as reasonably achievable (ALARA).

On arrival at an emergency department, immediate monitoring of the patient and rescue personnel for radioactive contamination is begun. Contaminated clothing is removed, bagged, tagged, and held for later radiation survey. The nurse measures with the Geiger counter and documents the amount of the patient's contamination. Swab cultures of body orifices are obtained. Urine, feces, vomitus, and wound secretions are collected and radioassayed for contamination.

Decontamination process is started after ensuring protection of the staff. Any pregnant staff and those of childbearing age are omitted if possible. The decontamination process is begun on wounds prior to contact with intact skin. Copious, gentle irrigation with water, physiologic saline, or a 3 percent solution of hydrogen peroxide will remove most wound contaminants. If eyes are affected, they are irrigated next with copious amounts of sterile water or physiologic saline. If ears are contaminated, the ear canal is gently swabbed and then flushed with water or physiologic saline using an ear syringe. Intact skin is cleansed last by gentle scrubbing with a soft sponge under a warm stream of water to avoid splashing. A mild soap or detergent can be used. For more aggressive treatment, the nurse uses a paste mixture of powdered detergent, cornmeal, and water. Care is taken not to abrade the skin. Chemical treatment with a 3 percent hypochlorite bleach solution is used only if the soap scrubs are ineffective. If hair is contaminated, it is shampooed several times, then rinsed with lemon juice. If this process is ineffective, all hair is removed with an electric razor.

Internal contamination must be treated urgently to prevent incorporation, which is time dependent, occurring when a radioactive material has crossed the cell membrane. Treatment is then aimed at hastening elimination or excretion of the contaminant. Agents readily available are emetics, laxatives, and diuretics. Expert advice is requested for therapeutic modalities after identification of the type and amount of contaminant.

Decontamination is completed when the radioactive count rate is at a near-normal level. Patients and staff must be free of contamination before leaving the area. All contaminated clothes, waste, and water used for irrigation are properly disposed. The patient is transferred to a clean stretcher. If appropriate expertise for decontamination or disposal is unavailable onsite, assistance or advice is solicited from other sources. Burn wounds from radiation are treated as other thermal injuries after decontamination, but the radionuclide usually will remain in the burn eschar.

The irradiated patient mishap is usually due to a therapeutic misadventure. Prior to the initiation of radiotherapy, patient teaching includes information on what will occur, misconceptions regarding radiotherapy, equipment that must be used, and reinforce-

TABLE 3-9. Skin Care Guidelines for Radiotherapy

For accurate positioning of treatment, indelible ink marks are placed on skin by the therapist. These may not be washed off.

The treated area is kept dry. Gentle washing is permitted. Pat dry.

Treatment area is not shaved.

If a reaction occurs from radiation and the area becomes red and itchy, it is kept dry and lightly dusted with corn starch.

The use of alcohols, creams (especially metal-based creams), soaps, deodorants, ointments, or lotions is prohibited unless prescribed by a radiologist.

The patient wears light cotton clothing to avoid irritation or friction in the treated area. Wools can be an irritant and are avoided. The patient may not wear bra, girdle, belt, or other restrictive clothing directly over the treatment area.

Direct constant sunshine on the treated area is avoided. Sunbathing is restricted until after consultation with a radiologist.

The treated area is protected from further damage, such as pressure, creating more vascular compromise. The use of tape in or near the treated area is also avoided.

ment of the radiologist's explanation of the treatment. The necessity of following specific skin care guidelines (Table 3-9) is explained.

SUMMARY

Burn injuries can be caused by dry heat, moist heat, chemicals, electricity, and radiation. The causative agent has major implications for both the prognosis and the treatment of the burn injury.

Common to all types of burns is the importance of immediately managing the patient's airway, breathing, and circulation when indicated. Cooling of the wound and a thorough head-to-toe assessment for concomitant injuries are also crucial.

While much of the management of burns may have similarities in the early emergency treatment, the differences are many. The burn nurse uses knowledge of the special pathophysiologic processes of each type of burn in assessing the injury as well as planning, implementing, and evaluating the care.

REFERENCES

1. Artz, CP, Moncrief, JA, and Pruitt, BA: Burns: A Team Approach. WB Saunders, Philadelphia, 1979, p 17.
2. Ibid, p 19.
2. Ibid, p 19.
4. Katcher, ML: Scald burns from hot tap water. JAMA 246:1219, 1981.
5. Moritz, AR and Henriques, FC, Jr: Studies of thermal injury II. The relative importance of time and surface temperature in the causation of cutaneous burns. Am J Pathol 25:695, 1947.
6. Bakalar, HR, Moore, JD, and Hight, DW: Psychosocial dynamics of pediatric burn abuse. Health Soc Work, 6(4):27-32, 1981.
7. Saydjari, R, Abston, S, Desai, MH, and Herndon, DN: Chemical burns. Journal of Burn Care and Rehabilitation (5):397, 1986.
8. Boswick, JA. The Art and Science of Burn Care. Aspen Publishers, Rockville, MD, 1987, p 241.
9. Ibid, p 242.

10. American Medical Association: A Guide to the Hospital Management of Injuries Arising From Exposure to or Involving Ionizing Radiation. AMA, Chicago, 1984, p 4.
11. Pratt, M, et al: The Price of a Beautiful Tan: A Case Report. Journal of Burn Care and Rehabilitation 8(2):125, 1987.

BIBLIOGRAPHY

Artz, CP, Moncrief, JA, and Pruitt, BA: Burns: A Team Approach. WB Saunders, Philadelphia, 1979.
Burkhalter, P and Donley, D: Dynamics of Oncology Nursing. McGraw-Hill, New York, 1978.
Cooper, JS and Pizzarello, DJ: Concepts in Cancer Care. Lea & Febiger, Philadelphia, 1980.
Dressler, DP, Hozid, JL, and Nathan, P: Thermal Injury. CV Mosby, St. Louis, 1988.
Hills, SW and Birmingham, JJ: Burn Care. Fleschner Publishing, Bethany, CT, 1981.
Jelenko, C: Chemicals that burn. J Trauma 14(1):65, 1979.
Jones, CA and Feller I: Burns, what to do during the first crucial hours. Nursing '77, 7(3):22, 1977.
Pelias, ME and Parry, SW: Thermal injuries. Current Concepts in Wound Care 10(3). 1987.
Salisbury, RE, Newman, NM, and Dingeldein, GP: Manual of Burn Therapeutics. Little, Brown, & Co, Boston, 1983.
Saydjari, R, Abston, S, Desai, MH, and Herndon, DN: Chemical burns Journal of Burn Care and Rehabilitation 7(5):404, 1986.
Stratta, RJ, et al: Management of tar and asphalt injuries. Journal of Surgery, 146(6):766, 1983.
Sykes, RA, Mani, MM, and Hiebert, JM: Chemical burns: Retrospective review. Journal of Burn Care and Rehabilitation 7(4):343, 1986.
Travis, EL: Primer of Medical Radiobiology, U.S. Government Publication, 1985.
Tribble, CG, et al: Lightning injury. Current Concepts in Trauma Care, 1984.
Wagner, M: Care of the Burn Injured Patient: A Multidisciplinary Approach. Publishing Sciences Group, Littleton, MA, 1980.
Wilkens, EW, Textbook of Emergency Medicine. Williams & Wilkins, Baltimore, 1982.

Chapter 4

DOREEN J. KONOP

GENERAL LOCAL TREATMENT

Local treatment of burns encompasses a variety of therapies. Depending upon the extent and type of burn injury, a single treatment may be selected or a combination of treatments used.

Topical agents are one type of local treatment used to control the proliferation of microorganisms at the burn wound. These agents may be applied directly to the burn injury and left open or covered with an occlusive dressing. When treatment requires the wound to be covered, dressings in a variety of forms may be selected. Hydrotherapy is used as a treatment modality to cleanse wounds, assist in fighting infection, assist in removing nonviable tissue, and promote both healing and patient comfort. Debridement, another type of local treatment, involves the removal of nonviable tissue also to promote healing, prevent outgrowth of bacteria, and prepare the site for grafting. In circumferential burns, an escharotomy may be needed to allow for expansion of the skin to accommodate edema and restore circulation to distal areas. Escharotomies can be performed in various ways, but all methods result in disrupting the eschar to alleviate constriction. Finally, skin grafting is another method that may be used alone or in conjunction with other modalities to treat burn wounds locally.

General local treatments of burns injuries encompass a variety of techniques. Used alone or in combination with one or more other methods, all share common goals. These treatments are employed to promote patient comfort and healing, preserve or restore both function and appearance, and prevent sepsis. A thorough physical, psychosocial, and developmental assessment of the patient serves as the basis for selecting and implementing the treatment modality for the optimum outcome.

DRESSING TYPES

Various dressing techniques are available for management of burn wounds. Each has its advantages, disadvantages, and special indications for use.

Open Method

The open method is a popular form of treatment for burn wounds. It involves application of topical agents without the use of gauze dressings. This allows for constant daily observation of the burn wound to assess healing and diagnose infection. It facilitates physical therapy insofar as range of motion exercises are *not* restricted by bulky dressings. This open technique also reduces possible hyperthermia. The open method is particularly helpful in treating burns of the face, neck, ear, and perineum. Disadvantages of this technique include a patient's predisposition to hypothermia and increased discomfort from exposure of wounds. It also may require frequent reapplication of the topical agents and frequent bed linen changes. Finally, the open method often cannot be used effectively on children or uncooperative adults, as wound management is made more difficult.

Closed Method

The closed method of wound management involves the application of occlusive dressings over the burn wound. These occlusive dressings offer protection of the burn from outside contamination and provide for the absorption of fluid and exudate from the wound into the dressing. In addition, it also aids in immobilizing injured areas. Dressings help to reduce evaporative fluid loss and often increase patient comfort. This closed method technique is frequently used in infants, children, and uncooperative adults. It is used frequently to facilitate debridement of the burn wounds and to prepare the wounds for grafting. Dressings protect freshly grafted areas from trauma and are also useful in securing splinting, immobilization, and pressure devices. Occlusive dressings consist of an inner layer of fine mesh or coarse mesh gauze and an outer layer of roll gauze to keep the dressings intact. Topical creams or ointments are usually impregnated into the inner dressings or they can be applied directly to the wound and then covered with a gauze bandage. Dressings (unless otherwise indicated) are light, simple, easy to apply and remove, and nonrestrictive so that range of motion is not severely limited. These types of dressings are changed at least once or twice a day or more often if indicated.

Biologic Dressings

The use of biologic dressings has proved to be a most beneficial tool in the treatment of burn injuries. The term "biologic dressings" refers to tissue obtained from living or deceased humans (homograft-allograft) or deceased animals (heterograft-xenograft). Pigskin is currently a widely used product in addition to human skin. However, the preference between pigskin and cadaver skin depends upon the availability and consideration of cost (cadaver skin costs more than pigskin). Biologic dressings can be used in a variety of situations. It can be used to cover a clean, excised burn wound prior to autografting; in managing a partial-thickness burn; and as a donor site dressing. In partial-thickness burns, biologic dressings have been found to stimulate epithelialization, and hasten wound healing. It is important, however, that prior to its application all blisters and loose skin be removed. The homograft or heterograft is then placed directly on the burn wound. No topical antibiotic therapy is indicated. Wounds are observed for pus formation which indicates infection. If this occurs, the dressing is removed at once. As the wound heals, the biologic dressing begins to lift off, allowing for the exposure of the epithelial buds. When used as a temporary graft, however, the pigskin is changed every 2 to 3 days, whereas cadaver skin can be left in place much longer. The biologic dressing reduces pain, promotes mobility, reduces evaporative fluid loss, and protects the wound from trauma and infection.

Synthetic Dressings

Synthetic dressings are also used in the treatment of partial-thickness burns. These dressings function the same as biologic dressings by promoting epithelialization, improving mobility, and reducing pain. Synthetic dressings have several advantages in that they are less costly, more readily available, and easier to store. Synthetic dressings can be used quite successfully in the management of donor sites and superficial partial-thickness wounds. These dressings exist in many shapes and forms and are made from a variety of materials. One such dressing is a biosynthetic skin substitute that consists of a nylon fabric bonded to a silicone rubber membrane. This particular product adheres well to wound surfaces and is used by many burn centers for the treatment of partial-thickness wounds and excised wounds that are awaiting grafts. Generally, synthetic dressings contain no antimicrobials, although some can be used in conjunction with topical creams or ointments. Other synthetic dressings consist of adherent elastic films, hydroactive dressings, or colloidal suspensions that are usually permeable to air, vapor, and fluids. Again, it is important to note that the burn wounds must be thoroughly cleansed and be free from any loose skin or blisters before the dressing is applied. The nurse also watches for symptoms of infection as the healing process is monitored. These symptoms include temperature elevation as well as the presence of foul drainage, erythema, or cellulitis surrounding the burn wound. These observations are reported to the physician immediately, and the product is then discontinued. Synthetic dressings are becoming increasingly popular with a variety of products currently on the market to meet the growing demands.

Epithelial Cell Cultures

An alternative approach for providing permanent coverage for full-thickness wounds is the use of epithelial cell cultures or "cultured skin." This technique is fairly new but is increasing in popularity because of the advantages it offers. Essentially, the cell cultures are obtained from full-thickness skin biopsies taken from the patient's unburned skin. The epithelial cells from the epidermal layer are then "spun off" and cultured in a nutrient medium. This process results in small sheet grafts, which are then applied to clean, excised full-thickness burn wounds. Epithelial cell culture grafts are useful in that they represent a potential, unlimited source of autografts in patients with extensive burns and limited donor sites. Histologic studies and long-term followup studies are currently being done to determine pathologic changes and functional properties of the cultured skin. Results thus far are promising.

TOPICAL AGENTS

Modern advances in burn care have resulted from the recognition that burn wound infection and its complications are a major cause of mortality in the burn patient. Wound care is aimed at controlling sepsis through the use of topical agents, diligent cleansing, and early excision and grafting of full-thickness burns. Burn wound sepsis is defined as more than 100,000 organisms per gram of tissue in burn tissue, and the presence of organisms in underlying unburned tissue. Surface colonization is present with every burn wound and begins within hours following a burn injury. Initially, gram-positive organisms (usually *Staphylococcus* and *Streptococcus*) are predominant. However, after several days gram-negative organisms also begin to proliferate and invade the burn tissue, although national trends are now showing a decrease in the incidence of *Pseudo-*

TABLE 4-1. Topical Agents

Frequently Used	Less Often Used
Silver sulfadiazine	Povidone
Bacitracin	Gentimicin
Mafenide	Nitrofurazone
Silver nitrate	Neomycin

monas infections. Because a full-thickness burn leads to a coagulation necrosis of skin and thrombosis of nutrient blood vessels, the resulting ischemia provides an excellent medium for bacterial growth. In addition, systemically administered antibiotics are ineffective because of poor delivery to the site of the infection. Therefore, the importance of local wound care cannot be overstated. Topical antimicrobial agents have played a major role in reducing the incidence of burn wound sepsis; however, topical agents do not prevent infection. They merely serve to control or limit the bacterial population until such time that wound healing takes place or excision of the burn wound is performed. Although the search for the ideal topical agent continues, a variety of antibacterials are used effectively in burn wound management. Desirable qualities for topical agents include broad-spectrum antimicrobial activity, the ability to penetrate eschar, minimal absorption, limited metabolic complications, and the promotion of re-epithelialization. In addition, its application and removal should be as comfortable for the patient as possible. The medications that are the most frequently used topical agents and other, lesser used topicals are listed in Table 4-1. They may be used alone or in combination, depending on the type of burn and method of treatment. No single agent should preclude the use of another. Sensitivity studies may also be helpful in determining the appropriate topical antibacterial agent. Table 4-2 summarizes the advantages and disadvantages of each of the topical agents discussed in subsequent sections.

Silver Sulfadiazine

Action. Silver sulfadiazine is a water-soluble cream with broad-spectrum activity. It is bactericidal for many gram-negative and gram-positive bacteria, as well as against yeast. Its antibacterial action is accomplished via its action on the cell wall and cell membrane. Silver sulfadiazine does not have deep penetrative action into burn eschar.

Indications. Silver sulfadiazine is a topical antimicrobial drug indicated as an adjunct for the prevention and treatment of wound sepsis in patients with partial- and full-thickness burns.

Contraindications/Precautions. Because sulfadiazine therapy is known to increase the possibility of kernicterus, silver sulfadiazine cream should not be used on pregnant women at term, on premature infants, or on newborn infants during the first month of life. The safe use of silver sulfadiazine during pregnancy has not been established. Therefore, the preparation is not recommended for pregnant women unless, in the physician's judgment, the therapeutic benefit outweighs possible risks to the fetus.

Adverse Reactions/Side Effects

- Dermatologic: rash, itching, burning
- Genitourinary: interstitial nephritis
- Hematologic: leukopenia

TABLE 4-2. Advantages and Disadvantages of the Topical Agents Used in Burn Care

Topical Agent	Advantages	Disadvantages
Silver sulfadiazine	Can be used with or without dressings Is painless Can be applied to wound directly Broad-spectrum Effective against yeast	Does not penetrate into eschar
Silver nitrate	Broad-spectrum Nonallergenic Dressing application is painless	Poor penetration Discolors, making assessment difficult Can cause severe electrolyte imbalances Removal of dressings is painful
Povidone-Iodine	Broad-spectrum Antifungal Easily removed with water	Not effective against *Pseudomonas* May impair thyroid function Painful application
Mafenide Acetate	Broad-spectrum Penetrates burn eschar May be used with or without occlusive dressings	May cause metabolic acidosis May compromise respiratory function May inhibit epithelialization Painful application
Gentamicin	Broad-spectrum May be covered or left open to air	Has caused resistant strains Ototoxic Nephrotoxic
Nitrofurazone	Bactericidal Broad-spectrum	May lead to overgrowth of fungus and *Pseudomonas* Painful application

NURSING CONSIDERATIONS

Assessment

- Assess wounds for infection and monitor progress of wound healing.
- Monitor white blood cells—transient leukopenia may occur. This will reverse itself on its own or when the drug is discontinued.
- Use with caution in patients with a history of hypersensitivity to sulfonamides. Discontinue using if allergic reaction occurs.
- Monitor hepatic and renal function. If impaired elimination of drug occurs and accumulation results, silver sulfadiazine is discontinued.
- If using silver sulfadiazine in conjunction with topical proteolytic enzymes, be aware that the silver in this compound may possibly deactivate the enzyme, rendering it ineffective. However, this is not the case when silver sulfadiazine is used with Travase.

Implementation

- Apply once or twice daily using sterile technique. The agent itself is painless, but wound manipulation is not. Patient is premedicated for pain.
- Before application, wounds are washed, debrided, and free of previously applied creams or ointments.
- Silver sulfadiazine can be used with or without occlusive dressings. It can be applied directly onto the burn wound or impregnated into gauze bandages that will be applied to patient. If open technique is used, a thickness of approximately 1/16 inch to 1/8 inch (enough to visually occlude the wound) is applied with a sterile gloved hand. The drug should be reapplied as often as necessary to areas from which it has been removed because of patient activity (Color Plates 11 and 12).

Silver Nitrate

Action. Silver nitrate is an antibacterial solution that is bacteriostatic and effective against the entire spectrum of burn wound organisms. Mode of action is achieved by precipitation of bacterial proteins by the silver ions. Silver nitrate is essentially non-allergic.

Indications. Silver nitrate is a topical antibacterial used in the treatment of partial- and full-thickness burns. Because it is effective against surface colonization yet has poor penetration into the burn wound, it is not indicated for management of infected burn wounds.

Contraindications/Precautions. No known contraindications.

Adverse Reactions/Side Effects

- Hematologic: hyponatremia, hypochloremia
- No sensitivity to silver nitrate has been reported

NURSING CONSIDERATIONS

Assessment

- Use of silver nitrate solution will lead to a blackish-brown discoloration of every-thing it comes in contact with. As a result, burn wounds may be difficult to assess, particularly progression and healing of deep partial-thickness burns.
- Monitor blood and urine electrolytes daily. Silver nitrate solution reduces evapor-ative water loss but also can cause severe electrolyte imbalances secondary to absorption of large volumes of free water. Sodium chloride supplements can be given orally or intravenously. Assess for signs and symptoms of hyponatremia and hypochloremia.

Implementation

- Silver nitrate is prepared as a 0.5 percent solution using distilled water as a diluent.
- Dressings applied to the burn are saturated with the solution and are moistened every 2 hours. The dressing application is painless.
- Dressings are changed twice a day. The removal of dressings can be painful due to the rapid debridement of eschar that results from the twice-a-day wound care. Patient is premedicated with appropriate pain medication.
- Dressings must be kept moist, or silver nitrate concentration can reach a caustic level.

Povidone-Iodine

Actions. Povidone is a water-soluble ointment with broad-spectrum bacteriocidal and fungicidal activity. It is a topical agent, active against gram-positive and gram-negative organisms.

Indications. Povidone has been used extensively as an antiseptic and disinfectant agent for wounds, lacerations, abrasions, and ulcers, and as a skin preparation for operating procedures. It is also used to some degree in the treatment of full- and partial-thickness burns although it is currently less popular than other topical ointments and its use is not widely documented. Most experts agree that povidone is not the agent to be used on wounds infected with the *Pseudomonas* organism.

Contraindications/Precautions. Povidone should not be used in patients with hypersensitivity or allergy to povidone or iodine.

Adverse Reactions/Side Effects

- Dermatologic: local sensitivity (i.e., rash, burning, irritation).
- Hematologic: occasionally increased blood iodine levels have been reported.

NURSING CONSIDERATIONS

Assessment

- Assess wounds daily for signs of infection and the progression of wound healing. Povidone has been shown in some studies to retard or inhibit epithelialization.
- Absorption of high levels of iodine may occur which can interfere with normal thyroid function.
- Povidone has limited penetration into burn eschar. It is not the treatment of choice if wound sepsis is present.

Intervention

- Apply a thin layer directly to burn wound, or impregnate into gauze dressings and change once or twice a day. It is easily washed off with water. It should always be wrapped in an enclosed dressing, as heat can cause the drug to "melt" off the body.
- Povidone is extremely painful in its application and for a period of time after application. Therefore, the patient should be premedicated accordingly.

Mafenide Acetate

Actions. Mafenide is a water-soluble broad-spectrum antibacterial cream, which, when applied topically, produces a marked reduction in the bacterial population of burn wounds. It exerts bacteriostatic action against many gram-positive and gram-negative organisms and has active penetration into the burn eschar.

Indications. Mafenide is a widely-used topical agent indicated for the treatment of full and partial thickness burns.

Contraindications/Precautions. Safe use of mafenide has not been established for pregnant women or nursing mothers.

Adverse Reactions/Side Effects

- Dermatologic: pain, burning, excoriation of new skin, bleeding.
- Allergic: rash, itching, facial edema, swelling, hives, blisters, erythema, and eosinophilia.
- Respiratory: hyperventilation, decreased pCO_2.
- Metabolic: acidosis, increase in serum chloride.

NURSING CONSIDERATIONS

Assessment

- Assess wound appearance, monitor for symptoms of infection, monitor progress of wound healing.
- Mafenide, a carbonic anhydrase inhibitor that decreases renal reabsorption of bicarbonate, can cause a metabolic acidosis.
- Hyperventilation leading to respiratory alkalosis may occur as a compensatory mechanism for metabolic acidosis.

- Acid base studies of the patient must be closely monitored, especially in patients with extensive burns, the very young, the elderly, and individuals predisposed to pulmonary complications. This includes serum electrolytes and arterial blood gases. Mafenide should be discontinued if respiratory function is compromised. Absorption of mafenide results in an osmotic diuresis. It is used with caution in patients with renal failure.
- Mafenide can inhibit epithelialization and thus is discontinued when burn wounds are clean and epithelial buds appear.

Implementation

- Mafenide must be applied twice to three times daily because it is broken down by tissue enzymes 8 to 10 hours after application. Mafenide may be used with or without occlusive dressing. If applied directly to wound, it is done with sterile gloves at a thickness of approximately $\frac{1}{16}$ inch. The burns are covered with mafenide cream at all times. Patients may experience pain or burning sensations with application and are therefore appropriately premedicated for adequate pain control.
- Some burn units may also use homemade preparations of mafenide soaks and find this to be an effective irrigating solution.

Gentamicin

Action. Gentamicin is an aminoglycoside with broad-spectrum bactericidal properties. It is prepared as a 0.1 percent cream and ointment and is effective against a wide variety of gram-positive and gram-negative organisms.

Indications. Gentamicin is indicated for treatment of primary and secondary bacterial infections of the skin. It is also effective in treating infected skin ulcers, infected lacerations and abrasions, and minor surgical wounds. At one time it had been one of the topical drugs of choice in the treatment of burns. However, it has been responsible for the early development of resistant strains of bacteria and is now recommended only for the treatment of small superficial burns. Gentamicin cream is no longer used as a topical agent in the treatment of deep extensive burn wounds.

Contraindications/Precautions. Gentamicin is contraindicated in those patients with a history of hypersensitivity to any components of the preparation.

Adverse Reactions/Side Effects

- Ototoxic and nephrotoxic when used over large body surface area.

NURSING CONSIDERATIONS

- Apply gently to affected areas three to four times a day. Wounds may be covered with gauze or left open to air.

Nitrofurazone

Action. Nitrofurazone is a topical antibacterial agent that is bactericidal for most pathogens causing surface infection.

Indications. Nitrofurazone is indicated for adjunctive therapy of patients with partial- and full-thickness burns when bacterial resistance to other agents is a real or potential problem.

Contraindications/Precautions. Nitrofurazone's safe usage in pregnant women, nursing mothers and children has not been established.

Adverse Reactions/Side Effects. Dermatologic: contact dermatitis, rash, pruritis, local edema.

NURSING CONSIDERATIONS

Assessment

- Assess wound healing, watching for possible signs and symptoms of wound infection.
- Nitrofurazone occasionally allows overgrowth of nonsusceptible organisms including fungi and *Pseudomonas*. If this occurs—or if irritation, sensitization, or super-infection develops—the nitrofurazone is discontinued immediately.

Implementation

- Apply a thin layer of nitrofurazone directly to wounds or impregnate into gauze.
- Nitrofurazone is extremely painful in its application; therefore, the patient is premedicated accordingly.
- Change dressings twice a day, or as directed by physician.
- Avoid exposure of the agent to direct sunlight, strong fluorescent lighting, and excessive heat.

HYDROTHERAPY

The evolution of burn care has brought about major advances in understanding the complexity of the body's response to an extensive burn injury. As a result, wound management now focuses on prevention and early recognition of infection, as well as aggressive treatment with early excision and grafting of full-thickness burns. Hydrotherapy can play an important role in the overall care of a burn patient. For purposes of discussion, hydrotherapy specifically refers to the treatment also known as "tubbing" or "tanking." This involves placing the patient in a large Hubbard tank or whirlpool, which enables him or her to perform wound care procedures and range of motion exercises as well as total body bathing. The warmth of the water and gentle whirlpool action have a therapeutic effect in facilitating physical therapy, removal of dressings, and cleansing of the burn wounds.

Procedure for Hydrotherapy

Hydrotherapy is usually performed once a day and involves much time and preparation on the part of the nursing and physical therapy staff. Initially, the procedure is carefully explained to the patient to ensure understanding of this treatment and to help minimize fears and anxieties. Because wound manipulation and exercise can be quite painful, the patient is adequately premedicated with analgesics as ordered. The tub is also thoroughly cleansed before and after use by the patient to prevent cross-contamination. Disposable plastic tub liners are also used to offer added protection. In addition, the nurse performing wound care is acutely aware of principles of infection control. This includes the use of hair caps, masks, gowns, and gloves as well as the practice of sterile technique during the hydrotherapy procedure.

The environment is kept warm for the burn patient in order to avoid hypothermia. The range of the water temperature in the tub is between 96° and 102°F and regulated for the patient's comfort. Various additives such as salt, disinfectants, and detergents are used to convert water into an isotonic, cleansing solution. Examples of these include Hibiclens, povidone, and Dreft. The tubbing procedure lasts 20 to 30 minutes.

Once the dressings are removed, the patient's burn wounds are gently cleansed with gauze pads or sponges and then inspected. Any loose skin or eschar can be removed with the gauze pad or debrided with scissors and forceps or scalpel if necessary (Color Plate 13). When washing wounds, the nurse uses a gentle but firm circular motion to cleanse creams, ointments, loose skin, or crusts from the patient. Excessive force will cause bleeding and increased pain and may also interfere with epithelialization of healing wounds. The nurse maintains the treatment within set time limits.

The patient's unburned areas are then washed, hair is shampooed, and male patients are shaved. This is important for it decreases the bacteria present on surrounding skin, improves hygiene, and gives the patient a sense of comfort and well-being. Physical therapy exercises are performed with qualified personnel at the end of the hydrotherapy procedure.

After the tubbing, the patient is thoroughly rinsed with warm water and then placed on clean warmed linens and covered to prevent chilling. Portable heat lamps, shields, or ceiling heating elements are very beneficial in maintaining a warm environment for patients during and after wound care procedures. Sterile dressings are then applied and the patient is returned to his/her room.

Nursing Considerations

Disadvantages of hydrotherapy include autocontamination and electrolyte imbalances.

Contraindications to hydrotherapy include invasive lines, fresh grafts, donor sites that must be kept dry, and patient conditions requiring bed rest. While the Hubbard tank has long been a useful and popular method of providing wound care and therapy to burn victims, other products are also available that allow for easy provision of wound care. Portable shower trolleys or tables are currently being used in many burn centers. They differ from Hubbard tanks in the following ways:

- Patients are not submerged in water; rather they are washed and showered with a fine water spray.
- Creams, ointments, and debris from wounds are immediately rinsed from the patient. Therefore, the risk of autocontamination of burn wounds is diminished.
- The shower units are smaller, thus taking up less space. They allow close assess to patients, permit ease of transfer in and out of treatment rooms, and are also easy to clean and maintain (Color Plate 14).

With the shower technique there is no benefit from whirlpool action or therapeutic effect from the water in promoting patient relaxation for physical therapy. What is important, however, is not the differences in equipment and technique but the common goals in the care of burn wounds. These goals are listed in Table 4–3.

Patient Education

There are several important issues to consider in the nursing care previously described. Again, patient teaching is essential, not only in informing patients of the methods of treatment but also in developing a trusting relationship. The patient's privacy is respected and protected during wound care procedures. Traffic in and out of

TABLE 4-3. Goals of Hydrotherapy

Cleansing of the burn wound
Removal of nonviable tissue
Prevention of infection
Patient comfort
Promotion of wound healing

rooms is kept at a minimum. Also, patients are allowed to participate in their own care if possible. This helps give the patient some sense of control and is emotionally and physically beneficial. Diversion such as music and videotapes can also be used in the treatment rooms. Favorite music and tapes can be played to direct a patient's attention away from the pain and discomfort of the treatments to familiar relaxing sounds and sights. Other nonpharmacologic measures such as imagery, relaxation, and breathing exercises can also be effective.

Finally, the plan and implementation of care must be individualized to meet the patient's needs. This will go a long way in helping to make an uncomfortable procedure more easily tolerated and accepted.

DEBRIDEMENT

Debridement is the removal of nonviable tissue (eschar). The purpose of the debridement is to promote healing, prepare the burn wound for grafting, and prevent the overgrowth of bacteria in, around, and under the eschar. Removal of this burned tissue reduces the risk of infection and burn wound invasion. Debridement can be accomplished by various methods including enzymatic, surgical, and mechanical techniques.

Enzymatic Debridement

Enzymatic debridement involves the use of chemical agents which act by digesting necrotic tissue, thus facilitating removal of burn eschar. One of the more widely used topical enzymes is sutilains ointment (Travase). Travase can be very useful in management of second- and third-degree burns, but it must be used judiciously.

There have been discussion and controversy related to the use of enzymatic debriding agents in preparation of wounds for grafting and increased incidence of infection. There is a belief by some that enzymes (such as Travase) do not debride and clean burn wounds sufficiently for grafting and that the subsequent "take" of these grafts is not optimal due to the condition of the granulation bed. Some also believe that the use of Travase over large burned areas brings about a higher risk of infection in the following way. The enzyme, while digesting necrotic tissue, also opens up thrombosed blood vessels. This causes oozing of blood at the site, which results in bacterial contact with the bloodstream; its use with antibiotics is therefore recommended. In many burn units Travase has generated good results when used in combination with silver sulfadiazine, which provides antibacterial protection, when used on burned areas no greater than 10 percent of the body surface; and when used on partial-thickness wounds in order to hasten removal of the thin film of eschar. Travase should not replace necessary surgical excisions of full-thickness wounds. It can be rotated on various burn sites to aid in debridement and is reapplied three to four times a day.

PROCEDURE

PROCEDURE

Travase ointment is applied in a very thin layer directly to the burn wound. It has a selected action on necrotic tissue only. It has no effect on normal intact skin. Travase is activated by water and therefore must be used with wet dressings or in conjunction with other water-based compounds. As previously mentioned, a water-based antibacterial agent commonly used with travase is silver sulfadiazine.

NURSING CONSIDERATIONS

The nurse must be aware of side effects or adverse reactions which include bleeding, pain, and dermatitis. Pain is variable and usually subsides after 1 or 2 hours. The patient is premedicated with appropriate analgesia. Enzymatic agents are discontinued if excessive pain or bleeding occurs or if skin irritation develops. The use of Travase can increase evaporative fluid loss. Therefore, the patient's intake and output is monitored. Travase is not used on burns of the face as it can cause severe irritation to the eyes. If this occurs, the eyes are rinsed immediately with large amounts of water. Finally, some enzymes may be rendered inactive when used in combination with certain antibacterial agents. The drug interactions are checked to verify the compatibility of enzyme and antibiotic.

PATIENT EDUCATION

The nurse teaches the patient about the side effects associated with this agent. The patient is also instructed to report pain.

Surgical Debridement

Surgical debridement or excision of burn wounds is indicated in the treatment of full-thickness burns and in deep partial-thickness burns of special areas. Aggressive early excision of full-thickness burns is desirable because it decreases the patient's risk of wound infection, provides for coverage and closure of the open wound, and hastens wound healing. Excision is usually followed by the application of skin grafts when possible or temporary grafts if donor sites are not available. Though necessary, surgical excision is not without risks, for it generally results in a significant blood loss and requires the patient to undergo general anesthesia. Optimally, surgery is performed within several days of admission. However, there are several reasons why it may be delayed. Surgeons will frequently postpone elective excision if the patient has a significant inhalation injury, cardiac or pulmonary complications, or other pre-existing or coexisting conditions that put the patient at risk for surgery and general anesthesia.

Full-thickness burns involving more than 20 percent of body surface area will be difficult to excise in just one operation; consequently, multiple surgeries are necessary. It is also not always possible to graft a freshly excised burn wound immediately after the excision. The full depth of the burn wound may be difficult to assess initially and there are frequently areas of mixed second- and third-degree burns, which can alter the type and outcome of the surgical procedure.

PROCEDURE

Full-Thickness Burns. Excision of full-thickness burns involves removal of the entire layer of skin until viable tissue is reached. This may also include excisions into subcutaneous tissue or fascia if deep wound necrosis is present. Again, blood loss is an inevitable result of burn excision and may extend the planned duration of surgery. After excision the wound is then grafted or covered with a temporary graft or dressing until autografting is possible.

Deep Partial-Thickness Burns: Tangential Excision. As mentioned earlier, excision is also recommended in certain deep partial-thickness burns, especially in those involving the hands. The procedure, referred to as "tangential excision," is different from the conventional excisions just described. Tangential excision is the removal of superficial nonviable burn tissue with preservation of a viable dermal layer. This technique requires a great deal of skill for the purpose is to shave only necrotic tissue until punctate or pinpoint bleeding is observed. The surgeon must be able to make a determination that the excision of necrotic tissue is complete and that the remaining dermis is clean enough to accept a graft. The blood loss incurred during the surgery can make this determination difficult. Once hemostatis is achieved, the excised area is then grafted. Tangential excision and grafting is the treatment of choice in deep partial-thickness burns of the hands for many reasons:

1. Although spontaneous healing of these wounds is possible, the injury heals slowly (sometimes over several weeks).
2. The tissue, once healed, is very thin and fragile. It later is predisposed to hypertrophic scar formation, which will interfere with normal range of motion.
3. Finally, tangential excision and grafting allows for quick and complete closure of the burn wound. This results in earlier mobility and offers superior cosmetic and functional results for the burned hand.

NURSING CONSIDERATIONS

(Refer to Chapters 20, page 385, and 21, page 402.)

PATIENT EDUCATION

(Refer to Chapters 20, page 381, and 21, page 406.)

Mechanical Debridement

Mechanical debridement is the removal of eschar, nonviable tissue, and debris from burn wounds which takes place during daily wound care procedures or with dressing changes. It causes a significant amount of pain, trauma, and anxiety for the patient not only in the endurance of this treatment but also in the anticipation of it. However, the approach of early surgical excision has significantly decreased the need for this type of debridement. If a patient's excisional surgery is delayed or if mechanical debridement is necessary, the patient must be adequately prepared and premedicated.

PROCEDURE

Mechanical debridement is performed primarily by the nursing staff and involves the use of scissors and forceps to manually excise loose tissue from the burn area. It is accomplished most easily during or after hydrotherapy. The nurse judiciously lifts loose, necrotic skin with forceps and cuts the tissue with debridement scissors. The eschar will appear blackish brown in color and may or may not be accompanied by pus formation. Mechanical debridement is not performed if the eschar is firmly adherent to the wound bed or if attempts to remove the eschar prove too difficult or traumatic. The procedure lasts no longer than 20 minutes and is stopped if excessive pain or bleeding occurs. Topical anticoagulants or electrocautery may be required if small areas of bleeding do not stop with manual pressure. Any areas of pus accumulation are cleansed and surrounding tissue debrided.

Another type of mechanical debridement is the use of wet-to-moist or wet-to-dry dressing changes (Color Plate 15). In burn wounds that have been excised but not yet grafted, the wet-to-moist, coarse mesh gauze dressing helps prepare the granulation bed for subsequent skin grafting. It stimulates the granulation tissue and also helps to remove any remaining necrotic tissue. The gauze dressing on excised wounds is kept moist at all times with either saline or an antibiotic solution. If allowed to dry, neoeschar formation will result.

NURSING CONSIDERATIONS

The nurse enlists the patient's help and cooperation by providing thorough explanations and emotional support throughout the procedure. Impending signs of infection or cellulitis are reported to the physician.

In relation to the coarse mesh gauze dressings, the changes are painful and may also cause bleeding. The dressings are moistened prior to their removal, and the new dressings are reapplied wet. If new dressings are too wet, they will not debride; if too dry they will destroy the new epithelialization. Dressing changes are generally performed every 4 to 8 hours a day and the patient is premedicated as needed. The patient's bed is well padded because of the frequent wetting of the dressing. Furthermore, the patient's room temperature is adjusted to ensure warmth and comfort since chilling may result from exposure with wet dressings. Wet-to-dry dressings function much the same as wet-to-wet dressings in the debridement of burn wounds. This technique, however, is used more often in partial-thickness burns to facilitate the removal of necrotic tissue. With this method, the gauze dressings are applied wet and removed dry. Once clean, the burn wound then epithelializes and healing takes place.

PATIENT EDUCATION

The patient is instructed to inform the nurse if the pain is excessive, as the procedure then discontinued. Diversions such as music can be used to shift the patient's attention away from the pain and discomfort. Play therapy can be effective with the pediatric patient.

ESCHAROTOMIES

Many physiologic changes occur in response to a burn injury. One of the earliest, most noticeable, and most important is edema formation resulting from alterations in the cardiovascular system. A thermal injury produces a marked increase in capillary permeability. This leads to a fluid shift with loss of fluid from the intravascular space to the extravascular space. This fluid accumulates not only in the burned area but in surrounding tissues as well. The more extensive the burn, the more generalized the edema.

Normally, the skin is soft, supple, elastic, and able to adjust to movement and growth. However, a circumferential full-thickness burn creates an increase in tissue pressures because the skin lacks the ability to expand and accommodate the swelling that occurs. The burn acts as a tourniquet not only by impeding arterial blood flow, but also by causing an increase in venous congestion. The most common site for tissue compromise secondary to tissue edema are the extremities. However, circumferential full-thickness burns to the chest and trunk can lead to respiratory insufficiency because of the restriction of the chest wall expansion. These conditions require the immediate inter-vention of an escharotomy to alleviate the pressure caused by the tight, thick, leathery eschar.

An escharotomy is a linear incision extending through the burn eschar down to superficial fat (Color Plate 16). It is a sterile procedure performed by the physician using a scalpel or electrocautery device. Escharotomies allow for the expansion of skin in order to accommodate the swelling and permit unrestricted blood flow to the distal area of the extremity.

Procedure

Escharotomies can be performed with or without the aid of analgesia, but always with adequate premedication. Even though nerve endings are destroyed in a full-thick-ness burn, the procedure does seem to cause apprehension and some discomfort. The incisions are made medially and/or laterally through the length of the circumferential burn. Chest escharotomies consist of incisions to the right and left arterior lateral chest wall extending from the clavicle to the bottom of the rib cage as well as across the midchest in a "W" or "H" formation. This alleviates the restriction of chest expansion and helps ensure the achievement of adequate respiratory volumes. Slight bleeding may occur with escharotomy procedures, which can be controlled with manual pressure, pressure dressings, or topical anticoagulants. The escharotomy itself is treated with topical antibacterial agents to protect it from infection. Monitoring the neurovascular status of extremities continues throughout the period of edema formation.

Enzymatic debriding agents can also be used in some instances as a type of "chemical escharotomy." It is particularly helpful in the prophylactic treatment of circumferential deep partial-thickness burns, especially those involving children. While edema can be anticipated, much uncertainty can exist as to whether escharotomies may be needed in the deep second-degree burn. A chemical escharotomy involves the direct application of sutilains (Travase) or a similar agent in one or two thin strips down the length of the extremity. This is done prior to the application of the topical antimicrobial cream. The chemical debriding action of the enzyme on the burn tissue can aid in alleviating or preventing excessive pressure formation in the involved area.

Nursing Considerations

All burned extremities, including one burned circumferentially, are elevated to limit edema formation. Neurovascular checks are performed every hour to monitor adequate circulation. If distal pulses are fleeting or not palpable, a Doppler ultrasonic flow detector can be used. Escharotomies may even be done on admission in anticipation of massive edema formation or in response to symptoms of impaired circulation. These symptoms include an increase in size and tightness of the limb, diminishing pulses, poor capillary refill, deep aching muscle pain, distal cyanosis, and sensory numbness and/or paresthesias. Direct monitoring or periodic direct monitoring of tissue pressure in areas of full-thickness injury can aid in the determination of need for escharotomy procedure. After the escharotomy has been performed, it is still necessary for the nurse to maintain elevation of the burned extremity and to continue hourly circulatory checks of distal pulses.

Patient Education

The patient is instructed to inform the nurse of any numbness or tingling sensations in the affected extremity. The patient is thoroughly prepared for this procedure. Ratio-nale for the use of no anesthesia is fully explained in order to help alleviate anxiety and gain cooperation.

GRAFTING

Skin grafting is the final step in the treatment of a full-thickness burn wound. A graft refers to tissue that is used to cover or close an open wound. Grafts may be applied as a temporary dressing or as a permanent closure for a clean, excised burn wound. The type of graft used depends on the type of surgery performed; the size, location, and depth of the burn wound; and the availability of suitable donor sites.

A skin graft, whether temporary or permanent, is a valuable tool in the management of open burn wounds. It functions by decreasing the patient's evaporative water loss as well as loss of proteins and electrolytes from the burns. This helps to reverse the patient's catabolic state and improves the nutritional status — steps that are essential in the recovery process.

Temporary Grafts

Temporary grafts have become very popular in their use as biologic dressings in burn wound care. These grafts may consist of homografts or heterografts. In addition to reducing fluid and electrolyte loss, the temporary graft has other functions as well. It protects the open wound by providing a physical barrier against infection and preventing the wound from drying out. Temporary grafts improve the patient's mobility and lessen the discomfort associated with painful dressing changes. They are used to cover excised areas, granulation tissue, and exposed tendon or bone prior to the time that autografting can take place. Temporary grafts or biologic dressings also help in preparing wounds for permanent grafting through the mechanical debriding action of the graft change. If donor sites are unavailable or in short supply, they allow one to "buy time" until autografting is possible.

HOMOGRAFT

A homograft is skin obtained from another human being, alive or recently deceased. Cadaver skin is the most common type of homograft used. It is usually procured from the thighs, abdomen, and back, so that tissue donation does not interfere with common burial practices. With family permission, skin is procured from the donor within 36 hours after death. The skin is placed in an antibiotic solution and then stored frozen. It can be used for an extended period of time, when it must be thawed prior to use. However, the earlier the skin is used, the better it will function. Certain conditions preclude the use of skin from a cadaver: cancer, hepatitis, dermatologic pathologies, sepsis, AIDS, and other communicable diseases. Adequate screening of cadaver donors must be mandated to ensure the continued safe use of this product.

HETEROGRAFT

A heterograft refers to skin obtained from another species. It is used in the same manner as a homograft. The most common and easily obtained heterograft is pigskin. It is available in a variety of forms which now include pigskin impregnated with silver.

PROCEDURE FOR TEMPORARY GRAFTS

The application of homografts and heterografts is simple and easy. The grafts are placed on the excised wound dermal side down, meaning the dermis of the donor skin is next to the patient's wounds. The graft is then cut or trimmed so that it covers the burn wound only. Care is taken to avoid overlapping or bunching of the graft. Air pockets or folds in the grafts are removed to make sure that the graft is in total contact with the open burn wound. Steri-strips may be used to secure the grafts in place as sutures or staples are usually not necessary. The grafts are then left open to air or are wrapped with occlusive dressings, depending on the size and location of the burn. Topical antibiotic creams are no longer needed when biologic dressings are used, although dressings can be impregnated with antibiotics to provide penetration into the wound if so desired. A meshed homograft or heterograft allows for drainage of fluid or exudate through the openings in the graft so that accumulation cannot occur.

Temporary grafts gradually become adherent to the excised wound. However, they can be changed every 3 to 5 days to prevent rejection as well as an excessive "take." Removal and reapplication of the grafts may require general anesthesia, especially if large burn wounds are involved. Homografts do become vascularized from capillaries in the granulation tissue. Removal of these temporary grafts mechanically debrides the excised wounds and is thus painful and may cause bleeding and tissue destruction. If the temporary graft is left in place too long, it may lead to excessive adherence, which can result in considerable bleeding when removed. This can interfere with planned auto-grafting and may require a complete surgical excision. The ability of a temporary graft to "take" signifies that the excised area is clean and ready for permanent grafting.

NURSING CONSIDERATIONS

Rejection of homografts or heterografts is signified by excessive pus formation and temperature elevations. Therefore, close monitoring is essential in order to detect early signs of infection or rejection. Grafts are removed and reapplied every 3 to 5 days, or as otherwise indicated. Since removal is usually painful, patients are premedicated.

PATIENT EDUCATION

Grafting, especially in terms of temporary grafts, may be a foreign concept to the patient, and is to be fully explained. Terms such as "take" and "rejection" are adequately discussed.

Permanent Grafts

The final step in the treatment of a full-thickness burn wound is the application of permanent grafts or autografts. An autograft is a skin graft that is taken from an un-burned area and placed on a clean excised wound. It involves using the patient's own skin to cover the open wound. This procedure, when successful, results in permanent closure and healing. Permanent grafts may be applied immediately after excision or they may be delayed until the recipient bed has been sufficiently prepared.

Various grafting procedures and techniques are used by surgeons in treating burn patients. Factors involved in determining the procedure of choice include the size, location, and depth of the burn wound, as well as the availability of suitable donor sites. In addition, the patient's cosmetic and functional results are important considerations in wound grafting because they are vital to the success and outcome of the care of the burn patient.

Autografting is performed as early as possible in the patient's hospitalization. Although all wounds may not be able to be grafted at once, there are priority areas for skin grafting, depending on the patient's condition and extent of burn. For example, major joint surfaces and burns of the hand, face, and neck are preferential sites for early excision and grafting in order to hasten healing, establish function, and improve the patient's sense of well-being. Grafting these areas first also ensures that they will be covered with the highest-quality donor skin. On the other hand, in patients with extensive full-thickness burns, the priority shifts from function and mobility to patient survival. Wounds are excised and grafted in order to remove large areas of eschar and provide coverage as soon as possible. Valuable donor skin is used where it provides the most benefit to the patient. In this case, grafts are used from any available donor site to close large open wounds quickly. The physician is able to predict when the excised tissue is ready for grafting. Because there are no guarantees of graft "take," an error in judgment could mean the loss of important donor skin.

Success or failure of graft take depends on many factors. These factors include the presence of bacteria and necrotic skin on the graft site, adequate hemostasis, the location of the graft site, the suitability of the donor skin, the securing of the graft, the immobilization of the grafted area, and nutritional status. Certain areas of the body are more difficult to graft than others. For example, burns of the axilla, perineum, and buttocks pose special problems because of their contour, location, and difficulty with immobilization. Meticulous attention is given to any of these variables that can affect the outcome of a graft. Success, therefore, depends on proper preoperative, intraoperative, and postoperative care by the burn team. (Refer to Chapters 20, page 385, and 21, page 402.)

SPLIT-THICKNESS SKIN GRAFT

Split-thickness skin grafting (STSG) is the most commonly used method of covering open burn wounds. This procedure involves obtaining a specimen of donor skin that includes the epidermis and a partial layer of the dermis and applying it to the recipient site. An STSG can vary in thickness depending on the donor site and the area to be grafted. Thin grafts (0.006 to 0.012 inch) are indicated when the donor site must be reused, and they generally result in a good "take." However, thin grafts are also more prone to chronic breakdown and hypertrophy. Thicker grafts (0.012 to 0.016 inch) are preferred for grafting areas where elasticity is essential. These areas include the hands, feet, and joint spaces. Thicker grafts tend to contract less but produce a donor site that requires a longer period of time to heal. The thickness of skin varies with age and its location on the body. For example, the skin on the medial thigh is very thin in comparison to the skin on the back, which is much thicker. This is considered when choosing donor sites with relationship to coverage of specific burned areas.

A STSG can be applied as a sheet graft or as a meshed graft. A sheet graft is not altered or expanded but is placed on the open area as a full sheet. This may be the preferred method of grafting a face or neck burn because it results in a smooth, even appearance that is more cosmetically acceptable than other types of grafts. However, a partially meshed graft may be used for the forehead to give the normal appearance of lines and wrinkles rather than the masklike appearance of a sheet graft.

A mesh graft is an STSG that is passed through a mesher that produces tiny slits in the skin. The meshing allows the skin to expand 1½ to 3, 6, or 9 times its original size. Mesh grafts have several advantages over sheet grafts. First, since they can be stretched and expanded, they are extremely valuable in the treatment of patients with extensive full-thickness burns. Mesh grafts allow coverage of larger areas than is possible with unexpanded sheet grafts, a feature that is important when few donor sites are available. The meshing of the graft also prevents fluid, blood, or wound drainage from accumulating and collecting under the graft and interfering with graft "take." The mesh allows fluid or exudate to escape via the openings onto the surface of the graft and into the dressings. With expansion, the graft takes on a "fishnet" appearance with the openings resembling diamonds (Color Plate 17). These interstices epithelialize from surrounding skin and eventually close and heal. The graft itself "takes" or vascularizes as capillaries from the granulation bed grow into the graft and provide it with a blood supply. This process begins within hours of the graft placement and is necessary for healing to occur. Any conditions interfering with capillary growth into the graft can result in full or partial loss of the skin graft. These conditions include infection, bleeding, incomplete excisions, mechanical trauma, poor nutritional state, and shock.

Mesh grafts may or may not be expanded depending on the area grafted and how much coverage is needed. Generally, grafts to the hands are not expanded because of the need for a thicker, more pliable graft.

Procedure. Once the recipient bed has been completely excised, it is important to achieve hemostasis prior to the application of the skin graft. This can be accomplished with electrocautery, manual pressure, or the use of thrombin, epinephrine, or saline-soaked pads. The skin grafts are then placed on the wound and are secured with staples, sutures, or steri-strips. Sheet grafts, which cover the entire open burn, may be managed by the open method or with dressings if so desired. Mesh grafts must always be dressed initially to prevent the wound and graft from drying out. Furthermore, dressings are also useful in absorbing drainage, immobilizing the area and protecting the graft from accidental movement and trauma. Dressings usually consist of a layer of fine mesh gauze, coarse mesh gauze, gauze rolls (e.g., Kerlex), and elastic bandages. Fluffs may be used to add bulk to the dressings. The dressing may have a layer of gauze impregnated with an antimicrobial ointment or cream, or may be wetted at intervals with saline or with an antibiotic solution. If this method is used, the dressing should feel damp, not saturated; otherwise, maceration of the grafts will occur.

Nursing Considerations. All grafted areas are immobilized to prevent slippage or movement of the newly placed grafts. Traction, bulky dressings, or individual splints are used, not only to immobilize the joint above and below the graft but also to maintain the affected area in a position of function. The first dressing change takes place 2 to 3 days after surgery. The dressing is removed very carefully as the grafts are usually not fully adherent at this time. The grafted areas may be gently cleansed and then redressed in the same manner. Dressings are used until the openings or interstices in the mesh graft have epithelialized and healed. At this time the grafts can then be left open to air. Sheet grafts are commonly left exposed. In this case the nurse frequently assesses the graft for collections of fluid or pus beneath the surface. Pooled secretions can be removed by gently rolling over the fluid collection with a sterile cotton swab to bring secretions to the graft edge where they may be absorbed into the cotton swab.

Patient Education. Grafting, as previously mentioned, may be a concept that is foreign to the patient. It is essential that the nurse provides for the patient an appropriate knowledge base related to the procedure, as well as the healing stages of the graft and donor sites is essential. The importance of immobilization and positioning in the healing process are included in the patient's teaching plan. The patient is told that postoperative pain usually occurs at the donor sites and not the graft areas.

FULL-THICKNESS SKIN GRAFTS

Full-thickness skin grafts are those that include the entire thickness of the dermal layer and are used primarily in reconstructive surgery or in small burns that result in deep defects. A full-thickness skin graft is 0.035 to 0.040 inch thick and thus includes

TABLE 4-4. Comparison of Split-Thickness and Full-Thickness Skin Grafts

	Split-Thickness	Full-Thickness
Layers	Epidermis Partial layer of dermis	Epidermis Entire dermal layer
Advantages	Donor site may be reused Healing of donor site is more rapid Results in good "take"	Allows more elasticity over joints Can reconstruct cosmetic defects Soft, pliable Gives full appearance Provides good color-match Less hyperpigmentation May allow hair growth
Disadvantages	Prone to chronic breakdown Likely to hypertrophy More likely to contract	Donor site takes longer to heal Requires split-thickness graft to heal or closure from wound edges

the hair follicles, sweat glands, and sebaceous glands—skin elements not generally present in split-thickness skin grafts. The grafts "take" by growth of capillaries from the granulation bed. As with split-thickness skin grafts, this process may be affected by conditions that hinder the grafts from obtaining an adequate blood supply.

Full-thickness skin grafts result in donor sites which require a split-thickness skin graft or closure from skin edges in order to heal. Therefore, they are not used for primary coverage of extensive third-degree wounds. They have been used to treat deep burns of the hands and feet accompanied by exposure of tendons or bone. They are also used over areas of muscle mass or soft tissue loss to provide a more natural contour to defect areas. These defects will not accept split-thickness skin grafts and therefore must be closed with a soft tissue flap. Full-thickness skin grafts have also been used in plastic surgery for reconstruction of eyebrows and for release of eyelid contractures. Donor skin taken from the scalp will have the potential for hair growth and has been successful in restoring a more natural appearance in a patient with severe facial burns. Full-thickness grafts are preferred for eyelid releases because they are less likely to contract than are split-thickness skin grafts. Stent dressings are commonly used for the immobilization and protection of full-thickness skin grafts and for grafting in concave areas of the body such as the leg, ankle, or underarm. They exert slight pressure and prevent movements that may interfere with the security of the graft. Full-thickness grafts can be obtained from the scalp, supraclavicular region, inner aspect of the upper arm, thigh, chest, groin, or back. The closer the donor site is to the grafted area, the better the skin texture and color match.

Table 4-4 compares the clinical advantages and disadvantages of split- and full-thickness skin grafts.

Procedure. (Refer to Split-Thickness Skin Grafts, page 59.)

Nursing Considerations. (Refer to Split-Thickness Skin Grafts, page 60.)

Patient Education. (Refer to Split-Thickness Skin Grafts, page 60.)

PEDICLE GRAFTS

A pedicle graft or flap is a full-thickness graft that is also used primarily in reconstruction and in deep tissue defects resulting from severe burns. This type of graft is performed as an adjacent flap or distant flap, which means the skin graft is transferred

TABLE 4-5. Factors Affecting Graft Viability

Factors Inhibiting Graft "Take"	Factors Promoting Graft "Take"
Infection	Adequate hemostasis
Necrotic skin (tissue)	Anatomic location of graft
Anatomic location of graft	Smooth contour
Perineum	Nonjoints
Axilla	Graft secured well
Buttocks	Immobilization of graft area
Poor-quality donor skin	Good nutritional status
Poor nutritional status	
Bleeding	
Mechanical trauma	
Shock	

from one part of the body onto another. However, the flap includes not only skin and subcutaneous tissue but an artery and vein as well. These subcutaneous vessels are presented in the pedicle portion of the graft in order to maintain an adequate blood supply to the flap, especially its most distal portion.

Procedure. Pedicle flaps can be performed for revisions of scar defects from surrounding healthy tissue. This involves excising the scar and transferring a flap by raising and swinging the tissue up to cover the defect. The area from which the flap was taken is then covered with a split-thickness skin graft. If this adjacent transfer of skin is not possible, then distant skin pedicle flaps can be performed. With this surgery, a skin flap from one area of the body is attached to the area in need of grafting. Once the distal part of the graft has taken, it will remain in place as the flap is divided and the remainder is returned to the original site. The open portion of the original donor is then covered with a split-thickness skin graft. Pedicle flaps are becoming less widely used while free skin flap procedures are gaining in popularity. Free skin flaps are less traumatic and complicated because they require only one surgery, they hasten healing, and the donor sites can usually heal by primary closure.

Nursing Considerations. All grafted areas must be immobilized to prevent movement or slippage of the newly placed grafts. Care of the dressing is similar to that of split-thickness skin grafts. (Refer to Nursing Considerations: Split-Thickness Skin Grafts page 60. Additionally, involved areas need to be assessed as to circulatory status; note color, warmth, sensation, and capillary refill. All involved extremities are elevated to promote proper circulation. Factors affecting graft viability are summarized in Table 4-5.

Patient Education. (Refer to Patient Education: Split-Thickness Skin Grafts, page 60).

Donor Sites

A donor site is an area of the body used to provide a skin graft to resurface a burn wound. Any area of the body can be used as a donor site including the chest, back, buttocks, legs, arms, and even scalp. However, it is preferable not to graft skin from joint surfaces. Selection of the donor site is dependent upon the availability of skin, the thickness of the skin needed, the area to be grafted, color match-up, and cosmetic concerns. In patients with extensive full-thickness burns, there may not be a luxury of selecting preferred donor sites. It is then a case of using whatever skin is available.

Procedure. Donor skin can be obtained using a variety of instruments called "dermatomes." Regardless of the method used, the removal of a split-thickness skin graft essentially creates a partial-thickness wound. Healing time varies, as it usually depends upon the thickness of the donor graft and the method of donor site management. Once the donor skin has been procured, hemostasis is achieved prior to the application of dressings. A mixture of epinephrine and thrombin is useful in controlling the bleeding from the donor site.

Many methods are used in the treatment of donor sites. The ideal dressing promotes healing, offers comfort to patients, and is easy to remove. Open fine mesh gauze, scarlet red, or xeroform gauze coupled with heat lamp treatments have been used with satisfactory results in donor sites; however, once the gauze dries, it forms a hard protective crust that is painful with movement.

Biologic dressings such as Biobrane may be used in the same way. As the donor site heals, the gauze dressings can be trimmed and then finally removed once the wound has epithelialized. Op-site or similar transparent wound dressings used in moist wound healing are also used in donor site management. The semipermeable membrane allows air to reach the donor site but holds in the fluid that initially oozes from the donor area. The donor site eventually dries and heals with a minimum of pain or trauma. The donor area may also be dressed with a topical cream or ointment and treated as a partial-thickness burn.

Regardless of the method of treatment, the donor site will usually heal in about 10 to 14 days and can be used to reharvest more donor skin. Subsequent skin grafts taken from the sites will be thinner and of lesser quality.

Nursing Considerations. The dressing over the donor site is trimmed as the wound heals; otherwise, the patient may pull at the dressing and further traumatize the skin.

Patient Education. The nurse instructs the patient that the donor site will be more painful than the graft site. Stages of wound healing are reviewed with the patient. The patient is taught not to pull at any dressings. As healing occurs, the donor site may be itchy. The patient is told not to scratch the donor site. Appropriate antipruritics are usually prescribed.

Wound Healing

Partial-thickness wounds have the ability to heal spontaneously from epithelialization that occurs from the sweat glands, hair follicles, and sebaceous glands. These wounds are treated knowledgeably in order to recognize symptoms of complications and to assess the progression of wound healing. A superficial partial-thickness burn will generally heal within 2 weeks. However, the deeper the burn extends into the dermis, the longer it will take for wound healing to be complete. Once healed, the wound appears dry, flaky, and pinkish. The patient often complains of itchiness, which may be difficult to control even with the use of antihistamines. Lanolin, cocoa butter, or other moisturizers are used on healed wounds until the initial dryness subsides. Partial-thickness wounds gradually fade and return to a normal skin color over a period of months. Hypertrophic scarring may occur, but this is difficult to predict. As a rule, the deeper the partial-thickness burn, the more propensity it has for hypertrophy. Pressure garments are indicated in instances where this scarring is anticipated.

The wound healing process of full-thickness burns is lengthy as it continues through the maturation of the skin graft. Although a split-thickness skin graft is a permanent closure of an open burn wound, it has characteristics that differ from normal skin. A skin graft, whether a sheet or mesh graft, has an appearance that cannot match that of unburned skin. Skin grafts, especially thin grafts, may break down, contract, or hypertrophy. This may cause contractures, which limit normal range of motion and result in an unsightly appearance.

Skin grafts may develop areas of hyperpigmentation, which are aggravated by exposure to sunlight. Also, there are variances in the return of sensation to the grafted areas. If grafting is delayed or heavy scar tissue develops under the graft, return of sensation may be delayed or spotty. Split-thickness skin grafts have few sweat glands and hair follicles and, once healed, tend to be dry and scaly. Daily cleaning with soap and water is of great importance not only for hygienic reasons but also to prevent infection and promote wound healing. Small areas where grafts may not have "taken" are debrided and allowed to heal from closure of surrounding tissue. Wound healing is also dependent upon good nutrition to meet the body's increased calorie and protein needs. The use of pressure garments is a necessity in helping to help keep scars soft and flat in an attempt to prevent hypertrophic scar formation.

SUMMARY

The care of a burn patient encompasses more than just local wound care. It involves attention to the patient's physical, emotional, and spiritual needs—all of which are necessary in the recovery process. The nurse's role as a burn team member is a vital one, for his or her skills of observation, assessment, and knowledgeable intervention can certainly make a remarkable difference in the patient's recovery from a traumatic, life-threatening injury.

NURSING CARE PLAN: GENERAL LOCAL TREATMENT OF BURNS

Nursing Diagnosis: Skin Integrity, Impairment of: Actual

May Be Related To:

- Burn wound
- Graft site
- Donor site

Possibly Evidenced By: Disruption of skin surface and destruction of skin layers.

Desired Patient Outcomes: Closure of wounds and donor sites. Complete "take" of skin grafts.

Interventions	Rationale
INDEPENDENT	
• Observe and assess wounds daily, noting adherence of grafts as well as pus or exudate on or under grafts.	• Grafts will gradually adhere to granulation tissue. Any necrotic tissue remaining on recipient bed may become infected.

Interventions	**Rationale**
• Maintain bedrest and immobilization of grafted area as appropriate. Patients with grafts to lower legs should remain on bedrest for 7 days; upper legs, 5 days.	• Patient movement may cause shearing of graft or may dislodge or disrupt graft placement, all of which could lead to loss of graft.
• Maintain dressings to mesh grafts. Maintain moisture to grafted area as ordered; e.g., wet dressings every 4 hours with appropriate solutions; *or* gentamicin ointment on fine mesh gauze; *or* Omiderm.	• Dressings must be intact and graft must be prevented from drying out to protect granulation tissue for widely meshed grafts.
• Protect donor site from trauma. Use bed cradle to prevent irritation from bed sheets if exposure method is used. Position donor site away from external pressure from bed, pillows, and the like.	• Donor sites are painful and easily traumatized. Bed cradles facilitate contact with air and promote comfort.
• Use heat lamp treatments to dry donor sites as appropriate. Protect from moisture.	• Rapid drying of donor sites promotes faster healing.
• Observe for the presence of edema, redness, tenderness, or unusual exudate on donor site.	• These symptoms are indicative of wound infection and will necessitate a change in treatment of the donor.

COLLABORATIVE

Temporary Grafts

• Temporary grafts must be changed every 3 to 5 days.	• Frequent changing of grafts aids in wound debridement and reduces risk of excessive "take" or rejection of grafts.
• Using sterile technique, remove old temporary graft from the patient slowly and carefully.	• Adherence of grafts may cause pain, bleeding, and trauma to the patient during removal. For large wounds, the procedure may require a surgical operation with general anesthesia.
• Allow grafted areas to be open to air or wrap in occlusive dressings as ordered (with or without antibiotics).	• Open method allows constant observation of graft site. Occlusive dressings absorb drainage, protect the grafted area, and are usually necessary with children and uncooperative patients.
• When the graft is removed, observe granulation tissue for cleanliness, color, and gross appearance.	• Clean granulation tissue that has a good "take" of the temporary graft will likely have success with permanent graft "take."

Permanent Grafts

• Assist physician with first postgraft dressing change. Nursing staff may perform subsequent dressing changes.	• Physician performs first change because of familiarity with graft location. At this time, physician also needs to assess graft "take" and note appearance of site.

Nursing Diagnosis: Skin Integrity, Impairment of: Actual (*Continued*)

Interventions	Rationale
• Hydrotherapy is avoided until graft "take" is ensured. Wound care and bath are performed in bed or on shower trolley if movement is permitted.	• Until grafts are adherent, patient is not immersed in water. Whirlpool action may disrupt grafts.
• With daily wound care, assess graft "take," cleanse wounds gently, and debride loose crusts or scabs from grafted areas. Trim excess grafts that have overlapped onto an unburned skin.	• Grafts must be cleansed well, with removal of necrotic tissue and exudate to aid in the healing process.
• Resume hydrotherapy and range of motion exercises on the fifth through seventh postoperative days if grafts are adherent.	• Splinting and immobilization result in stiffness. Hydrotherapy and physical therapy help the patient gradually return to full function without jeopardizing the adherent grafts.
• Use open technique on mesh grafts once epithelialization of interstices has taken place.	• Graft will no longer be in danger of drying and sloughing once grafts "take" and interstices close. Removal of dressings will also facilitate range of motion exercise.
• Use lanolin or other moisturizer of choice on healed grafts after wound care and p.r.n.	• Grafted areas are prone to dryness because of lack of oil-producing glands in the newly grafted skin. A moisturizer will help keep the skin soft and supple.

Donor Site

• If using fine mesh gauze on donor sites, trim loose edges daily to prevent accidental pulling of the gauze.	• As donor site heals, gauze will lift off to expose areas of epithelialization.
• When donor site is completely healed, remove dressing material, wash well with soap and water, and apply moisturizing cream to the area.	• Complete healing will usually take place within 2 weeks. Dressing will lift off easily and painlessly. Cleansing removes dried exudate, and moisturizer will improve the dry, flaky appearance of a newly healed donor site.

Nursing Diagnosis: Injury, Potential for Infection and Sepsis

May Be Related To:

• Loss of skin integrity
• Decreased resistance to infection
• Multiple dressing changes and tubbings, which increase opportunity for contamination

Possibly Evidenced By: Elevated temperature, positive wound cultures, and changes in wound drainage (odor, redness, tenderness, swelling, and amount of drainage).

Desired Patient Outcomes: Prevention of wound infection and sepsis.

Interventions	**Rationale**
INDEPENDENT	
• Observe grafts and dressings for presence of foul odor, redness, induration, cellulitis, or excessive wound drainage. Notify physician at once.	• These signs are indicative of infection and signal the need to change dressings and check graft site.
• Maintain aseptic technique during wound care procedures. Maintain protective isolation practices. Wash hands before and after patient care.	• Burn patient is susceptible to infection. Aseptic technique and isolation help protect patient from introduction of organisms and cross-contamination. Handwashing reduces the chance of cross-contamination.
• Monitor vital signs noting trends and reporting temperature elevations above 38.5°C to physician. Monitor respiratory status and observe for changes in level of consciousness.	• Temperature elevations may indicate sepsis or rejection of biologic graft. Early recognition of infection allows for prompt treatment.
• Accumulation of pus under graft must be removed by cutting graft and expressing infected material or "rolling" the graft with a cotton swab.	• Exudate or debris from burn wounds must be cleansed from the site to protect the open wounds from infection.
COLLABORATIVE	
• Obtain culture of purulent drainage if present on wounds. Obtain blood, urine, and sputum cultures for patients with temperature elevations above 38.5°.	• Identifies source of infection as well as sensitivities for topical and/or antibiotic therapy.
• If infection is present, remove dressing if possible, culture wounds, and apply an antimicrobial agent.	• Infection can cause delayed healing of a graft or donor site. It then requires treatment similar to a full- or partial-thickness wound using topical antibiotics to control bacterial proliferation.

BIBLIOGRAPHY

Artz, CP, Moncrief, JA, and Pruitt, BA (eds): Burns: A Team Approach. WB Saunders, Philadelphia, 1979.

Bayley, E and Smith, G: The three degrees of burn care. Nursing '87, March 1987.

Boswick, JA: The Art and Science of Burn Care. Aspen Publishers, Rockville, MD, 1987.

Chi-Chun, Y, Wei-Shia, H, and Tsi-Siang, S: Treatment of Burns. Shanghai Scientific and Technical Publishers, New York, 1982.

Coche, W, White, R, Lynch, DJ, and Verheyden, C: Wound Care. Churchill-Livingstone, New York, 1986.

Gaisford, JC, Slater, H, and Goldfarb, IW: The Management of Burn Trauma, A Unified Approach. Synapse Publications, Pittsburgh, 1983.

Hummell, RP (ed): Clinical Burn Therapy, A Management and Prevention Guide. John Wright & Sons, Boston, 1982.

Wachtel, T, Kahn, V, and Frank, H: Current Topics in Burn Care. Aspen Systems, Rockville, MD, 1983.

Wise, DL (ed): Burn Wound Coverings. Vols 1 and II. CRC Press, Boca Raton, FL, 1984.

Chapter 5

JANET A. MARVIN

INFECTION CONTROL

Infection is the leading cause of morbidity and mortality in burn patients after the first 72 hours. Infection control must be a consideration for these patients in every treatment and in every contact with them. Infections come from two sources: (1) endogenous sources, which include those organisms contained in or on the patient's own mucous membranes and skin, and (2) exogenous sources, which include the patient's environment and the people who come in contact with the patient.

ENDOGENOUS SOURCES OF INFECTIONS

Endogenous sources usually cause infectious problems in burn patients because of some physical or physiologic change that allows the invasion of common microorganisms. The most obvious of these changes is the loss of the intact skin as a result of the injury itself. In patients with minor injuries this loss is small and the morbidity is usually minimal (i.e., extending the length of time required for healing by a few days) but in more severe cases may cause increased functional or cosmetic deformities. For the patient with extensive injuries such infections may cause prolonged morbidity and increase mortality significantly. In addition to the obvious physical or physiologic changes which occur with loss of intact skin, burn patients are subject to other assaults from their own microbial flora. Examples of these are infections associated with indwelling catheters and tubes to include intravenous lines, Foley catheters, nasogastric tubes, and endotracheal tubes. Each of these tubes or catheters necessary for survival may cause local irritation and may predispose the burn patient to additional infectious risk from the normal flora of their skin or mucous membranes.

EXOGENOUS SOURCES OF INFECTIONS

Exogenous sources may compound the infectious problems in burn patients. Within the environment animate as well as inanimate objects may be the sources of contamination and infection. Exogenous infections are often far worse than endogenous infections because the organisms causing these infections have survived the usual aseptic hospital environment and may have become resistant to one or more of the standard antibiotics used to treat such infections.[1-3] These organisms are most frequently carried on the hands and apron area of health care personnel and are transmitted during therapeutic encounters with the patient.

Thus, adherence to strict aseptic procedures such as hand washing; gloving for contact with indwelling catheters, tubes, or open wounds; and wearing of impervious garments to prevent contact with the apron area of health care personnel can lead to significant reduction in the spread of exogenous organisms.

SPECIFIC ORGANISMS

A number of pathogens plague the burn patient and may include not only bacteria but also fungi and viruses. The most common organisms to colonize the burn wound include the organisms commonly found on the skin, such as *Streptococcus* and *Staphylococcus*; the normal enteric organisms such as the *Proteus* species and *Escherichia coli*; and common hospital nosocomial organisms such as the *Pseudomonas* and *Serratia* species. Common pathogens are summarized in Table 5–1.

The incidence of specific organisms is unit specific and varies over time as reported by several investigators.[4-7] Those that appear in almost every report include *Staphylococcus aureus*, *Pseudomonas aeruginosa*, *Serratia marcescens*, and *Klebsiella pneumoniae*. Yet reports of other organisms causing wound infection periodically appear in the literature.[8-11] Such organisms include group A *Streptococcus* or *S. pyogenes*,[8,9] *Staphylococcus epidermitis*,[10] and *Providencia stuartii*,[11] to name a few. Mason and coworkers[12] have also reported a high incidence of yeastlike organisms. Desai and associates have reported a similar incidence in *Candida* infections,[13] while Grube reported a much lower incidence from the University of Washington Burn Center.[14] Thus, it is relatively impossible to quote statistics for any one organism and the role that it plays in the causation of burn wound infections. A careful review of each unit's bacterial ecology over time is the most important information the burn team can have in assessing the type, spread, and virulence of the various organisms. Close attention to antibiotic sensitivities is also important to the appropriate treatment of these organisms.

TABLE 5–1. Common Pathogens of Burn Patients

Normal Skin Flora
  Streptococcus
  Staphylococcus
Normal Enteric Flora
  Proteus
  Escherichia coli
Common Nosocomial Pathogens
  Pseudomonas aeurginosa
  Serratia marcescens
  Klebsiella pneumoniae
Other Bacterial Organisms
  Group A *Streptococcus*
  Providencia stuartii
Yeastlike Organisms
Fungi
Viruses

Although textbooks of the past abound with the signs and symptoms associated with gram-positive and gram-negative infections, more recent reviews suggest that the specific symptoms exhibited by the individual patient have more to do with systemic factors such as immune response and volume status than they do with the specific organisms. Thus, with any infection the assessment parameters are those as listed later under objective signs of systemic infections.

IMMUNE RESPONSES

Also responsible for the increased risk of infection noted in the burn patient are the major physiologic derangements that occur in the specific immune responses of these patients. These include both alterations in humoral and cell-mediated immunity. Changes in humoral immunity are noted in decreased levels of immunoglobulins such as IgG, IgM, and IgA.[15-18] These immunoglobulins are proteins that have antibody activity against microorganisms that invade the body. It is suggested that the circulating level of each of these globulins decreases significantly soon after injury and then returns to normal over weeks or months. The levels of IgA and IgM return to normal more quickly than does that of IgG.[19-21] These antibodies play multiple roles in host defense to include toxin neutralization, bacteriolysis in the presence of complement, and opsonization of bacteria resulting in enhanced phagocytosis. Thus, these globulins are important to both complement and white cell function, and a defect in any of the three may lead to compromise in the function of each. Likewise, the complement system has a major role to play in the inflammatory process by neutralizing viruses, increasing vascular permeability, and enhancing leukocyte chemotaxis, as well as through opsonization leading to phagocytosis of microorganisms. A number of investigators have described decreases in C3a and C5a and other parts of the complement system after burn injury.[22-26] Thus, if complement activity is depressed then the response of chemotaxis cells and subsequent phagocytosis is likely to be depressed. Others have demonstrated defects in cell-mediated immunity to include neutrophils, monocytes, and macrophages.[27-32] These defects, along with those just mentioned, lead to decreased chemotaxis, phagocytosis, and intracellular killing. These altered complex interactions of the immune system, in addition to the metabolic alterations seen in burn patients, lead to a decreased ability of the host to defend against infection.

PROTECTIVE ISOLATION: TO ISOLATE OR NOT

Protective isolation (reverse isolation) has often been suggested as a way to prevent the spread of nosocomial infections to burn patients. The questions are:

- How much protective isolation is needed in the immunologically compromised patient?
- Are all burn patients sufficiently immunocompromised to need protective isolation?
- What should protective isolation include? Laminar air flow units? Gowns? Masks? Gloves? Shoe covers? Aprons? Individual rooms?

A number of reports suggest that the most elaborate protective system (i.e., laminar flow system) is the ultimate in protection.[33,34] Yet others would suggest otherwise.[35,36] A review of burn unit isolation practices reported at the American Burn Association in

1985 showed that the current use of protective isolation ran the gamut from complex laminar flow systems to the simple use of gloves for dressing changes.[37]

A review of the literature suggests that the spread of nosocomial infections in burn patients is due to two primary sources: the hands and the apron area of personnel.[38-40] Thus, the most simple, least time-consuming, least-expensive system that puts a barrier between the patient and the personnel's hands and apron area would seem to be the most effective way to protect the patients. If hands were washed before and after each patient contact, if gloves were worn for each contact with body secretions, and plastic aprons were worn each time the personnel came in contact with the patient or patient's immediate environment, it may be assumed that there would be a decrease in unit-acquired nosocomial infections. This is in fact true as evidenced by the decrease in unit-acquired nosocomial infections reported by the University of Washington Burn Center at the 1986 meeting of the American Burn Association.[41] Thus, when the questions are asked—To isolate or not? How to isolate? Whom to isolate?—the answers can be quite simple. Wash hands frequently and provide the best barrier to hand- and clothes-bourne infection as possible with gloves and aprons.

NURSING ASSESSMENT

The nursing assessment in relation to infection control in the burn patient focuses on two different aspects: the first is assessment of the patient for signs of local or systemic infection, and the second is assessment of the environment to prevent the spread of exogenous organisms. Figure 5-1 presents an infection control assessment tool.

Patient assessment includes initial assessment/history; status of tetanus immunizations; history of recent previous infections to include cold sores, rashes (with pustules) and boils, and so forth; and local and systemic signs of infection. Objective local signs of infection include redness extending beyond wound margins, purulent exudate, swelling and edema around the wound; warmth around the wound margins; and microbiologic culture showing significant growth ($>10^5$ organisms per gram of tissue) of pathogens. The subjective local signal of infection is the complaint of pain in and around the wound, especially throbbing pain unrelated to movement. Systemic signs of infection include both subjective complaints and objective parameters. As just noted under local signs, complaints of pain in and around the wound unrelated to movement may be elicited. In addition, the patient may complain of general achiness and malaise. The objective signs of infection include:

- Tachycardia
- Tachypnea
- Hypothermia or hyperthermia
- Confusion
- Unexplained acidosis
- Unexplained glycosuria
- Ileus or nausea
- Decreased blood pressure
- Decreased urine output
- Decreased platelet count
- WBC <5000
- Surveillance cultures (wound, sputum, blood, urine) showing significant colonization with pathogens

High WBC counts are usually seen in burn patients, and are more likely related to the injury itself than to a specific infection. Many of the signs or symptoms may occur in

INFECTION CONTROL ASSESSMENT

Name _____ Age _____

History   **Previous infections:**
_____ impetigo
_____ cold sores
_____ rashes with pustules
_____ boils
_____ other _____
_____
_____

Immunizations
_____ Tetanus _____ year _____ booster
_____ other _____

Current   _____ erythema beyond wound edges
local   _____ purulent exudate
manifes-   _____ swelling and edema around wound
tations   _____ warmth around wound
_____ culture $> 10^5$ organisms/gram of tissue
_____ complaints of pain, tenderness, and throbbing

Current   _____ tachycardia (___ rate)
systemic   _____ tachypnea (___ rate)
manifes-   _____ hypothermia (___ °C)
tations   _____ hyperthermia (___ °C)
_____ confusion
_____ acidosis
_____ glycosuria
_____ ileus
_____ nausea
_____ hypotension (___ / ___ mmHg pressure)
_____ decreased urinary output (___ cc/hour)
_____ decreased platelet count (_____ /cc)
_____ leukopenia (_____)
_____ culture showing significant colonization with pathogens

FIGURE 5–1. Infection control assessment: a brief review.

the burn patient in relation to other problems or complications, but the occurrence of three or more of these concurrently should be considered indicative of sepsis until proven otherwise.

Environmental assessment consists of regular methods to note compliance of personnel with aseptic procedures, isolation techniques, and continued surveillance of the nursing unit's microbial ecology by the infection control officer to note patterns of spread of specific organisms and development of resistant organisms. This surveillance includes a review of individual patient profiles as well as the attack rate for various organisms within the total population of the nursing unit. Routine environmental cultures are expensive and rarely useful in surveillance. Environmental cultures are only useful in tracing a source when a specific problem has been noted. In this case, this should include both animate objects (personnel) and inanimate objects in the environment.

NURSING CARE PLAN: INFECTION CONTROL

Nursing Priorities

Nursing priorities for these patients are:

1. Provide aseptic environment for patient
2. Monitor patient for signs of local and systemic infectious complications and notify physician of specific evidence of local or systemic infections
3. Monitor microbial ecology of the nursing unit

Nursing Diagnosis: Injury, Potential for Infection

May Be Related To:

- Burn injury causing loss of intact skin.
- Immunoincompetence of the patient with a significant injury (>20 percent total body surface area [TBSA]).
- Multiple invasive procedures necessary to treat the burn patients to include, but not limited to:
  - Intravenous cannulation, central or peripheral (multiple)
  - Intra-arterial cannulation
  - Endotracheal intubation/tracheostomy
  - Nasogastric intubation
  - Urinary catheterization
  - Escharotomies
  - Burn wound debridement (daily)
  - Surgical removal of eschar and autografting
  - Application of biologic and synthetic dressings
  - Improper application of aseptic technique

Possibly Evidenced By:

- Changes in wound drainage
- Positive wound and/or blood cultures

- Tenderness/Pain
- Hypothermia or hyperthermia
- Tachycardia
- Tachypnea
- Decreased blood pressure
- Changes in WBC

Desired Patient Outcomes:

- Remains free of signs and symptoms of infection.
- Surveillance cultures demonstrate normal flora or no significant growth of pathogens.
- In minor burns verbalizes strategies to minimize risk of infection and verbalizes knowledge of signs or symptoms of infection.

General Unit Outcomes:

- Frequent monitoring of unit microbial ecology will not reveal:
  - Spread of organisms from patient to patient or
  - Increase in colonization of patients with resistant organism

---

Interventions	Rationale
INDEPENDENT	
• Maintain isolation precautions appropriate for the patient's extent of injury.	• Use body substance isolation and protective isolation as appropriate to prevent the spread of infection.

Nursing Diagnosis: Injury, Potential for Infection (*Continued*)

Interventions	Rationale

Interventions

- Use strict aseptic techniques with wound care and all invasive procedures.

- Explain appropriate infection control procedures to patient and family (for home care also instruct concerning the recognition of infection).

- Monitor overall compliance with isolation procedures by all staff.

- Monitor patient for signs and symptoms of local infection by frequent wound inspection at time of dressing changes.
- Cleanse wound to remove exudate and debris in and around wound.
- Initially and periodically remove hair from and adjacent to wound sites (never shave eyebrows).
- Debride loose eschar and scabs from wounds during daily cleansing.

- Cleanse nonburned areas, especially hair-bearing areas, under nails, and perineal area.

COLLABORATIVE

- Apply topical antibacterial agents as prescribed. These may include but are not limited to:
  - Silver sulfadiazine
  - Mafenide cream
  - Mafenide solution
  - Silver nitrate
  - Povidone-iodine
  (Refer to Chapter 4, pages 44–49.)
- Administer tetanus toxoid or tetanus hyperimmune globulin as prescribed.

Rationale

- Strict aseptic technique should prevent the occurrence of iatrogenic infections associated with invasive procedures.
- *For minor burns:* Wound care may be given by the patient or the family; thus, they are instructed in appropriate home care techniques to prevent infection and also the recognition of infection (Refer to Chapter 8, page 121).
  For major burns: The family is instructed in appropriate hand washing and other infection-control measures.
- Breaks in technique are always brought to the attention of the offending health care worker in a discrete manner to prevent the spread of infection.
- This assists in the identification of infectious processes.

- This decreases bacterial contamination.

- Hair left in or near wound sites becomes matted with exudate and may promote infection.
- Eschar or scabs should be removed gently so as not to cause bleeding. Necrotic tissue provides a medium for bacterial proliferation.
- These areas may harbor bacteria and predispose the patient to increased infection risk.

- Antibacterial agents are used to prevent the microbial invasion of the burn wound. The nurse is aware of the advantages and disadvantages of each therapy used and specific side effects associated with their use.

- Tetanus infection remains a prime concern in any open wound; thus, protection through appropriate immunization is imperative.

Interventions	**Rationale**
• Administer prescribed antibiotics. Monitor for side effects and draw appropriate blood levels as prescribed.	• Burn patients have been shown to have altered antibiotic metabolism; thus, it is necessary to monitor serum levels of many antibiotics, especially the aminoglycosides.
• Obtain routine or prescribed cultures as appropriate for culture and sensitivity. Monitor culture reports and report significant changes in type or quantity of organisms or changes in sensitivity patterns.	• Routine wound and sputum cultures allow early detection and treatment of wound or pulmonary infection.
• Note similarity of organisms and resistance patterns between patients.	• Monitoring of unit microbial ecology will help prevent cross-contamination.
• Avoid placing intravenous lines in leg veins of adults to avoid later complications of thrombophlebitis.	• Intravenous lines and catheters in leg veins of adults increases the risk of thrombophlebitis and sepsis because of reduced peripheral blood flow and stagnation in nonambulatory patients.

REFERENCES

1. Hambraeus, A and Ransjö, U: Attempts to control clothes-borne infection in a burn unit. J Hyg Camb 79:193, 1977.
2. Ransjö, U: Attempts to control clothes-borne infection in a burn unit, 3. An open-rooted plastic isolator or plastic aprons to prevent contact transfer of bacteria. J Hyg Camb 82:385, 1977.
3. Ransjö, U: Attempts to control clothes-borne infection in a burn unit, 2. Clothing routines in clinical use and the epidemiology of cross-colonization. J Hyg Camb 82:369, 1979.
4. Hansbrough, JF, et al: Identification and antibiotic susceptibility of bacterial isolates from burn patients. Burns 11(6):393, 1985.
5. Mason, AD, McManus, AT, and Pruitt, BA: Association of burn mortality and bacteria: A 25 year review. Arch Surg 121(9):1027, 1986.
6. Lee, JJ, et al: Infection control in a burns unit. J Burn Care and Rehab. In press.
7. Ward, CG: Bacterial opportunists: A 20-year survey. Report at Symposium: Burns and Infection, Dallas, Feb 14–16, 1985.
8. Webster, A, Scott, GMS, Ridgeway, GL, and Grüneberg, RN: An outbreak of group A streptococcal skin infection: Control by source isolation and Teicoplanin therapy. Scand J Infect Dis 19:205, 1987.
9. Whitley M, Sleigh JD, Reid W, et al: Streptococcal outbreak in a regional burns centre and a plastic surgery unit. J Hosp Infect 5:63, 1984.
10. Demling, RH and Maly, J: The treatment of burn patients in a laminar airflow environment. Ann NY Acad Sci 353:294, 1980.
11. Curreri, PW, et al: Providencia stuartii sepsis: A new challenge in the treatment of thermal injury. Ann Surg 177(2):133, 1973.
12. Ibid, 5.
13. Desai, MH, Herndon, DN, and Abston, S: Candida infection in the massively burned patient. Program and Abstracts of the 18th Annual Meeting of the ABA, Chicago, Apr 11, 1986.
14. Grube, BJ, Marvin, JA, and Heimbach, DM: Candida: A decreasing problem for the burned patient? Arch Surg 123(2):194, 1988.
15. Arturson, G, Johansson, SGD, Högman, CF, and Killander, J: Changes in immunoglobulin levels in severely burned patients. Lancet 1:546, 1969.
16. Kohn, J and Cort, DF: Immunoglobulins in burned patients. Lancet 1:836, 1969.

17. Munster, AM, Hoaglund, HC, and Pruitt, BA: The effects of thermal injury on serum immunoglobulins. Ann Surg 172:965, 1970.
18. Ninnemann, JL, Fisher, JC, and Wachtel, TL: Effect of thermal injury and subsequent therapy on serum protein concentrations. Burns 6:165, 1980.
19. Ibid, 15.
20. Ibid, 16.
21. Ibid, 18.
22. Heideman, M: The effect of thermal injury on hemodynamic, respiratory, and hematologic variables in relation to complement. J Trauma 19:239, 1979.
23. Heideman, M, Kaijser, B, and Gelin, L: Complement activation and hematologic, hemodynamic, and respiratory reactions early after soft tissue injury. J Trauma 18:696, 1978.
24. Hill, JH and Ward, PA: C3 leukotactic factors produced by tissue protease. J Exp Med 13:505, 1969.
25. Alexander, JW, McClellan, MA, Ogle, CK, and Ogle, JD: Consumptive opsoninopathy: Possible pathogenesis in lethal and opportunistic infections. Ann Surg 184:672, 1976.
26. Bjornson, AB, Altemeier, WA, and Bjornson, HS: Changes in hormonal components of host defense following burn trauma. Ann Surg 186:88, 1977.
27. Warden, GD, Mason, AD, and Pruitt, BA: Suppression of leukocyte chemotaxis in vitro by chemotherapeutic agents used in the management of thermal injuries. Ann Surg 1181:363, 1975.
28. Warden, GD, Mason, AD, and Pruitt, BA: Evaluation of leukocyte chemotaxis in vitro in thermally injured patients. J Clin Invest 54:1001, 1974.
29. Curreri, PW, Heck, EI, Browne, L, and Baxter, C: Stimulated neutrophil antibacterial function and prediction of wound sepsis in burn patients. Surgery 74:6, 1973.
30. Miller, CL: Alterations in Macrophage Function Following Thermal Injury. In Ninneman JL (ed): The Immune Consequences of Thermal Injury. Williams & Wilkins, Baltimore, 1981, pp 49–65.
31. McManus, AT, Lescher, TJ, Mason, AD, and Pruitt, BA: Altered human granulocyte glucose metabolism following severe thermal injury. Proceedings of the American Burn Association, New Orleans, 1977.
32. Demarest, GB, Rosen, H, and Altman, LC: Chemiluminescence of polymorphonuclear leukocytes in patients with thermal injury. Proceedings of the American Burn Association, New Orleans, 1979.
33. Burke JF, et al: The control of a bacterially isolated environment to the prevention of infection in seriously burned patients. Am Surg 186(3):377, 1977.
34. Ibid, 10.
35. Choctau, WT: Is there a need for barrier isolators with laminar air flow in managing adult patients with major burns? J Burn Care and Rehab 5(4):331, 1984.
36. May, SR, Ehleben, CM, and DeClement, FA: Delirium in burn patients isolated in a plenum laminar air flow ventilation unit. Burns 10(5):331, 1984.
37. Lee, JJ, Marvin, JA, and Heimbach, DM: Survey of Isolation Techniques. Presented at the 17th Annual Meeting of the ABA, Orlando, FL, 1985.
38. Ibid, 1.
39. Ibid, 2.
40. Ibid, 3.
41. Marvin, JA, et al: Comparison of burn unit microbial colonization before and after two efforts to improve isolation techniques. Presented at the 18th Annual Meeting of the ABA, Chicago, 1986.

Chapter 6

MELVA KRAVITZ

NUTRITIONAL CARE

The nutritional support required by burn patients is dependent upon two factors: the patient's preburn nutritional status and the extent of the total body surface area (TBSA) burn. Adequately nourished patients with minor burns need no nutritional support beyond a regular diet. Patients with adequate preburn nutrition and moderate burns require a high-calorie, high-protein oral diet. Patients with minor or moderate burns in combination with preburn malnutrition require assessment of the patient's nutritional status and an individualized plan to restore positive nitrogen balance. Patients with poor preburn nutritional status are classified as having a critical injury, regardless of burn size, because of the body's decreased ability to resist infection, heal the burn, and tolerate operative procedures. All patients with major burn injuries require nutritional support above normal daily requirements in order to survive the injury. In particular, nutritional deficiencies contribute to immune defects which may lead to failure of immune defenses. Cell-mediated immunity, antibody production, the reticuloendothelium system, neutrophil function, and fibronectic and opsonic capacity are all affected by nutritional defects.[1]

RESPONSES TO A BURN INJURY

The four major nutrition-related responses to a burn injury are hypermetabolism, catecholamine elevation, hyperglycemia, and nitrogen imbalance. An understanding of these responses provides rationale for interventions and an improved evaluation of treatment outcomes.

Hypermetabolism

Hypermetabolism characterizes the metabolic response to burn injury, with the magnitude of the physiologic alteration being related to the extent of injury. Negative nitrogen balance, loss of intracellular components, and a rapid decrease in body weight are consequences of the increase in metabolic activity. The extensive loss of protoplasmic mass results in severe erosion of energy and protein stores essential to optimal body function. Studies have suggested that energy expenditures may be increased from 40 to

100 percent above basal levels in patients with burns exceeding 30 percent TBSA.[2] Following severe burn injury, metabolic rates increase in a linear manner in patients with up to 40 to 50 percent TBSA burns. Recent studies using indirect calorimetry indicate that there appears to be an upper limit to the calories required at near twice the predicted basal metabolic rate.[3] This suggests that the maximal level of heat production is reached with a 50 percent TBSA burn, and patients with larger burns are not capable of achieving a greater increase in metabolic rate; thus, metabolic rate rarely exceeds twice normal levels regardless of the source of stress. The metabolic rate also varies with the time postburn. Oxygen consumption is near normal during the emergent resuscitation phase, followed by rises and peaks in the presence of infection or stressful operative procedures during the acute healing phase. Decreases in the metabolic rate occur in a curvilinear manner as infections are resolved or wound coverage is achieved and the metabolic rate returns toward a predicted basal level.

The etiology of the hypermetabolic response following thermal injury has been studied extensively but the precise mechanism has only recently been defined. In the 1960s, it was thought that increased water loss from the burn wound resulted in surface cooling and stimulated metabolic heat production in order to generate more heat and maintain body temperature. Since the metabolic rate in thermally injured patients treated in a warm (32°C) environment is lower than the rate of patients treated in a cooler (22°C) environment, this evidence was initially interpreted to support the hypothesis that hypermetabolism in burn patients was in response to increased surface cooling due to increased evaporative water loss.[4] However, Zawacki and associates[5] in 1970 reported that covering the wound with a semipermeable membrane, thus blocking evaporative water loss, produced no consistent alteration in the hypermetabolic rate in burn patients studied at 25°C ambient temperatures. Additionally, when burn patients were placed in rigidly controlled conditions in an environmental chamber, a curvilinear relationship between metabolism and burn size, along with a direct linear relationship between evaporative water loss and percent TBSA burn, was demonstrated. Thus, evaporative water loss in a burn patient was found not to be the primary stimulator of the hypermetabolic response but a contributing factor of only approximately 20 percent. The hypermetabolic response is not due to the patient being externally cold but, rather, to an increased heat production related to an endogenous reset in core metabolic activity. At any ambient temperature, the core and mean skin temperatures of the burn patient are well above that of unburned individuals. The increase in core temperature and metabolic rate seems to be the result of a reset of the hypothalamic-adrenal axis and an accompanying increase in catecholamine release.[6]

Catecholamine Elevation

Catecholamines are elevated following thermal injury with the adrenergic activity related to the magnitude of the injury and to oxygen consumption of the patient. Carefully controlled adrenergic blockage by Wilmore and coworkers[7] in patients with large surface area burns demonstrated a consistent decrease in metabolic rate, suggesting that increased catecholamines and adrenergic activity are the major calorigenic mediators responsible for the hypermetabolic response following burn injury. Burn patients with injuries greater than 40 percent TBSA appear to maintain maximal or near-maximal rates of catecholamine synthesis and utilization until wound closure is accomplished. Exposing patients to a cool environment (21°C) results in a mild cold stress, ordinarily a stimulus for elaboration of additional catecholamines. Patients who eventually survived their burn injury responded to cold stress by increasing heat production as a result of increased catecholamine elaboration. In contrast, patients with very large burns who lacked catecholamine reserves or tissue responsiveness to cold stress failed to generate sufficient additional heat to maintain internal heat balance in 21°C ambient temperature and became hypothermic. All of the nonresponding patients in this study subsequently died from complications of their injury.[7] Thus, comparing burn size with metabolic rate, it would appear that there is a limit to the physiologic response in extensively burned patients lacking the sympathetic physiologic reserve to compensate for further physiologic stresses such as infection, operative procedures, or the environmental stress of ambient temperature changes.

Stratta and colleagues[8] reported the occurrence of burn injury in an adrenalectomized patient receiving long-term steroid replacement therapy, thus illustrating the role of adrenal hormones in the systemic response to thermal injury. The patient, a 29-year-old white man, had a bilateral adrenalectomy 13 years prior to the burn injury for presumed Cushing's disease, with maintenance on replacement corticosteroids. The patient sustained a 35.5 percent TBSA burn, 3.5 percent of which initially appeared to be full-thickness, and a serious inhalation injury. He exhibited defective thermogenesis, maintaining his body temperature at or below 37°C despite the environmental control of the burn unit and constant use of a heat shield. In addition, he was unable to respond to stressful episodes (i.e., surgical procedures) and developed marked hypothermia that was difficult to control. Although his initial catecholamine levels were elevated, they were significantly lower than those of burn patients with intact adrenal function. Another aspect of the patient's metabolic response was a complete lack of glucose intolerance, with normal to low levels of serum glucose throughout postburn convalescence. He demonstrated remarkably poor wound healing and ultimately required autografting of most of his wound. Healing of both the wound and the donor sites proved to be his major clinical problem. The patient survived and was discharged on postburn day 114.

Hyperglycemia

Glucose kinetics are also altered following burn injury. Hyperglycemia is a common occurrence in critically ill patients with the elevation of fasting blood sugar above normal being related to the severity of the injury or the presence of systemic infection. Oral or intravenous glucose tolerance tests in patients following burn shock or systemic infection demonstrate prolonged elevations of serum glucose concentrations that are characteristic of "diabetes in injury" or "stress diabetes." Long and associates[9] demonstrate an increase in the flow of glucose through the extracellular fluid compartments in critically ill patients and hepatic catheterization studies demonstrated inhibition of hepatic gluconeogenesis is dampened. Wilmore and coworkers[10] demonstrated that glucose disappearance is increased following burn injury in spite of persistent hyperglycemia and that glucose flow is related to the extent of body surface burn, with return toward normal as burn wound closure is accomplished.

The insulin response to glucose is dampened during burn shock resuscitation; however, the response is comparable to that of a normal individual's when the glucose is elevated during the height of the burn patient's hypermetabolic phase. During the emergent phase, insulin levels decrease and the patient develops hyperglycemia, an effect probably due to the early postburn elevation of catecholamines which inhibit insulin action. During the acute phase, although insulin levels rise to meet the demands of the hypermetabolic state, the patient remains hyperglycemic. The hyperglycemia appears to result from increased gluconeogenesis rather than decreased insulin effectiveness.[11] Thus, while it is apparent that glucose kinetics are altered, it appears that the increase in glucose flow is due to a decreased insulin inhibition of hepatic gluconeogenesis while glucose utilization in the peripheral tissues remains at normal levels.

Nitrogen Imbalance

Nitrogen imbalance is associated with major burn injury, with one effect of major trauma being an increase in the excretion of body nitrogen. Major injury and infections lead to weight loss and severe alterations in body composition even when calories and protein are supplied in substantial amounts. Tissues appear to have an obligatory glucose demand for maintaining metabolism and for energy production aimed at tissue repair. Protein degradation may be the body's only recourse to glucose stores when a major injury occurs.[12]

The mechanism and mediators of the increased nitrogen loss following major burn injury have only recently been clarified. Cahill and colleagues[13] studied proteolysis and glyconogenesis in starvation and found that amino acids, primarily analine, are released from the muscle bed, transported to the liver, and converted to glucose. This provides a constant source of readily available fuel to maintain function of essential glucose-dependent tissues. Because glycogen stores are limited and fatty acids cannot be converted to new glucose, this alanine cycle provides an ongoing supply of glucose at the expense of body protein. Thus gluconeogenesis and ureagenesis reflect the body's protein catabolic response to injury.

This same sequence of metabolic events occurs with infection, hypermetabolism, and cold exposure. The signal regulating muscle proteolysis is again catecholamines which stimulate an outpouring of lactic acid from the muscle followed by an efflux of 3-carbon amino acid fragments to shuttle 3-carbon intermediates to the liver for conversion to glucose. The 3-carbon nitrogen-containing alanine compound moves back into the liver with other 3-carbon intermediates and is converted into new glucose; the nitrogen released is simultaneously processed to urea. Thus, the rate of ureagenesis as reflected by urine excretion of urea generally correlates with the rate of gluconeogenesis.

Hepatic gluconeogenesis is directed by the interaction of the hormones: insulin promotes hepatic storage while catecholamines, augmented by glucagon and glucocorticosteroids, stimulate hepatic glucose production. In addition, the mobilization of substrate from the periphery is stimulated by catecholamines and this signal for mobilization is increased by an insulin deficiency. Increased adrenergic activity is a major mediator in the metabolic response following injury not only by stimulating calorigenesis but also by regulating substrate mobilization of the Cori and alanine cycles, thereby controlling hepatic gluconeogenesis.

ASSESSMENT

The most easily recognized and documented assessment of the nutritional needs of burn patients is the massive loss of body weight which occurs in the absence of significant nutritional support. Kinney and coworkers[14] noted that the ratio of fuel burned in stressed patients is remarkably constant, with fat contributing from 80 to 85 percent of the calories used and the remainder of the energy originating from the body's protein mass. Maintenance of body protein appears to be critical for survival. Loss of one fourth to one third of protein mass from the body is predictably fatal. This degree of negative nitrogen balance in humans is associated with a 40 to 50 percent body weight loss. Patients with greater than 40 percent TBSA burn demonstrate the maximal stress response within predictable ranges of body mass. The tissue breakdown associated with major burn trauma has been shown to liberate as much as 30 g of nitrogen daily.[15] Even in the presence of supranormal oral intake, weight losses of 25 percent of preadmission weight were found by 3 weeks postinjury. In these hypermetabolic patients, providing early protein and caloric support of at least the predicted energy requirements is necessary for optimal care and may be essential for survival. Weight loss following burn injury is not an obligatory component of the response to trauma but rather a reflection of the difference between the total energy requirements of the patient versus the ability to provide these requirements in the form of adequate intake. With early initiation of vigorous nutritional support, erosion of the total body mass and subsequent starvation leading to immunologic alterations is not inevitable in the massively burned patient.

Caloric Assessment/Caloric Formulas

The hypermetabolism in burn patients directly correlates with the extent of the burn injury; therefore, the caloric requirement also varies with the extent of the injury. Newsome and associates[16] demonstrated that weight stabilization follows definitive wound closure by almost 2 weeks and concluded that since both the magnitude and duration of the catabolic phase are related to the size of the injury, emphasis must be placed on supplying the patient with caloric intake adequate to achieve net balance until wound healing is complete. This appears to be the case in both conservative wound management and in early excision and grafting methods.[17]

Several predictive formulas are used to estimate the caloric requirements of burn patients and all are based on either preburn body weight and percentage TBSA or square meters of body surface area (BSA) and percentage TBSA burn. These are delivered in conjunction with fluids to meet daily evaporative water and basal metabolism needs. The two most widely used formulas are the Curreri formula for adult patients and the Polk formula for pediatric patients (Table 6–1). Curreri and colleagues[18] demonstrated that the daily caloric requirements for a group of adult burn patients could be expressed by a formula:

25 kcal × body weight in kilograms + 40 kcal × % **TBSA** burn

Polk predicted the daily requirement for children as

60 kcal × body weight in kilograms + 35 kcal × % **TBSA** burn

The Galveston formula[19] predicts the daily caloric needs of pediatric patients as:

1800 kcal per square meter of BSA +

2200 kcal per square meter of body surface burned

It is important to emphasize that these formulas represent more than just a total caloric intake: they also predict a positive nitrogen balance for the patient. The ideal ratio of kilocalorie to nitrogen is reported to be between 150:1[20] (16 percent of the kilocalories as nitrogen) and 100:1[21] (25 percent of kilocalories as nitrogen), since some investigators report that severely catabolic patients require a lower kilocalorie to nitrogen ratio (kcal:N) or higher protein intake. Optimal substrate (kilocalorie, carbohy-

TABLE 6–1. Predictive Formulas for Caloric Requirements

ADULT	
Curreri	25 kcal × body weight (kg) + 40 kcal × TBSA burn
PEDI	
Polk	60 kcal × body weight (kg) + 35 kcal × TBSA burn
Galveston	1800 kcal/M² BSA + 2200 kcal/M² TBSA burn

drate, protein, and fat) must be considered along with kcal:N ratios. Supplemental vitamins and minerals to meet minimum recommended daily requirements are also essential. In general, fat can contribute 30 to 40 percent of the total diet kilocalories. High-carbohydrate loads have been associated with increased stress to the pulmonary system as a result of increased carbon dioxide production, increased respiratory quotient (RQ) ratios over 1 indicating that some of the glucose was being converted to fat rather than energy, and hepatomegaly from fat deposition. In addition, carbohydrate oxidation produces water, so that when carbohydrate is administered in excess, fluid volume overload may occur.[22] Burke and coworkers[23] defined optimal glucose range as 4.7 to 6.8 mg/kg per minute. Thus, 45 to 55 percent of the total kilocalories may be carbohydrates without increasing carbon dioxide production or fatty acid infiltrates of the liver. The content of specific enteral formulas may be obtained by referring to product labels.

The assumption that nutritional intake equals utilization is not necessarily true in burn patients. If a patient is losing tremendous amounts of nitrogen or not absorbing glucose, the net caloric utilization will be much less than the amount provided. Daily calorie counts and meticulous intake and output records are essential, as is daily weighing. In addition, daily nitrogen balance studies and, whenever possible, indirect calorimetry measurements provide improved evaluation of therapy while providing nutritional support to hypermetabolic burn patients. The measurement of energy expenditure in burn patients using indirect calorimetry facilitates accurate assessment of each patient's nutritional status. Saffle and associates[24] studied 29 burn patients with a mean burn size of 35 percent TBSA burn, and found that the use of indirect calorimetry permitted tailoring of nutritional support for burn patients in an improved manner over that of using predictive formulas alone.

NUTRITIONAL MANAGEMENT

Three principles guide the nutritional management of patients with critical burns: (1) hypermetabolism follows burn injury and persists until the wounds heal or are closed by autografting; (2) the healing process occurs only in a state of positive nitrogen balance; and (3) any patient with a functioning gastrointestinal tract should receive enteral (intestinal) nutrition.

Immediately postburn, the body changes from an anabolic (or energy storage) mode to a catabolic (or energy utilization) mode. In addition to wound healing, the ability to forestall infectious processes depends greatly upon adequate nutrition. The majority of immune abnormalities following burn injury appear to be related to altered nutrition (Table 6–2). Alexander[25] compares the immune abnormalities associated with burn injury to those caused by protein malnutrition, and reports similar disturbances including decreased numbers of macrophages, T cells, and B cells; impaired antibody responses; depressed complement activity and T-cell function; impaired nonspecific inflammation; and impaired neutrophil function. Some immunologic abnormalities associated with malnutrition, such as antibody response, can be corrected within a short time with adequate nutritional support, whereas others, such as chemotactic response, may take 2 to 3 weeks to be corrected.

Wilmore and Aulick[26] describe glucose as the major metabolic fuel for all cellular components of the healing wound. This is true whether the wound is healing by reepithelialization or by incorporation of a split-thickness autograft. No healing will occur in the absence of adequate nutrition; prolonged wound closure time increases the risk of infection, burn wound sepsis, and death.

TABLE 6-2. Immune Defects Resulting from Altered Nutrition

Decreased numbers of macrophages, T cells, and B cells
Impaired antibody responses
Depressed complement activity and T cell function
Impaired nonspecific inflammation
    Impaired neutrophil function
Impaired chemotaxic response

Nutritional Routes

The routes for administering caloric support following major burn injury are enteral or parenteral or both. Any patient with a functional gastrointestinal tract should receive enteral nutrition. While acknowledging that meeting the nutritional requirements of burned patients remains one of the most essential factors in survival, the method used must be the most suitable for the patient (Table 6-3). In the past, methods were limited to nasogastric or intravenous feedings, both of which often lead to severe complications. The complications associated with nasogastric feedings are most often due to aspiration and subsequent pulmonary complications. Intravenous feedings using total parenteral nutrition (TPN) require a central venous access, and complications are related to catheter-associated infections and sepsis. Herndon and colleagues,[27] in a prospective randomized study of 28 adult patients with burn size greater than 50 percent TBSA, demonstrated that TPN supplementation of oral caloric intake was of no apparent benefit.

ENTERAL FEEDINGS

Because of the potential complications of both nasogastric tubes and TPN, an alternative method using the nasojejunal route and a small, mercury-weighted polyurethane feeding tube was developed. These tubes use a liquid formula diet delivered into the gastrointestinal tract, thus eliminating the infectious complications associated with TPN. The principal advantage of this method over the nasogastric method is that the feeding is not delivered into the stomach but rather to the duodenum or proximal jejunum. The location of the tube permits feeding comatose, confused, or intubated patients. The two criteria for use of this tube are an intact, functional gastrointestinal tract and radiologic fluoroscopy capabilities for tube placement. The tube, size 7 French, is available in both pediatric and adult lengths. The placement and use of the tube have been described in a study by Kravitz and associates,[28] in which the jejunal tube feeding method was evalu-

TABLE 6-3. Comparison of Enteral Feeding Methods

Method	Advantages	Disadvantages
Intermittent Bolus	Follows normal eating patterns; less chance of bacterial contamination	Requires checking placement every feeding; may lead to emesis, to aspiration, and to distension
Continuous Drip	Easier to administer; less time-consuming to the staff; less reflux and acute distension	Higher chance of bacterial contamination; gastrointestinal tract does not rest

ated in two groups of adult and pediatric patients. Group I received high-calorie, high-protein oral diets; group II received the same diet plus the jejunal tube supplement. Comparison of the caloric intake showed that the adults in group II received 45.9 percent more kcal/kg per day and 67.2 percent more protein than did those in the other group. Children in group II received 117 percent more kcal/kg per day and 91.1 percent more protein than those in group I. Thus, the use of tube feedings can significantly increase the amount of nutrition delivered to burn patients.

Enteral nutrition may be provided using either the intermittent or continuous drip method. In one comparison study of the two methods in 76 burn patients, the continuous drip method was preferred because of a lower incidence of gastrointestinal responses.[29] However, another study in neurologic patients reported no differences in the outcome of the methods.[30] Mechanic and Dunn[31] report the pros and cons of each method. Continuous drip is easier to administer, is less time-consuming to the staff, and minimizes acute gastric distention with reflux. However, the likelihood of bacterial contamination of the formula is greater with the continuous drip method and, because the stomach and intestine are constantly filled, there is little opportunity for the gastrointestinal tract to rest. The intermittent bolus method more closely follows normal eating periods, but use of a nasogastric tube is time-consuming to the staff because tube placement must be checked before each feeding to decrease the incidence of aspiration. Bolus feedings administered too rapidly can lead to emesis and/or aspiration or feelings of distention. Because the formula is kept at room temperature for short periods of time, the incidence of bacterial contamination is reduced.

Initiation of tube feedings requires an adjustment period for the patient during which a diluted formula and decreased rate of administration is gradually increased to full-strength formula at the desired rate. Failure to introduce the feedings gradually results in diarrhea or vomiting or both, which will be prolonged and difficult to reverse. When diarrhea and vomiting associated with tube feedings occur, this is often controlled by a reduction in intake for a few days, which avoids having to change to the parenteral route. The source of the intolerance should not be placed too quickly on the tube feeding, since certain antibiotics, a developing gram-negative infection, or adynamic ileus may be present.[32]

The actual type of commercial or hospital-prepared diet used is not as important as assessing the caloric needs of the patient and meeting them. If the patient cannot take anything by mouth, the administration of a 1 kcal per ml feeding at 200 ml per hour will provide 4800 kcal per day to an adult patient. However, since the ingestion of food by mouth begins a cascade of beneficial digestive actions, the ideal situation is an oral high-calorie, high-protein diet supplemented by tube feedings to reach the total required daily nutritional needs. An increase in protein intake (kcal:N ratio of 100:1) appears to have some benefit to the hypermetabolic burn patient. Fortunately, most patients with burn injury regain gastrointestinal function within 3 to 5 days after injury and can receive their nutritional needs enterally throughout the recovery phase. Patients who are taking oral diets but are not meeting caloric needs may be able to drink oral supplements in addition to oral intake to increase their total caloric intake without necessitating tube feeding. Because appetite loss is common, the feeding of frequent small meals and attention to food preferences help increase total intake. Encouraging family members to bring food to the patient helps the patient and family to feel more in control and may also increase overall caloric intake.

PARENTERAL FEEDINGS

In some patients, enteral feeding may not be possible, and TPN may become the only method available. Indications for intravenous TPN following burn injury include weight loss exceeding 10 percent of body weight; clinical status prohibiting adequate enteral nutritional intake; and a debilitated malnourished preburn state. Special requirements in delivering TPN to burn patients include allowing for the increased insensible fluid losses associated with the burn wound. Evaporative water loss from the burn wound is calculated as:

$$(25 \text{ ml} + \% \text{ TBSA burn}) (\text{M}^2\text{BSA}) = \text{ml per hour of evaporative water loss}$$

This is in addition to the normal requirement of 1500 ml/M^2 BSA daily. When the placement of intravenous lines is limited because of extensive burns, the concentration of the delivered TPN solution may be decreased and the hourly flow rate increased in order to meet both the free water and the nutritional requirements. Triple-lumen central venous catheters also facilitate the administration of large volumes of intravenous fluid. Central catheters are changed using a rewire procedure at 48 hours postplacement followed by discontinuation of the catheter after the second 48-hour period with subsequent placement at a different site. This frequent changing of both catheter and site greatly decreases the incidence of septic complications. Another requirement regards prevention of fatty acid deficiencies. Although the routine use of fat emulsions as a measure to preserve body protein mass has been shown not to be of benefit,[33] when TPN is to be the only source of nutrition for longer than 5 to 7 days intravenous fat emulsions are given to prevent a fatty acid deficiency.

NURSING CARE PLAN: NUTRITIONAL SUPPORT

Nursing Priorities

1. Maintain adequate nutrition to withstand the stress of trauma.

2. Maintain adequate nutrition to meet the demand for proper healing.

Nursing Diagnosis: Nutrition, Alteration in, Less Than Body Requirements

(Refer to Chapter 9, page 172, for care plan.)

REFERENCES

1. Hansbrough, JF, Zapata-Sirvent, RL, and Peterson, VM: Immunomodulation following burn injury. Surg Clin North Am 67:69, 1987.
2. Ireton, CS, et al: Evaluation of energy expenditures in burn patients. J Am Diet Assoc 86:331, 1986.
3. Bell, SJ and Wyatt, J: Nutrition guidelines for burned patients. J Am Diet Assoc 86:648, 1986.
4. Harrison, HN, et al: The relationship between energy metabolism and water loss from vaporization in severely burned patients. Surgery 56:203, 1964.
5. Zawacki, BE, et al: Does increased evaporative water loss cause hypermetabolism in burned patients? Ann Surg 171:236, 1970.
6. Burdge, JJ, Conkright, JM, and Ruberg, RL: Nutritional and metabolic consequences of thermal injury. Clin Plast Surg 13:55, 1986.
7. Wilmore, DW, et al: Catecholamines: Mediator of the hypermetabolic response to thermal injury. Ann Surg 180:653, 1974.

8. Stratta, RJ, et al: Thermal injury in an adrenalectomized patient. J Trauma 23:934, 1983.
9. Long, CL, et al: Carbohydrate metabolism in men: Effect of elective operations and major injury. J Appl Physiol 31:110, 1971.
10. Wilmore, DW, et al: Insulin response to glucose in hypermetabolic burn patients. Ann Surg 183:314, 1976.
11. Shuck, JM, et al: Dynamics of insulin and glucagon secretions in severely burned patients. J Trauma 17:706, 1977.
12. Lundholm, KG: Nutritional problems in trauma. Acta Chir Scand (Suppl)522:183, 1985.
13. Cahill, GF, et al: Hormone-fuel interrelationships during fasting. J Clin Invest 45:1751, 1966.
14. Kinney, JM, et al: Tissue composition of weight loss in surgical patients, I. Elective operation. Ann Surg 168:459, 1968.
15. Soroff, HS, Pearson, E, and Artz, CP: An estimation of nitrogen requirements for equilibrium in burn patients. Surg Gynecol Obstet 112:159, 1961.
16. Newsome, TW, Mason, AD, Jr, and Pruitt, BA, Jr: Weight loss following thermal injury. Ann Surg 178:215, 1973.
17. Rutan, TC, et al: Metabolic rate alterations in early excision and grafting vs. conservative treatment. J Trauma 26:140, 1986.
18. Curreri, PW, Richmond, D, and Marvin, J: Dietary requirements of patients with major burns. J Am Diet Assoc 65:415, 1974.
19. Hildreth, MA, et al: Evaluation of a caloric requirement formula in burned children treated with early excision. J Trauma 27:188, 1987.
20. Long, CL, et al: Parenteral nutrition in the septic patient: Nitrogen balance, limiting plasma, amino acids and calorie to nitrogen ratios. Am J Clin Nutr 29:380, 1976.
21. Bell, SJ and Wyatt, J: Nutrition guidelines for burned patients. J Am Diet Assoc 86:648, 1986.
22. Ireton, CS, et al: Evaluation of energy expenditures in burn patients. J Am Diet Assoc 86(3):331, 1986.
23. Burke, JF, et al: Glucose requirements following burn injury. Ann Surg 3:274, 1980.
24. Saffle, JR, et al: Use of indirect calorimetry in the nutritional management of burned patients. J Trauma 25:32, 1985.
25. Alexander, JW: Immunity, nutrition and trauma, an overview. Acta Chir Scand (Suppl) 552:141, 1985.
26. Wilmore, DW and Aulick, LH: Metabolic changes in burned patients. Surg Clin North Am 58:1173, 1978.
27. Herndon, DN, et al: Failure of TPN supplementation to improve liver function, immunity, and mortality in thermally injured patients. J Trauma 27:195, 1987.
28. Kravitz, M, et al: The use of the Dobbhoff tube to provide additional nutritional support in thermally injured patients. Journal of Burn Care and Rehabilitation 3:226, 1982.
29. Hiebert, JM, et al: Comparison of continuous vs. intermittent tube feedings in adult burn patients. JPEN 5:73, 1981.
30. Taylor, T: A comparison of two methods of nasogastric tube feedings. J Neurosurg Nurs 14:49, 1982.
31. Mechanic, HF and Dunn, LT: Critical care nursing technique. Nutritional support for the burn patient. Dimens Crit Care Nurs 5:20, 1986.
32. Sutherland, AB: Nutrition and general factors influencing infection in burns. J Hosp Infect (Suppl B):31, 1985.
33. Long, JM, et al: Effect of carbohydrate and fat intake on nitrogen excretion during total intravenous feeding. Ann Surg 185:417, 1977.

Chapter 7

MADELEINE T. MARTIN
ROSLYN SELIGMAN

PSYCHOSOCIAL CARE OF THE BURN PATIENT AND SIGNIFICANT OTHERS

In caring for the burned patient, the nurse provides holistic care. The physical, psychosocial, and spiritual needs of the patient are viewed as equally important and are addressed. Psychosocial care involves the stages of the nursing process: assessing, planning, intervening, and evaluating. This chapter includes parameters for consideration for each of these steps.

While meeting the emotional needs of the patient has basic underlying principles, there are developmental differences between the adult and child. Therefore, for purposes of organization, the adult and child will be discussed separately. Interventions and rationale listed in each section, however, may be considered for both groups.

PSYCHOSOCIAL ASSESSMENT: ADULT

Burn injury, large or small, represents an alteration that requires a period of adjustment. A number of factors have been identified that affect this psychosocial reaction to physical injury, and the nurse considers these in assessing the patient's response.

One factor is the characteristic of the injury itself. Location (such as the face), severity, and reversibility of this injury, for example, will influence the patient's reaction. Also, the situation surrounding the burn incident may result in differing responses. If the injury was sudden or spontaneous, the response may be different from that of a prolonged injury, such as is seen in an entrapment. If the injury was arbitrary or an "act of God," the individual may view it differently from an event with personal significance, such as a faulty piece of equipment about which the person repeatedly complained, or a careless or neglectful situation.

The significance of the injury may vary emotionally, socially, and occupationally from victim to victim. It may be psychologically more damaging if the individual interprets the injury as punishment for some real or imagined transgression. Similarly, permanently disfiguring injuries or ones causing permanent occupational impairment demand more psychologic adjustment.

Situational factors may occur throughout the course of treatment that facilitate or delay psychosocial adjustment. The sudden, unexpected assault on the patient and subsequent disruption of roles take the person almost instantaneously from a functional contributing adult to someone dependent on others for care and survival. The manner in which care is provided as well as the surroundings all affect the development of the trust relationship necessary for movement through psychosocial adjustment. The nature and adequacy of the rescue and subsequent medical and nursing interventions may also have long-term psychologic implications.

General personality factors of the individual preburn are not minimized. Culture and ethnic background have been found in some research to play a part not only in psychosocial adjustment but also in overt emotional response patterns. Past general health, including previous hospitalizations, is a part of the individual's history that will color his or her ultimate reaction to the burn.

Therapeutic emotional care involves observing, assessing, interacting, and intervening, with the ultimate nursing goal of maximizing psychosocial recovery. Lee[1] has identified four stages of psychosocial responses that can be anticipated postburn: impact, retreat or withdrawal, acknowledgment, and reconstruction (Table 7–1). Impact is the initial response of shock, and disbelief is experienced immediately postinjury. Depersonalization is frequently seen, in which the patient or family, or both, may be aware of what is happening but do not believe it could be happening to them. The family and patient may be overwhelmed by the many decisions to be made, and nursing interventions are directed toward decreasing anxiety and beginning a trusting relationship.

As the patient and family begin to move on in their adjustment, the phase of mistrust or withdrawal may be seen. At this time the patient may try to minimize the seriousness of the injury by suppression or repression. The third phase is acknowledgement, which is when mourning can begin, followed by the reconstructive phase wherein the patient and family accept limitations and begin to build a new future.

The patient's passage through each of these phases and overall acceptance of the injury is the ultimate goal of nursing care.

TABLE 7–1. Lee's Stages of Psychosocial Responses

Impact
    Immediately postburn
    Shock
    Disbelief
    Depersonalization
Retreat or Withdrawal
    After initial impact
    Suppression
    Repression
    Mistrust
Acknowledgment
    Following retreat
    Mourning
Reconstructive
    Final phase
    Acceptance of limitations
    Beginning of rebuilding

NURSING CARE PLAN: PSYCHOSOCIAL CARE OF THE BURNED ADULT

Nursing Priorities

1. Minimize pain and discomfort
2. Minimize loss of self-concept
3. Encourage healthy family interactions
4. Support effective coping mechanisms

Nursing Diagnosis: Pain

(Refer to Chapter 9, page 169)

Nursing Diagnosis: Self-Concept, Disturbance In

May Be Related To:

- Physical loss
- Disfigurement
- Loss of role functions

Possibly Evidenced By: A negative response to changes in body image, self-esteem, role performance, or personal identity; refusal to look directly at injured area or in a mirror; denial of disfigurement; withdrawal or signs of grieving such as crying or anger.

Desired Patient Outcomes: Patient will verbalize feelings about self-concept and will relate how changes have been integrated into self-perception, with the ultimate goal of feeling comfortable with who he or she is.

Interventions	Rationale
INDEPENDENT	
• Provide an atmosphere of acceptance.	• Acceptance provides for testing reality and reactions of others, which is important for an individual's self-identity.
• Encourage expression of feelings about loss of previous self-perceived identity.	• Development of a realistic self-concept is based on identification of those qualities compatible with a person's perception preinjury.
• Encourage realistic perception of changed body image.	• Person's self-concept incorporates others' perception. Honest responses by the nurse are also necessary for reality testing.
• Assess coping strategies, building on those used successfully by the individual in the past, and recommend alternative coping strategies when necessary.	• The use of appropriate coping mechanisms is necessary to maintain homeostasis. Coping mechanisms that have been used successfully in the past can be applied to this new situation.

Nursing Diagnosis: Self-Concept, Disturbance In (*Continued*)

Interventions

- Listen to the patient and observe for nonverbal communication.

- Encourage expression of what the body changes mean to the patient.

COLLABORATIVE

- Involve family in interacting with patient.
- Work with family to provide support and positive comments.

Rationale

- Patient may express developing remarks or behaviors about self related to physical changes.
- People respond to alterations/changes differently. The nurse does not assume how the patient feels but gathers objective data on the significance of the event to each patient.

- Withdrawal of family may reinforce low self-concept.
- Patient's ultimate self-concept will include feedback from significant others.

Nursing Diagnosis: Social Isolation

May Be Related To:

- Alterations in interpersonal relations related to hospitalization
- Loss of previous role functions
- Alterations in appearance
- Bulky dressings
- Infection control
- Loss of or impaired sensory motor functions

Possibly Evidenced By: Verbalizations; moving away from interactions with others; withdrawal; hostility; insufficient or unsatisfactory responses from social interactions.

Desired Patient Outcomes: Patient uses withdrawal only as a means of coping in selected situations. Patient moves increasingly toward positive interactions with family and others. Ultimately, patient will be able to interact with the environment and people, as in preburn state.

Interventions

INDEPENDENT

- Establish a positive nurse-patient relationship.

- Talk with the patient, using therapeutic communication techniques.

- Explore alternative ways in which the patient who has sensory-motor impairment can communicate with others nonverbally such as nodding, writing, blinking, or touching.

Rationale

- The patient's trust and ability to relate positively to the nurse is the basis for subsequent nursing interacting.
- Hearing verbal comments assures the person of the nurse's concern, decreases isolation, and provides stimulation.
- A substitute method of communication is necessary for feelings of comfort and security.

Interventions	Rationale
• Observe for evidence of reduced withdrawal.	• Watching surrounding activities, talking, and asking questions are all evidence of interest in the environment and attempts at intervening.
• Interact in an unhurried manner.	• Psychologic and physiologic comfort are promoted through effective communication. An unhurried approach demonstrates the nurse's respect and caring for the patient.
• Offer feedback to the patient's comments and expression of feelings.	• Comfort is promoted through effective communication with others. Feedback clarifies the person's perception of messages given.
• Encourage expression of feelings.	• Expressing feelings allows for ventilation and supports an objective and honest appraisal of those feelings by the patient and nurse.
• Be consistent in approach to patient.	• Trust and comfort are promoted through predictable situations and behavior and by having a sense of control over situations.
• Encourage visitors as tolerated by patient's physical condition.	• Comfort is promoted by interaction with others. Anxiety is decreased for both family and patient when they are allowed to be near each other.
• Offer environmental stimuli through contact with people, environmental change, and involvement in daily routine.	• External stimuli encourage the patient to be aware of and/or respond to the environment even if unable to interact as in preburn state.
• Provide frequent contact with the patient, including touch.	• Frequent contact reassures the patient that he or she is cared for and not alone. It also allows opportunity for frequent observation of the patient.
• Explain noises, treatments, and other unfamiliar elements in the patient's environment.	• When the patient's normal sensory input is impaired, environmental stimuli may be unclear or threatening. Knowledge of the surroundings decreases anxiety.

COLLABORATIVE

• Support the family during their interactions with the patient.	• Patient's inability to communicate may frighten or confuse family members, leading to their avoidance and further patient isolation.
• Involve other staff in interactions with patients as patient tolerates.	• Once the patient is comfortable with the one-to-one relationship, this trust can be transferred to others involved in his or her care, increasing comfort and feelings of security.

Nursing Diagnosis: Social Isolation (*Continued*)

Interventions	Rationale
• Encourage visits by family and significant others.	• A sense of comfort and security is promoted through interacting with others who care.

Nursing Diagnosis: Coping, Ineffective Family

May Be Related To:

- Role changes due to hospitalization
- Prolonged hospitalization and rehabilitation that exhausts supportive capacity of family

Possibly Evidenced By: Verbalizations; withdrawal of family; less than supportive behavior of family; hostility; anger; anxiety; conflict or lack of communication among family members.

Desired Patient Outcomes: Family actively and appropriately participates in patient's physical and psychosocial care. Family members are supportive of each other.

Interventions

INDEPENDENT

- Assess anxiety and coping behaviors.

- Assess family's knowledge level of the situation.

- Identify other stressful factors that the family is experiencing.

- Establish a therapeutic relationship with the family.

- Provide brief, simple explanations of procedures and equipment. Answer questions honestly.
- Include family in planning and caring for the patient.
- Assist family in initiating therapeutic communication with patient.
- Encourage family to deal with the situation gradually.

Rationale

- Anxiety must be dealt with prior to other interventions. Problem-solving abilities may be at a lower level due to regression related to crisis.
- Provides a basis for teaching and determines readiness of family to be involved in care of the patient.
- Other factors may be contributing to ineffective behaviors (e.g., financial difficulties; an illness occurring out of town).
- Family must be able to trust and relate positively to nursing staff in order to become more involved in patient care.
- Shorter explanations will be more readily retained due to emotional stress the family is experiencing.
- Involvement enhances feelings of usefulness, control, and self-worth.
- Encourages involvement and helps to decrease anxiety.
- Family may be unable to cope with entire situation, but may be able to deal with in small increments.

Interventions	Rationale

COLLABORATIVE

- Refer to appropriate resources as necessary: families of burn patients' support group; psychologist; psychiatrist; social workers.

- Provide expert help and consultation as needed.

Nursing Diagnosis: Post-Trauma Response

May Be Related To:

- Burn incident

Possibly Evidenced By: Nightmares; verbalizations; confusion; amnesia regarding traumatic event; detachment; depression; anxiety; headache; nausea; palpitations.

Desired Patient Outcomes: Patient will express decreased anxiety when flashbacks occur, and deal with this emotional reaction appropriately. Physical complaints are absent.

Interventions	Rationale

INDEPENDENT

- Assess patient for emotional changes and physical reactions in excess of physical injuries.
- Provide opportunities for patient to talk freely about the traumatic incident. Allow patient to progress at own pace; do not force issue; accept silence. Assist patient in identifying and utilizing ego strengths and coping mechanisms.
- Assist patient in dealing with stress.

- Provides baseline data for individual reaction to trauma.

- Assists patient in dealing with situation. Rushing patient may cause more isolation. Allows patient to work through own adjustment. Allows patient more control; helps patient handle situation that exists.
- Allows patient to manage stress appropriately.

COLLABORATIVE

- Consult with trained counselors, therapists, and psychiatrists regarding such therapies as medications, cognitive restructuring, relaxation, and so on.
- Encourage patient and significant others to participate with an appropriate support group.

- Permits appropriate therapies; assists nurse in planning of interventions.

- Assists patient and significant other(s) in understanding these reactions and dealing with them appropriately.

Nursing Diagnosis: Fear

May Be Related To:

- Pain (burn; treatments; procedures)
- Knowledge deficit
- Hospitalization
- Environment of burn unit (rules; caps, gowns, masks; isolation procedures)
- Threat of death or disability

Possibly Evidenced By: Crying; verbalizations; apprehension; nausea; heart palpitations; diarrhea; diaphoresis; aggression; increased pulse; increased respirations; withdrawal.

Desired Patient Outcomes: The patient will acknowledge and cope with the fear; associated physical symptoms and signs are alleviated.

Interventions	Rationale
INDEPENDENT	
• Assess patient and significant other(s) for signs and symptoms of fear (as previously noted).	• Provides baseline data for plan of care.
• Provide constant explanations and information about care: verbal and written.	• Allows patient and significant other(s) to understand the progression of care and clarifies misconceptions.
• Encourage questions and expression of feelings.	• Assists patient and significant other(s) to deal more effectively with fear.
• Encourage patient and significant other(s) to become appropriately involved in patient's care.	• Promotes acceptance and control.
COLLABORATIVE	
• Consult with entire burn team in care from admission to discharge.	• Provides a wider support system and promotes coordination of activities.

Nursing Diagnosis: Grieving, Anticipatory/Dysfunctional

May Be Related To:

- Physical disfigurement due to burn injury
- Loss of normal way of life (e.g., family, job)
- Uncertainty of body image (i.e., outcome of wound healing and future plastic surgery)
- Loss of possessions during burn event

Possibly Evidenced By: Denial; anger; changes in activity level and communication patterns; sleep disturbances; crying; regression; verbalizations of loss; withdrawal; changes in eating habits.

Desired Patient Outcomes: The patient (and/or significant others) identifies problems and progresses in dealing with states of grief at own rate.

Interventions	Rationale

INDEPENDENT

- Assess patient and significant other(s) for cues as to how they are dealing with the present situation.

- Provides baseline data in further identifying the problem and its causative factors. Helpful in beginning resolution and acceptance without forcing patient to face too much at one time.

- Provide frequent opportunities for verbalizations without excessive confrontation about realities.
- Permit expression of feelings within appropriate limits.
- Acknowledge appropriate expressions of grief.

- Patient needs the opportunity to express feelings openly in nonjudgemental environment.
- Allows patient some control while avoiding destructive behavior.
- Allows patient and significant other(s) to know that these feelings are normal and need to be expressed.

- Provide explanations of treatment and care as well as outcomes.

- Patient and significant other(s) can better deal with situation with truthful explanations; allows patient and significant other(s) to clarify situation and begin to cope.

- Assist patient and significant other(s) in using previously learned coping strategies as well as appropriate new strategies.

- Allows patient and significant others to deal with current situation and prepare for future outcomes.

COLLABORATIVE

- Assist patient and family in planning for the future and/or funeral.

- Provides support system to patient and others. Outcomes will differ (e.g., change in occupation, death).

- Provide appropriate referrals (e.g., support groups, social services, psychologist, occupational and physical therapists).

- Assists patient and significant other(s) in resolving situation.

Nursing Diagnosis: Adjustment, Impaired

May Be Related To:

- Inadequate support systems
- Loss of career or job
- Changes in role
- Environmental conditions: burn unit, intensive care unit (ICU)
- Assault to self-esteem

Possibly Evidenced By: Verbalizations; lack of cooperation; lack of progress in recovery; lack of future goals; anger; withdrawal.

Desired Patient Outcomes: The patient will identify the problem and demonstrate interest in care. The patient will identify changes in personal life to permit proper adjustment.

Nursing Diagnosis: Adjustment, Impaired (Continued)

Interventions	Rationale
INDEPENDENT	
• Assess the extent of the patient's limitations and strengths.	• Provides baseline data.
• Encourage expression of feelings regarding impaired function.	• Allows patient to perceive limitations in order to work toward adjustment.
• Assess prior coping strategies and recommend alternatives as appropriate.	• Most previous coping strategies can be applied to present situation. Identifies patient's strengths.
• Assist patient in identifying attainable goals.	• Patient will require guidance in this area.
• Assist patient and significant other(s) in plan of action to meet physical and emotional needs (e.g., feeding, bathing, looking at burns, ambulating).	• Helps patient and significant other(s) to adjust appropriately.
• Implement plan of care focusing on smaller activities, gradually increasing as appropriate. Pace activities according to patient's needs and provide continual feedback and reinforcement.	• Allows patient and significant other(s) the appropriate time to adjust. Again, provides time for adjustment as well as building the patient's self-esteem.
COLLABORATIVE	
• Organize a burn team conference to focus on causes of impaired adjustment and to initiate plan of care.	• The patient's problems will be multifocal due to the very nature of the burn injury.
• Support the family and significant other(s) in their interactions with the patient.	• Impaired adjustment may lead to avoidance and isolation.
• Document appropriate referrals upon discharge (e.g., Visiting Nurses Association, social services, occupational and physical therapists).	• Promotes continued adjustment and wellness at home.

Nursing Diagnosis: Powerlessness

May Be Related To:

• Critical care environment
• Burn care regimen
• Insecurity about outcome
• Necessity for multiple procedures and treatments

Possibly Evidenced By: Verbalizations; depression; lack of participation in care; dependency; passivity; frustration; crying; anger.

Desired Patient Outcomes: The patient will express, and provide evidence of, control over present situation and future. The patient will participate in care.

Interventions	Rationale

INDEPENDENT

- Identify locus of control: external (noting expressions of lack of control); internal (noting expressions of responsibility and control).

- Provides data on whether control is internal or external; this data provides for a better plan of care and helps patient and others deal more effectively with powerlessness. (For example, if internal control, encourage patient to take control of own care; if external control, begin with small tasks and increase appropriately.)

- Assess patient and significant other(s) for related behaviors (e.g., anger, frustration, "giving up").
- Avoid use of confrontation or logic.

- Provides baseline data to indicate degree of powerlessness.

- When the patient feels helpless and hopeless, these tactics will not be effective.

- Assess and deal with manipulative behavior.
- Provide opportunities for communication; demonstrate concern and caring attitude.
- Assist patient in defining short-term goals and routines for meeting needs. Assist patient in identifying self-care deficits and capabilities.
- Encourage involvement of significant others in care of patient.
- Provide timely explanations to patient and significant others.

- Assign scheduled visits to patient.

- The patient may be manipulative of staff and others in an attempt to gain control.
- Assists patient in feeling more hopeful, less isolated.

- Manageable steps allow more control and patient identifies abilities; reduces helpless behavior; permits as much control as appropriate.
- Reduces feelings of helplessness and enhances sense of control.
- Reduces hopelessness of situation; helps patient to deal with present situation, thereby increasing control.
- Demonstrates concern to the patient; reduces hopelessness and helplessness.

COLLABORATIVE

- Refer patient and significant other(s) to support groups and/or counseling as appropriate.
- Consult with therapist, counselors, and psychiatrists as appropriate.

- Assists in dealing with situation; reduces helplessness.

- Helpful in setting goals and implementing care.

Nursing Diagnosis: Family Process, Alteration In

May Be Related To:

- Crises resulting from burn injury
- Disturbances in normal functions

Possibly Evidenced By: Inability to meet family needs; inability to accept help from burn team; family expressions of confusion; inability to accept feelings of burned family member; ineffective decision making; ineffective communication; inappropriate boundary maintenance.

Nursing Diagnosis: Family Process, Alteration In (*Continued*)

Desired Patient Outcomes: Family will be able to communicate and interact effectively to meet psychosocial and physiologic needs.

Interventions	Rationale
INDEPENDENT	
• Assess for causes and contributing factors.	• Establishes data base for effective plan of care.
• Note family components, including extended family.	• Helps direct effective interventions to key members.
• Identify communication techniques.	• Identifies strengths and weaknesses, which can help direct effective communication among family members.
• Assess role expectations of family members, including burn patient.	• Helps in support of roles the burn patient can no longer assume and identifies key family functions important to the patient.
• Assess energy expenditure of family.	• Determines if energy is conserved and used to maintain homeostasis.
• Evaluate cultural and religious influences.	• Adds to understanding of family functions and expectations.
• Assess community and other support systems.	• Helps to plan for support of lost or impaired functions.
• Encourage open communication among family members.	• Assists all members of the family in effectively performing expected functions.
• Identify previous family coping mechanisms.	• Assists family in using these to cope with present crisis.
• Teach stress management techniques.	• Assists family in reducing anxiety and other stressors.
• Allow and encourage frequent visiting.	• Permits maximum opportunity to continue some role functions and provides support to burn patient.
COLLABORATIVE	
• Refer to appropriate community resources as needed.	• Provides for followup care in the community for support systems to promote positive functioning.

Nursing Diagnosis: Anxiety

May Be Related To:

• Crisis of burn injury
• Threat to self-concept
• Threat of death
• Threat to health status
• Threat to socioeconomic status

Possibly Evidenced By: Complaints of uneasiness, helplessness, or apprehension; worry; sleeplessness; restlessness; trembling; decreased eye contact; quivering voice; increased wariness.

Desired Patient Outcomes: Patient will have adequate rest and sleep periods.

Patient will express a decrease in apprehension.

Interventions	Rationale

INDEPENDENT

- Assess level of anxiety.
- Evaluate physical causes: pain, adverse drug reactions, steroid therapy.
- Encourage patient to identify sources of anxiety.
- Monitor physical signs and symptoms: palpitations, tachycardia, increased blood pressure.
- Assess coping and defense mechanisms.

- Establish therapeutic relationship and encourage patient to communicate.
- Do not give false reassurances or discourage patient's verbalizations.
- Provide accurate information about anxiety-producing subjects.
- Assist the patient to develop new coping mechanisms if previous ones are ineffective.

- Helps establish data base and priorities.
- Cause should be treated directly whenever possible.
- Permits interventions to be directed at cause.
- Quantifies response to anxiety in nonverbal or withdrawn patient.

- Assists in guiding effective use to conserve energy.
- Permits patient to deal with feelings openly and to work toward resolution.
- Patient needs to know nurses are empathetic and supportive.
- Helps patient deal realistically with fears.
- Patients who are stressed may have difficulty identifying new effective mechanisms.

PSYCHOSOCIAL ASSESSMENT: CHILD

Comprehensive nursing care of burned children involves knowledge of biopsychosocial issues in addition to knowledge of specialized medical-surgical treatment and technical skill in wound care (see Chapter 14). Factors related to the child's personality and family background, the circumstances of the trauma, hospitalization, therapy, and issues of separation from home and family interrelate in a complex way with each other and with demographic variables of age, sex, race, and socioeconomic status. In addition, the subtle and elusive interactional responses of institutional caretakers and family members with each other and with the patient are important.

In order to assist the nurse in delivering planned and rational therapeutic management, examples are provided in this chapter to focus on clinical data illustrating the interaction within the patient (child)–nurse dyad and to elaborate on that interaction within the context of the illness (child-nurse-burn triad). These examples aim to sensitize caretakers of burned children to their own reactions, to the reactions of the patient, and to how these interrelate. In persons under age 18, the trauma of a severe burn is vividly described in their verbalizations.

A 5-year-old girl said, "Bang." She repeated to the nurse, "Bang, you shot off all my fingers. All my fingers are off." A 7-year-old boy, while thrashing about, screamed out, "I'm on fire. See the smoke." A 13-year-old girl dreamed her mother and sister were burned and died in the fire. She awakened crying and then stated, "It is better that I am the one who was burned." A 14-year-old boy suddenly awakened and said he could see a lot of dead bodies (his friends) moving around. A 6-year-old girl yelled during debridement, "Nobody likes me. Everyone always tries to hurt me. I am ugly." An anxious 8-year-old boy stated, "My arms are all purple and filled with blisters. If the skin comes off, I will die."[2]

Burn nursing personnel are in contact with the patients daily over a long, continuous period of time. Their observations, emotional experience, and responses differ from other members of the burn team who spend more limited time and their coping mechanisms need to be of a different nature and degree. For example, to understand that teeth grinding might be uncontrollable for a burned child is one thing; to tolerate the sound of it for 8 hours is quite another. Under most circumstances, the anxieties, apprehensions, misperceptions, loneliness, and mistrust in these children could not be missed. Yet, for those involved in the minute-to-minute care of these individuals, interactions occasionally occur that seem insensitive and perhaps even nontherapeutic. The following vignette illustrates this point.

A 8-year-old with burns covering 80 percent of her body called the nurses "goddam SOBs" during dressing change. Asked if this made her feel better, she replied, "Yes." When staff requested she use other words, she replied, "No." One week later she warned the nurses she would curse, using "goddam." Again, they indicated she should shout, cry, or use some other word. The surgeon responded that he would "spank her bottom." When the patient related her cursing to her parents, her mother told the nurses they should wash her mouth out with soap.

From these staff and parental responses, caretakers appear to be protecting themselves from the present traumatic and painful situation made more explicit by the patient's abusive language. The question, then, is whether exercising authority and power allows staff to function more effectively and whether these reactions foster adaptive modes in the patient or instead foster less effective staff functioning and make the patient feel more pain, rejection, loneliness, and mistrust followed then by nontherapeutic reactions? In contrast to the responses given, could those caring for this patient have shared her pain empathically and still have done an effective job which included inflicting pain?[3] Nurses can find coping mechanisms that will allow responses calming to the patient and thereby increase the patient's control and self-esteem. A system that supports nurses in understanding their emotions and the relationship of these to the patient would assist in this endeavor.

Whereas previous studies[4-16] have reported on reactions of the patient and management of these reactions, more recent reports by nurses have focused on the responses of nurses and also on techniques useful in helping them to function more effectively.[17-20] Reports such as these foster understanding and thereby improve the comprehensiveness and effectiveness of therapeutic management. For example, Fagerhaugh's description of pain expression and control on a burn unit permits a glimpse of the nurses' difficult tasks and strategies employed to cope.[21] Fagerhaugh states:

Where pain is irreducible, inevitable and cannot be completely relieved, there is a tendency for staff to focus on other concerns. The literature on the medical management of burns, for instance, indicates primary concern with the complexities of technical treatment and pain management, with psychosocial aspects receiving only fleeting attention. This is completely understandable; although the staff is immersed in and surrounded by pain, they are limited in their relief of it, and besides, they have more pressing priorities.[21]

This report describes the helplessness staff members sometimes experience and how they cope by using denial and minimization of psychosocial issues and maximize the technical care they can offer competently.

The following case vignette illustrates that sensitive humane responses can also be competently given. The nurse offered on-target responses that led to effective comprehensive care.

> Alice, a 15-year-old white girl, was burned in a house fire in which her older sister, brother-in-law, and friend died. On postburn day 18, while the nurse was reading her a depressing letter from her mother, Alice began to cry. Following her letter, the nurse also read a card that contained Bible verses, including Psalm 23. Alice then cried uncontrollably and asked the nurse to read no more. She began to vomit. As the nurse was cleaning up, Alice apologized, "I am sorry." The nurse replied, "You have nothing to be sorry about. I understand and, furthermore, I know being in the hospital is no fun." Alice then asked the nurse if she would mind if she cried more. The nurse replied, "No, I cry sometimes myself and always feel better afterwards." Following this, Alice cried for a long time and then said the card made her think of her sister who died in the fire. Nearly a week later on postburn day 24, Alice was noted to be more aware of her surroundings. She seemed surprised to learn the hospital had burned patients who walk. The nurse indicated all the patients walk before discharge. Alice then asked if she would be able to walk and how long it would be before she was transferred from the ICU to another room. The nurse explained certain details about the hospital's procedure. Then Alice requested that the nurse read her mail. The nurse noted that Alice's reaction on this occasion was quite different from that described 1 week earlier.

Nurses caring for burned children need an awareness of the totality of the situation. Knowledge includes what individual children of varying age, sex, and developmental levels bring to a traumatic situation. Information about how the patient was previously disciplined, and by whom, is important, as is information about the child's response to the discipline. Nurses also recognize that they appraise events objectively and realistically; in contrast, a child does so subjectively, irrationally, and emotionally.[22]

In caring for both adults and children, nurses are aware that in being human, they too will use certain strategies to cope with the tasks inherent in their work. In accomplishing tasks, the nurse's work includes painful procedures. During these procedures, nurses may be the recipients of angry outbursts. Only infrequently can patients thank nurses for their painstaking efforts and devotion. Rather, recognition of nurses' labors come from patients at other times or even from other sources.

The importance of close relationships in life-threatening circumstances is noted by Hamburg,[23] who states:

> The effectiveness of a coping behavior is strongly related to the feeling that one's presence is not only valued by significant other people, but is virtually indispensable to them."

Margaret Mead also noted this possibility and asked, "Does this feeling engender for the patient extraordinary hope for the future?"[24] Mead was referring to the feeling that one's presence is valued and is indispensable to his or her significant other, the caretaker. In a study of emotional factors in survival,[25] one possible trend noted was a better prognosis for children with hopeful parents.

What role the attitude of the nurse plays in the parents' feelings toward their child, or vice versa, awaits further study. Watson and Johnson[26] reported on the emotional significance of acquired physical disfigurement in five selected cases of children. They noted their findings corroborated those of Macgregor and her associates that the child perceives and imitates the defenses against anxiety used by the parents. Data reported here support the same application to the patient and caretakers. Another study[27] reported similar findings for acutely ill patients in an intensive care unit vis-a-vis each other.

For both the nurse and the patient, means of coping appear to mirror each other, that is, to have a similar nature. The patient uses mechanisms such as denial and splitting of the ego[28,29] in order to keep distress within bounds, maintain an integrated self, conserve energy, remain hopeful, and view himself or herself as wanted, worthwhile, and lovable. Similarly, some responses by the nurse appear based on denial of the patient as severely injured. Further, how does the patient view a particular response? As punitive and nonempathic? As helpful and reflective of what he or she received at home? As what the patient deserves for the "badness" he or she feels along with guilt? This list of possibilities could go on. Suffice it to say that in playing such a pivotal role in the life of these patients, nurses need to sensitize themselves to the means by which they cope and, hence, respond to the continuous trauma present.

Describing emotional symptoms such as anxiety, depression, delusions, delirium, and hallucinations is not enough to develop and nurture understanding. In addition, nurses must know in whom these symptoms occur, under what circumstances, and which interactional pattern(s) between patient and nurse foster coping and which do not.

Some children with a small burn do not cope well and, therefore, may be more difficult to manage than those with a large burn who cope effectively. Some patients, irrespective of the extent and degree of their burn, adjust better with the presence of their loved ones, whereas others perform poorly. Too little is known about the forces that contribute to these circumstances. The following nursing diagnoses are relevant to the issues previously raised. Many of those diagnoses discussed under "Psychosocial Care: Adult," p 89, also have application for the child. They should, however, be considered in light of the child as being different from the adult.

NURSING CARE PLAN: PSYCHOSOCIAL CARE OF THE BURNED CHILD

Nursing Priorities

1. Minimize pain and discomfort
2. Minimize disruptions in psychosocial development
3. Minimize disruptions in family patterns
4. Support effective coping mechanisms

Nursing Diagnosis: Pain

May Be Related To:

- Physical factors such as injury, treatments, immobility.
- Psychologic stressors.

sure, and respiratory rate (acute pain); decreased appetite; decreased involvement in therapy.

Possibly Evidenced By: Verbalizations, crying, screaming, thrashing, moaning, facial grimaces, withdrawal, resisting movement of affected area. Also increased pulse rate, blood pres-

Desired Patient Outcomes: The patient experiences minimization of pain through the use of a variety of drug- and nondrug-related interventions.

Interventions

INDEPENDENT

- Accept pain as what the child says it is.

Rationale

- Pain is a subjective response to discomfort or unpleasant stimuli. It varies from individual to individual.

Interventions	Rationale
• Assess the child's pain on a frequent basis.	• Effective nursing treatments are based on good assessment; use facial expression chart for assessment. Children may express pain verbally, behaviorally, and by facial expression.
• Be aware of the nurse's own feelings about nursing tasks that cause pain.	• Nurses' feelings often affect their perception of the environment. Feelings about inflicting pain may alter response to and assessment of the child's pain.
• Accept the patient's individual ways of expressing and coping with pain in a nonjudgmental manner.	• Acceptance promotes feelings of security and decreases anxiety. Response to stress is learned behavior, and individuals respond differently based on past life experiences.
• Talk with parents about their feelings concerning the child's pain.	• Verbal interactions promote comfort. Expression of feelings allows for ventilation and supports the nurse-family relationship.
• Explore alternative, nonpharmacologic methods of managing pain such as hypnosis, visual imagery, and diversion.	• Pain is a complex response to stress involving physiologic, psychologic, and social components. These same parameters should be considered in offering therapeutic interventions.

COLLABORATIVE

• Involve family in pain management strategies.	• Involvement gives the family a feeling of control, decreasing anxiety.
• Administer medications as ordered (morphine, methadone, Tylenol with codeine, Tylox).	• Narcotics disrupt the physiologic response to pain associated with painful dressing changes, grafting, and exposure of nerves.

Nursing Diagnosis: Growth and Development, Alteration In

May Be Related To:

- Stress of trauma.
- Resulting disruption to relationships with significant others.

Possibly Evidenced By: Regression.

Desired Patient Outcomes: Child will manifest behaviors appropriate for age and stage of development.

Interventions	Rationale
INDEPENDENT	
• Demonstrate acceptance of the child with caring behaviors and a secure environment.	• The child must feel secure and accepted in order to try new behaviors and progress to a higher development level.

Nursing Diagnosis: Growth and Development, Alteration In (*Continued*)

Interventions

- Assess the child's level of psychosocial development through the course of illness.

- Assess the physical-behavioral and psychologic parameters normally associated with chronologic stages of development.

- Provide children with concrete ways of knowing how long treatments will take, when family will arrive, and so on.
- Encourage and support independent behaviors by the child.

- Talk with the child, explaining procedures. Obtain information related to child's perceptions.

- Provide comfort and nurturing.

- Include various strategies in the nursing care to encourage expression of feelings (i.e., play therapy, art, and music).

Rationale

- Signs of regression may be indicators of increased stress or faltering ability to cope. Conversely, if the child continues to show developmental growth, this gives some reinforcement that the environment is perceived as secure by the child.
- Knowledge of the expected levels of functioning responses and cognitive abilities allows the nurse to plan realistic interventions. Deviations from these should be accepted, but efforts made to increase feelings of security and comfort for the child.
- Children, at differing developmental stages, have differing perceptions of time periods.
- It is a source of satisfaction and pride for children as they learn mastery over their environment at different stages. Allowing them to maintain this mastery and control supports self-esteem and prevents nurse-child conflicts.
- Children interpret health care intervention in a variety of ways, including as threats of mutilation or punishment or both. Explanations and caring behaviors may help give better understanding of what is happening in the environment.
- The child's development and comfort depend on a sense of nurturing by a caring "other." The nurse assumes this role in the absence of the mother.
- The younger the child, the less effective verbal expression is for communicating. Physical expressions of feelings provide an alternative for preverbal children and earlier cognitive developmental stages.

COLLABORATIVE

- Make referrals as appropriate (e.g., psychiatrist, psychologist, child development therapist).

- Provides comprehensive approach to meet psychosocial needs; provides a basis for interventions.

Nursing Diagnosis: Parenting, Alterations In

May Be Related To:

- Hospitalization and distance from home
- Stress of trauma
- Lack of knowledge
- Inability to cope with body disfigurements

Possibly Evidenced By: Verbalizations of child and parent; inattention to child's needs; inappropriate caretaking behaviors; abandonment.

Desired Patient Outcomes: Child and parent express and demonstrate satisfaction with their relationship and with appropriate parenting behavior such as communicating freely, expressing feelings, and providing guidance.

Interventions	Rationale
INDEPENDENT	
• Encourage expression of feelings.	• Expressing feelings allows for ventilation and supports movement toward a positive family-patient relationship.
• Involve parents in child's daily routine whenever possible.	• Some mutually shared responsibility promotes feeling of control for both parents and child, supporting an environment of comfort and safety.
• Provide time for parents to be alone with the child.	• Contact between the parent and child is important in maintaining attachment and communication among family members.
• Ask parents for input on child's home routine, likes and dislikes, and so on.	• Increased and accurate information about the child's preburn environment and routine can assist in providing a supportive hospital environment. Familiar routines provide some sense of security in a stressful hospital environment.
COLLABORATIVE	
• Provide referrals to other health care professionals as appropriate (e.g., family therapists, psychiatrists, psychologists).	• Provides a basis for nursing interventions. Ensures that complex psychosocial needs are addressed by appropriate members of the health care team.

Nursing Diagnosis: Family Process, Alteration In

May Be Related To:

- Trauma
- Separation
- Changes in family member roles and treatments

Possibly Evidenced By: Verbalizations by family; inability to cope with situation; ineffective decision-making ability; inability to meet needs of family.

Nursing Diagnosis: Family Process, Alteration In (*Continued*)

Desired Patient Outcomes: Family will develop alternative functioning patterns during hospitalization, modifying over time and ultimately preparing for the return of the child to the home.

Interventions	Rationale
INDEPENDENT	
• Talk with the family using therapeutic communication techniques.	• The verbal exchange with the family assures the family of concern, decreases loneliness, and supports positive interpersonal relationships.
• Provide the family with information about the child's progress.	• Knowledge about the child's treatments and responses to therapy help reduce incorrect perceptions, fear, and anxiety.
• Explain the possible need for family restructuring during illness phases.	• Changes in family relationships and roles during hospitalization may cause frustration and anxiety. Knowledge that this is a normal process and expression of feelings foster positive adaptation.
• Encourage expression of feelings.	• Listening to the family's expression of feelings shows interest and caring.
COLLABORATIVE	
• Involve multiple members of the care team in early predischarge planning.	• Reintegration of the child into the home with some changes and limits is stressful. Each member of the team has a unique contribution to make in educating the family and smoothing the transition process.

Nursing Diagnosis: Coping, Possible Ineffective

May Be Related To:

• Trauma
• Disfigurement
• Separation
• Sensory overload

Possibly Evidenced By: Inability to make decisions, changes in communication, inappropriate use of defense mechanisms.

Desired Patient Outcomes: Child and family will adapt previously used coping strategies and/or learn new ones to maintain effective interactions and decrease anxiety.

Interventions	**Rationale**

INDEPENDENT

- Determine how the child and family have coped with stress in the past.

- All individuals have coping strategies to maintain homeostasis. Using those healthy familiar strategies assists in adaptation, decreasing anxiety, and promoting a person's belief in his or her own resources.

- Accept the child's need to use coping mechanisms,* which might be socially unacceptable in other situations, as long as they are not injurious to his or her safety.

- Society has predetermined acceptable standards for behaviors (including coping behaviors) at selected stages of development. Regression is normal during hospitalization. The goal is to increase comfort and security and the nurse assesses personal feelings and responses to ensure a supportive attitude toward the child.

- Provide coping alternatives for the child such as play, diversion, and crying. Provide in a manner that supports acceptance of the child and expression of feelings.

- The goal of psychosocial nursing care is to support the child's adjustment to the stress. New coping methods not previously tried may increase the comfort level.

Nursing Diagnosis: Social Isolation

May Be Related To:

- Delay in accomplishing developmental tasks
- Alterations in physical appearance
- Unaccepted behaviors

Possibly Evidenced By: Verbalizations of loneliness, expressed feelings of rejection, discomfort in public, absence of support persons, withdrawal, poor eye contact, unacceptable behavior.

Desired Patient Outcomes: The patient will interact, exhibiting acceptable social behaviors with family and staff.

Possible Mechanisms Include:

Protest: May be demonstrated as yelling and fighting during treatments; also, often highly adaptive as resists submission to illness and death.

Identification With the Aggressor: Modeling behaviors and dress of physicians and nurses—may give sense of control and identification with environment. If rejected by staff, may be seen as personal rejection or exclusion.

Withdrawal: Adaptive for conservation of energy. Should be supported and allowed at some times. Maladaptive depressive withdrawal may ultimately end in lack of desire to live.

Denial: May be adaptive or maladaptive. At some points, exclusion of or refusal to deal with certain information/stressors may be necessary for conservation of energy.

Nursing Diagnosis: Social Isolation (*Continued*)

Interventions   Rationale

Refer to Chapter 7, page 90, for interventions and rationale.

Nursing Diagnosis: Post-Trauma Response

May Be Related To:

• Burn event

Possibly Evidenced By: Re-experience of the burn event, flashbacks, nightmares, survival guilt, verbalizations, flat affect, development of phobias, headache, impulsiveness, change in mood, confu-

sion, nausea, loss of memory, withdrawal, stuttering.

Desired Patient Outcomes: The patient will exhibit decreased anxiety when flashbacks occur. Coping behaviors will be appropriate to developmental stage.

Interventions   Rationale

Refer to Chapter 7, page 93, for interventions and rationale.

Nursing Diagnosis: Fear

May Be Related To:

• Inability to communicate
• Environmental stimuli
• Separation from support system
• Pain

Possibly Evidenced By: Impulsiveness; apprehension; terror; panic attacks;

tachycardia; pupil dilation; vomiting, diarrhea; aggression; withdrawal.

Desired Patient Outcomes: The patient will acknowledge and cope with the fear in behaviors appropriate to developmental stage. Physical signs and symptoms will be absent.

Interventions   Rationale

Refer to Chapter 7, page 94, for interventions and rationale.

Nursing Diagnosis: Grieving, Dysfunctional

May Be Related To:

• Loss of appearance
• Loss of previous activities of daily living

• Loss of physiopsychosocial well-being
• Loss of possessions in burn event

Possibly Evidenced By: Impulsiveness; apprehension; terror; panic attacks; tachycardia; pupil dilation; vomiting, diarrhea; aggression; withdrawal.

Desired Patient Outcomes: The patient and family will identify problems appropriate to developmental stage of patient and progress through grief stages at their own rates.

Interventions

Rationale

Refer to Chapter 7, page 94, for interventions and rationale.

REFERENCES

1. Lee, J: Emotional reactions to trauma. Nurs Clin North Am 5:577, December 1970.
2. Seligman, R: Emotional responses to burns in children. In Howells, JG (ed): Modern Perspectives in the Psychiatric Aspects of Surgery. Brunner/Mazel, New York, 1976, p 468.
3. Bernstein, NR, Sanger, S, and Fras, I: The functions of the child psychiatrist in the management of severely burned children. J Am Acad Child Psychiatry 8:620, 1969.
4. Seligman, R, MacMillan, BG, and Carroll, SS: The burned child: A neglected area of psychiatry. Am J Psychiatry 128(1):84, 1971.
5. Seligman, R, Carroll, SS, and MacMillan, BG: Emotional responses in a pediatric intensive care unit of children sustaining major burns. Psychiatry Med 3(1):84, 1972.
6. Seligman, R, Carroll, SS, and MacMillan, BG: The burned child: Emotional factors and survival. In Matter, P (ed): Research in Burns Transactions of the Third International Congress on Research in Burns. Hans Huber, Bern, 1971, p 655.
7. Seligman, R: The burned child. In Pattison, EM (ed): The Experience of Dying. Englewood Cliffs, Prentice-Hall, 1971, p 119.
8. Davidson, SP: Nursing management of emotional reactions of severely burned patients during acute phase. Heart Lung, 2:370, 1973.
9. Gladston, R: The Burning and Healing of Children. Psychiatry 35:57, 1972.
10. Hamburg, DA, Hamburg, B, and deGoza, S: Adaptive problems and mechanisms in severely burned patients. Psychiatry 16:1, 1953.
11. Holter, JC and Friedman, SB: Etiology and management of severely burned children. Am J Dis Child 118:680, 1969.
12. Kjaer, GC: Psychiatric aspects of thermal burns. Northwest Med 68:537, 1969.
13. Long, RT and Cope, O: Emotional problems of burned children. New Engl J Med 264:1121, 1961.
14. Nover, RA: Pain and the burned child. J Am Acad Child Psychiatry 12:499, 1973.
15. Woodward, JM: Emotional disturbances of burned children. Br Med J 1:1009, 1959.
16. Woodward, JM: Emotional reactions in burned children and their mothers. Br J Plast Surg 13:316, 1961.
17. Campbell, L: Special behavioral problems of the burned child. Am J Nurs 76:220, 1976.
18. Davidson, SP, and Noyes, R, Jr: Psychiatric nursing consultation on a burn unit: Use of the group method. Am J Nurs 73:1715, 1973.
19. Fagerhaugh, SY: Pain expression and control on a burn care unit. In Nurs Outlook 22:645, 1974.
20. Talabere, L and Graves, P: A tool for assessing families of burned children. Am J Nurs 76:225, 1976.
21. Fagerhaugh, SY: Pain expression and control on a burn care unit. Nurs Outlook 22:645, 1974.
22. Freud, A: Conclusion. In Bergmann, T: Children In the Hospital. International Universities Press, New York, 1965, p 137.
23. Hamburg, DA: Coping behavior in life-threatening circumstances. Psychother Psychom, 23:13, 1974.

24. Mead, M: Culture and Commitment. Natural History Press, Doubleday, New York, 1970, p XIX.
25. Seligman, R, Carroll, SS, and MacMillan, BG: The burned child: Emotional factors and survival. In Matter, P (ed): Research in Burns Transactions of the Third International Congress on Research in Burns. Hans Huber, Bern, 1971, p 655.
26. Watson, EJ and Johnson, AM: The emotional significance of acquired physical disfigurement in children. Am J Orthopsychiatry, 28:85, 1985.
27. Seligman, R, Carroll, SS, and MacMillan, BG: Emotional responses in a pediatric intensive care unit of children sustaining major burns. Psychiatry Med 3(1):84, 1972.
28. Seligman, R, MacMillan, BG, and Carroll, SS: The burned child: A neglected area of psychiatry. Am J Psychiatry 128(1):84, 1971
29. Seligman, R: A psychiatric classification system for burned children. Am J Psychiatry 131 (1):41, 1974.

BIBLIOGRAPHY

Bernstein, N: Emotional Care of the Facially Burned and Disfigured. John Wiley & Sons, New York, 1984.
Campbell, C: Nursing Diagnosis and Interventions in Nursing Practice. John Wiley & Sons, New York, 1984.
Carpentino, L: Handbook of Nursing Diagnosis. Philadelphia, 1984.
McLane, A (ed): Classification of Nursing Diagnosis. CV Mosby, St Louis, 1987.
Patterson, D, et al: Post traumatic stress disorder in hospitalized patients with burn injuries. Journal of Burn Care and Rehabilitation 11(3):181, 1990.
Tempereau, C, Grossman, A, and Brones, M: Volitional collapse (loss of will to live) in patients with burn injuries. Journal of Burn Care and Rehabilitation 10(5):464, 1989.

CARE ACCORDING TO SEVERITY OF BURNS

Chapter 8

PAT VACCARO
RITA BOLEK TROFINO

CARE OF THE PATIENT WITH MINOR TO MODERATE BURNS

The American Burn Association (ABA) has developed a method for classifying a burn injury into one of three categories — minor, moderate, or major. This classification is based upon the severity of the injury, which is determined by certain criteria. These criteria, or severity factors, include depth of tissue destruction, total body surface area (TBSA) affected, cause of the injury, age, pre-existing illness, location or area of the body affected, and any associated injuries occurring at the time of the accident. This classification enables medical personnel to more efficiently meet the patient's needs and to anticipate potential problems and complications. Table 8–1 identifies the severity grading system used for a burn injury as described by the ABA. According to this classification, a minor burn injury can be defined as any partial-thickness (PT) injury that involves less than 15 percent of the TBSA in adults and less than 10 percent TBSA in a child, or a full-thickness (FT) injury of less than 2 percent TBSA in an adult. A moderate burn injury involves a partial-thickness of 15 to 25 percent TBSA in adults and 10 to 20 percent TBSA in a child, or a full-thickness (FT) injury of 2 to 10 percent in an adult.

In addition to considering the depth and extent of a burn injury when determining classification, other severity factors must be considered. If the cause of the burn injury is electrical or chemical, this mechanism of tissue destruction varies from that of a thermal burn and therefore requires careful observation of the patient during the first 24 to 48 hours postburn. The age of the patient and the presence of any pre-existing illness, such as diabetes or peripheral vascular disease, might also contribute to reclassifying a minor or moderate injury as a major burn injury. If a burn injury involves any one of the special care areas such as the hands, feet, face, or perineum it may also be considered a more serious injury due to the possible complications associated with burns in any of these areas. Finally, if the patient has any associated injuries, such as an inhalation injury or fractures, or an improper psychosocial home environment, the presence of these factors may further complicate the patient's recovery and thus classify a minor or moderate injury as a major injury. In summary, then, the depth and extent of a burn injury classify

113

TABLE 8-1. Severity Grading System Adopted by ABA

	Minor*	Moderate	Major
Partial-Thickness	<15% TBSA — Adults <10% TBSA — Child	15–25% — Adults 10–20% — Child	>25% TBSA — Adults >20% TBSA — Child
Full-Thickness	<2% TBSA — Adult	2–10% TBSA — Adults	>10% of TBSA
Treatment	Usually outpatients, Children and elderly; Possibly 1–2 days' hospital admission.	Admission to hospital, preferably one with expertise in burn care (e.g., burn unit).	Admission to burn center.

*Minor burns exclude:
1. Burns of face, hands, feet, and perineum
2. Inhalation injury
3. Electrical burns
4. Burns complicated by other trauma
5. Poor-risk patients
6. Patients with improper psychosocial facilities
    The existence of any of these circumstances would further classify the patient as a moderate or major burn accordingly.

it as minor, moderate, or major; however, the presence of any additional severity factors may reclassify it as a more serious injury. Therefore, a 70-year-old patient with a 20 percent partial-thickness injury involving the face and hands may be classified as a major injury due to the presence of additional severity factors.

In addition to this severity grading system that aids in classifying a burn injury, the ABA has established admission criteria to help emergency rooms determine proper placement of burn patients. The presence of any one of these factors would warrant admission to a burn center. During the ABA's 20th Annual Business Meeting in Seattle, Washington, 1988, the burn center admission criteria were established as depicted on Table 8-2.

Over 1 million people sustain a burn injury in the United States each year. About 90 to 95 percent of all these burn injuries are minor burns and can be treated on an outpatient basis. Partial-thickness burns may be due to hot liquids, steam from a car

TABLE 8-2. Burn Center Admission Criteria of ABA

1. Second- and third-degree burns >10% total body surface area (TBSA) in patients <10 or >50 years old
2. Second- and third-degree burns >20% TBSA in other age groups
3. Second- and third-degree burns that involve face, hands, feet, genitalia, perineum, and major joints
4. Third-degree burns >5% TBSA in any age group
5. Electrical burns including lightning injury
6. Chemical burns
7. Burn injury with inhalation injury
8. Any burn patient with concomitant trauma (e.g., fractures) in which the burn injury poses the greatest risk of morbidity or motality
9 Burn injury in patients with pre-existing medical disorders that could complicate management, prolong recovery, or affect mortality

radiator, flash burns from the superheated ambient air of an explosion or house fire, or excessive exposure to sunlight or other sources of ultraviolet light. Contact with a hot object such as an iron or other appliance may also cause deeper partial-thickness injury, depending on length of contact time.

PATIENT HISTORY

When caring for a burn patient in the emergency room, obtaining an accurate history is of utmost importance. A burn injury is certainly a painful and frightening experience for any person. Providing a calm and reassuring environment generally will elicit a cooperative response from the patient. Determining the exact circumstances surrounding an injury can provide the medical personnel with essential information regarding the outcome of the patient's injury and hospitalization. A patient with a minor or moderate burn injury is generally less compromised hemodynamically, more alert and cooperative, and therefore better able to provide the necessary information. An observer or family member is also consulted regarding the circumstances of the accident.

First, the nurse determines whether the injury occurred within an enclosed space and how long the patient may have been entrapped. Patients who have a history of entrapment are closely examined for inhalation injury, regardless of the size of their burn.

Next, identify the etiology of the burn. Different burning agents cause different degrees of depth and injury. A 10 percent TBSA burn caused by an electrical source is more severe than one caused by a hot object or a scald. In addition to deeper tissue destruction, other abnormalities, such as spinal cord injuries and cardiac dysrhythmias, may be associated with an electrical injury.

Determine the patient's duration of contact time with the burning agent. The depth of the injury is directly related to the length of time the burning agent is in contact with the skin surface.

It is also important to ascertain whether the clothing caught on fire. Burning clothing usually indicates a burn of greater depth and possible presence of inhalation injury, due to products of combustion resulting from burning clothing.

Identify the immediate first aid treatment provided. If the patient's clothing was removed and the injury was cooled down immediately post-burn, this would aid in decreasing the depth.

Determine the patient's action at the time of injury, and therefore, any resulting associated injury. Did the patient leap from a window during a housefire? Was he or she thrown as the result of an explosion? Did he or she fall while running as an immediate response to the injury? Always remember that every burn patient is also a trauma patient, and even though the burn injury may be the most obvious injury at that time, another associated injury may be more life-threatening, and should be treated accordingly.

Finally, the nurse determines if the patient experienced any change in level of consciousness at the time of injury. If a loss of consciousness was experienced at the time of injury, another source such as hypoxia, head injury, intoxication, or drug overdose is sought.

In addition to obtaining an accurate history regarding the circumstances of the accident, it is also necessary to obtain a thorough patient history. If one were simply to look at the description of the injury alone — for example, a 15 percent partial-thickness burn — a true estimation of the severity of the injury would not be appreciated without considering the patient's personal history and the burn severity factors previously discussed.

The patient's age plays a major role in wound healing and the overall response to the injury. The very young (under age 1) and the older (over age 60) populations may experience more complications during hospitalization due to their immature immune systems and pre-existing illnesses, respectively. In addition, both age groups have very thin skin and tend to have deeper injuries. The patient's past medical history is carefully reviewed, since the presence of illnesses such as congestive heart failure or diabetes may complicate the patient's response to therapy. Additional information to include in the patient history is the presence of allergies, diet, daily medications (both prescription and over-the-counter), the date of their last tetanus immunization, and the patient's use and/or abuse of tobacco, alcohol, and drugs.

The psychosocial factors involving the patient and family are also considered. It is important to recognize their emotional response and its appropriateness in relation to the injury. Even a minor injury, depending on the location and cause of the burn, can create great anxiety. Other issues to be considered include:

1. Does the nature of the accident implicate the patient in any way (e.g., auto accident, drugs, alcohol, risk-taking behavior in adolescents)?
2. Were there other people more severely injured, or was there possibly a death?
3. Does the accident involve additional losses (e.g., home, pet)?
4. What does the injury mean to the patient in regard to place in the family and occupation?

Finally, the patient's level of pain tolerance is continuously assessed. The pain related to a burn injury will not be completely relieved until the wound itself is healed. With a partial-thickness burn injury, the pain is more prominent, due to the exposure of nerve endings as a result of tissue damage. A patient with full-thickness injury experiences minimal pain, since the nerve endings are destroyed. Although medication only minimizes the pain, it may also be effective in calming the patient. When assessing the patient's pain, it is also important to identify it as pain related to burn injury or pain related to possible associated injury. Again, a burn patient is also a trauma patient. Although the burn injury is the most obvious injury, the presence of other injuries may be more life threatening and need to be managed in order of priority.

PHYSICAL ASSESSMENT

The physical assessment of the burn patient is accomplished using the same techniques and format that would be used for any patient. Since burn wounds may interfere with certain aspects of this assessment, only slight adjustments in assessment skills are necessary to complete a thorough examination. For example, in auscultating breath sounds on a patient with chest dressings, it would be more advantageous to wait to do this during dressing changes. The following are key points to remember in assessing the burn patient with a minor or moderate injury.

Inspection

When assessing the patient's burn wounds, it is important to note any involvement of the special care areas: the face, hands, feet, and perineum. As previously discussed, if these special care areas are involved, the injury may be considered more serious. When examining the face, it is closely observed for singed nasal hairs and burns of the lips. The oral cavity is also closely inspected for redness, edema, and sooty sputum. Although the size of the dermal burn may be small, a significant inhalation injury may be present if the injury involved entrapment. In young children, the tips of the outer ear canal and the backs of the hands are examined for burns. Children may cover their faces with their hands to hide from the flames. Although the child may have no facial burns or singed nasal hairs, burns along the edges of the ears and dorsum of the hand may clue the nurse to the presence of an inhalation injury. The eyes also are carefully examined for singed eyebrows and eyelashes. The physician can determine corneal burns with the use of fluorescein dye. If corneal damage is present, an ophthalmology consult is necessary.

In addition to determining the location of the dermal burns, it is also necessary to estimate the extent of the body surface affected by the burn injury. In an adult, this can be quickly estimated in the prehospital setting, using the "Rule of Nines." However, the Lund and Browder chart is more commonly used for both children and adults in the hospital setting (refer to Chapter 2, page 23).

The depth of the burn injury is largely determined by the color and appearance of the wound. Initially, it is often difficult to make an accurate determination of the depth, due to tissue changes that may still be occurring. All affected areas are inspected, palpating eschar to determine level of pain, dryness or moisture, and type of eschar (soft and elastic or hard and leathery). In addition to the color of the wound, all these characteristics will help determine the wound's depth (refer to Chapter 2).

When inspecting a burn injury, it is most important to note the presence of a circumferential injury. This injury exists when the burn wound extends the entire circumference of an anatomic structure, such as an extremity or the trunk. The interstitial edema together with the tight outer eschar compress the nerves and vessels and can diminish the circulation to that part. If the trunk is involved, respirations may be affected. A circumferential injury of the arm can diminish circulation to the hand. If the circumferential injury is a partial-thickness injury, this can usually be remedied by elevating the extremity to decrease edema. Occasionally, Travase, a proteolytic enzyme, may be applied to produce a chemical escharotomy. A full-thickness circumferential injury may require a surgical escharotomy. This involves making a linear incision along the length of the extremity and down through the eschar until punctate bleeding is reached. This incision allows the eschar to expand, thus releasing the pressure on the vessels and nerves (refer to Chapter 4, page 55). Assessing color, capillary refill, and temperature of both burned and unburned extremities is also important in determining peripheral tissue perfusion.

Palpation

When assessing the burn patient, the presence of pain and sensitivity in the burn wound aid in determining the depth of injury. A partial-thickness injury is generally more painful than a full-thickness injury, due to the presence of exposed nerve endings in the dermis. In a full-thickness injury, the nerve endings in the dermis are destroyed. Various areas of the eschar are palpated to observe the patient's response. Also noted are dryness or moisture, type of eschar, and edema, as previously discussed.

Frequent assessment of peripheral pulses is essential to monitor peripheral tissue perfusion. Good perfusion is an indication of adequate fluid resuscitation. Although this is usually not a problem with a minor or moderate burn injury, a circumferential injury may exist. Therefore, it is essential to frequently monitor the circulation to the affected extremity. Peripheral pulses are palpated at least once an hour. If palpation is questionable, the nurse uses a Doppler device. The physician may also order intracompartmental pressures to be assessed (refer to Chapter 3, page 37). When palpating the pulse, capillary refill and temperature of fingers and toes are also assessed.

Core body temperature in addition to skin temperature is monitored. Because one function of the skin is to help regulate body temperature, when the integrity of the skin is altered, so is this function. However, maintaining normal body temperature in a patient with a minor or moderate burn injury is usually not a problem. A slight temperature elevation is not uncommon.

Percussion

Percussion is not applicable.

Auscultation

When assessing a burn patient, it is always necessary to assess for the presence of an inhalation injury. Both lung fields are auscultated for the presence of wheezing, rhonchi, and other abnormal breath sounds. These may indicate airway obstruction or inhalation injury. Additional signs and symptoms of inhalation injury are investigated. Even if the patient has only a minor or moderate dermal burn, this does not exclude the presence of severe inhalation injury.

When assessing the circulatory status of the burn patient, the blood pressure and heart rate reflect the hemodynamic status regarding fluid resuscitation. With a minor or moderate burn injury, the blood pressure is often slightly elevated, due to pain and discomfort. In a patient with a major injury, the blood pressure is more likely to be decreased due to hypovolemia. Both types of patients will be tachycardic in response to the injury, fluids, and pain. Blood pressure and heart rate are auscultated as needed, depending on severity of the injury.

When assessing the gastrointestinal system of the burn patient, absence of bowel sounds may indicate the presence of paralytic ileus, which may be due to a neurogenic response to the burn injury or to hypoperfusion of the gastrointestinal organs early postinjury. Generally, this is less common in minor burns but still occurs. Depending upon the extent of the injury, a burn patient may not be permitted anything by mouth for the first 12 to 24 hours postburn if intravenous fluids are being administered. Generally, a patient with a greater than 20 to 25 percent TBSA burn will have a nasogastric tube inserted. Bowel sounds are assessed, as are nausea, vomiting, and abdominal distention. Curling's ulcer, a duodenal stress ulcer, is another complication that can affect the gastrointestinal tract. These ulcers have been documented to occur as early as 5 hours postburn. The incidence of Curling's ulcer in a patient with a minor or moderate burn is not high. The patient's past medical history (e.g., gastric ulcer) and psychologic make-up, however, can contribute to the development of a Curling's ulcer. A patient with a moderate burn injury is usually placed on a regimen of antacid prophylactically.

DIAGNOSTIC STUDIES

Most patients with a minor burn injury (less than 15 percent PT TBSA) do not require any extraordinary laboratory studies. Patients with a moderate burn injury (15 to 25 percent PT-TBSA), who may be admitted to a medical-surgical or a burn unit, require the routine admission laboratory studies. Alterations in laboratory values generally reflect the degree of tissue damage and therefore are usually greater when a larger percentage of the body surface is affected by the burn injury. Changes also depend on the patients' pre-existing state of health. Therefore, variations in these values are usually less in a minor or moderate burn injury. The initial laboratory studies and variations that may be seen early postburn include the following:

Diagnostic Test	Rationale
• Arterial Blood Gas Levels (ABGs)	• ABGs aid in determining hypoxemia possibly related to inhalation injury. Hypoxemia and hypercapnea can be seen in carbon monoxide poisoning.
• Carboxyhemoglobin Level	• Elevation of greater than 15 percent indicates inhalation injury due to carbon monoxide poisoning. Heavy smokers can normally have up to a 5 percent carboxyhemoglobin level.
• Chest X-ray	• This is usually normal in the early postburn period, even in the presence of inhalation injury.
• Cervical Spine (C-spine) Series	• This is usually done on all trauma and burn patients to determine the presence of any associated injury sustained when the accident occurred. Also, patients with an electrical injury (moderate and major injury) can also sustain C-spine fractures due to the tetanic muscle contractions that may result from contact with electrical current.
• Bronchoscopy	• This diagnostic study may be indicated when there is a history of entrapment and other physical signs of inhalation injury are observed (e.g., facial burns, sooty sputum). It is not uncommon for a patient with a minor or moderate injury to also have inhalation injury. Edema, erythema, and carbonaceous sputum may be visualized in the airway with inhalation injury.
• Electrocardiogram (ECG)	• An ECG indicates the presence of myocardial ischemia or dysrhythmias, which may occur even with minor or moderate burn injury, depending on the patient's pre-existing state of health. A patient with an electrical injury is especially prone to cardiac dysrhythmias.
• Serum Potassium	• The serum potassium level tends to be elevated initially postinjury, due to the hemolysis of red blood cells (RBCs) and thus the loss of intracellular potassium. As fluid resuscitation progresses and the patient becomes better hydrated, the potassium in the bloodstream is excreted through the kidneys, leaving the patient with a low serum potassium level. However, in a minor or moderate burn injury, the hemolysis of red blood cells is less significant than in a major

Diagnostic Test	Rationale
	burn injury and therefore, a marked change in the serum potassium level may not be seen.
• Serum Sodium	• The serum sodium level may be normal or slightly decreased due to loss of extracellular fluid or body water. The sodium may also be trapped in the interstitial edema fluid at the injury site.
• Blood Urea Nitrogen (BUN)	• The BUN may be elevated due to decreased renal perfusion and the excessive catabolism of proteins resulting directly from the injury.
• Serum Glucose	• Blood sugar levels may be elevated due to the stress response.
• Hematocrit	• A falsely elevated hematocrit is usually present early postburn and suggests hemoconcentration due to the fluid shift from vascular spaces to interstitial spaces. As fluid resuscitation progresses and the patient becomes better hydrated, hematocrit may decrease, reflecting hemodilution.
• Hemoglobin	• A falsely elevated hemoglobin may also be seen early postburn due to hemolysis of RBCs which releases free hemoglobin into the bloodstream. Later, as fluid resuscitation progresses, hemoglobin may decrease.
• White Blood Cells (WBCs)	• Leukocystosis can occur due to the inflammatory response resulting from the injury.
• Urine Myoglobin	• A positive urine myoglobin, which indicates muscle damage, is often seen with an electrical injury. Myoglobin is a pigment that gives muscle its red color. When muscle is damaged, myoglobin is released into the bloodstream. When myoglobin is present, it may be necessary to increase intravenous (IV) fluid intake so that the kidneys are adequately perfused, thus decreasing the risk of tubular necrosis. A positive urine myoglobin is not common in a minor or moderate injury.
• Serum Albumin	• Serum albumin may be decreased due to loss of protein from the burn wound. Because of increased capillary permeability, there is a shift of protein from the intravascular space to the interstitial space, and thus, into the wound.

- Serum and Urine Osmolarity

- Both of these values help determine the patient's state of hydration.

PLACEMENT OF PATIENT

A patient diagnosed with a minor burn injury is usually treated in the emergency room and discharged, provided the patient's psychosocial environment, together with cognitive and motor skills, are adequate to facilitate healing and recovery. A minor burn, with proper treatment, heals without complications. A moderately burn injured patient is usually triaged to a burn unit or a medical-surgical unit, where the wounds can be monitored more closely for infection and treated more effectively. Although minor and moderate burn injuries are certainly not as severe as major injuries, inappropriate treatment of the former can cause delayed healing, infection, and possible conversion to a full-thickness injury.

OUTPATIENT SETTING

Most burns are minor and the majority of these burns are treated in an outpatient setting. However, the outpatient treatment of burns in this chapter encompasses not only those patients with minor burns but also those with moderate to severe burns who have recovered and are discharged from the hospital. The nursing priorities listed in the following care plan are for outpatient treatment.

NURSING CARE PLAN: BURN CARE IN AN OUTPATIENT SETTING

Nursing Priorities

1. Minimize and control bacterial contamination to promote healing
2. Minimize pain and discomfort
3. Provide emotional support to patient and significant others
4. Maintain adequate nutrition to meet caloric and protein demands for proper healing
5. Maintain joint mobility by providing range-of-motion (ROM) exercises and proper splinting (as applicable)
6. Provide assistance and referrals as necessary

Nursing Diagnosis: Knowledge Deficit, Wound Healing, and Burn Treatments

May Be Related to:

- Lack of knowledge of the healing process
- Lack of knowledge about the development of scar tissue
- Lack of knowledge about nutritional needs
- Lack of knowledge about musculoskeletal needs

Nursing Diagnosis: Knowledge Deficit, Wound Healing, and Burn Treatments (*Continued*)

Possibly Evidenced By: Inability to answer questions regarding outpatient regimen, inability to provide adequate return demonstration of procedures.

Desired Patient Outcomes: Patient can verbalize understanding of outpatient regimen and perform a return demonstration of procedures adequately.

Interventions	Rationale

INDEPENDENT

- Explain purpose of procedures and treatment in *lay terms*, both verbally and in writing. Require a return demonstration for all procedures.

- Patient will more likely adhere to regimen if the purpose is understood. Patients need to have written instructions to take home, because their anxiety may cause them to forget verbal instructions. Return demonstration provides evaluation of learning.

- Explain the purpose for washing the burn, using a good clean technique: To clean the burn; to loosen and/or remove dead skin; to promote exercising of the burned area (often it is easier to exercise in the shower or tub).

- For home care, unless otherwise indicated, good clean technique is adequate. Use nonmedical terms in explanations to increase patient understanding.

- Identify all equipment necessary for the bath or shower: clean washcloth; clean towel; mild soap (such as Ivory or Dove); plastic bag; scissors; bottle of rubbing alcohol, cotton ball; and dressing materials (as per physician order).

- It is necessary to be very specific so that the good clean technique is adhered to.

- Explain the entire washing procedure step-by-step:
  - Wash hands.
  - Clean scissors with cotton ball soaked in alcohol.
  - Prepare tub or shower; test water beforehand—not too hot, not too cold.
  - Remove old dressings, place in the plastic bag and discard; if some of the dressing sticks to the burn, soak off in the shower or tub.

  - Wash burns with the soap and washcloth or gauze pad; wash gently but firmly being sure to remove all creams, ointments, and loose skin.
  - Rinse thoroughly.

- All procedures must be very detailed for patient to perform correctly.

  - Avoids further injury.

  - Removing old dressings helps prevent reinfection. Soaking dressings that stick to the burn prevents the patient from destroying new epithelializations.
  - Patient must apply enough pressure to cleanse appropriately.

  - Prevents reinfection; provides a cleaner surface.

Interventions	Rationale

- ◦ Gently pat dry with a clean towel.
- ◦ Open and apply the dressings as ordered.
- Explain the purpose for the burn dressing: to promote healing, to prevent infections, to keep wound moist, to protect burned area from injury.

  • Patient will be more aware of the value of complying to regimen.

- Identify all equipment necessary for the dressing change: for example, gauze sponges (specify size); 6-inch gauze rolls (Kerlix); nonallergic tape; scissors; rubbing alcohol; tongue blade; cotton ball; sterile topical agent.

  • Specificity is necessary to ensure proper technique.

- Explain the entire dressing procedure in detail as per physician orders.

  • Encourages proper performance of procedure.

- Identify care of donor site (if applicable): wash with mild soap and water during bath or shower.

  • Allows proper healing of donor site.

- Encourage patient to eat foods high in proteins and calories. Provide helpful hints:

  • Promotes proper healing of skin. Instructions need to be explicit in order for patient to comply.

  - ◦ Make gravies with dinners.
  - ◦ Add skim milk powder to recipes.
  - ◦ Add a few eggs and/or peanut butter to milkshakes.
  - ◦ Eat foods such as meats, eggs, nuts, fruits, fish, poultry, cheese, vegetables, beans, milk, and cereal.

- Explain signs and symptoms of wound infection: redness, swelling, warmth (warm to touch), soreness or an uncomfortable feeling (different from when patient left the hospital), drainage (pus), unpleasant odor, color change to bluish-green or black, and fever (greater than 100°F).

  • Burn, graft, and/or donor areas are all in the process of healing and can therefore develop infections more easily. Since skin integrity is interrupted, the body has lost its natural defenses against infection.

- Explain the purpose of splints (if applicable):

  • Patient will be more apt to comply with the use of splints if properly explained.

  - ◦ Splints are devices especially molded for patient by occupational therapist (OT).
  - ◦ These devices help skin to heal properly and keep affected muscles in proper condition.

- Identify proper usage of splints (if applicable):

  • Improperly used splints will cause more skin and muscle damage.

  - ◦ Apply the splint exactly as shown in the hospital.
  - ◦ Call OT if skin becomes red or sore from wearing splints.

Nursing Diagnosis: Knowledge Deficit, Wound Healing, and Burn Treatments (*Continued*)

Interventions	Rationale

○ Wash splint once a day in cold water and a mild soap (usually after dressing change).

• Review all exercises that the patient may need to perform at home. Provide a list of specific exercises and how often they should be done. OT may have an illustration of each exercise, if needed.

    • Maintains ROM of all extremities.

• Review the care of healed skin (burn, graft, or donor):

    • Skin usually becomes dry, itchy, and flaky; gentle care is necessary to prevent further injury or infection.

○ Wash area thoroughly with mild soap and water.

○ Pat completely dry.

○ Apply moisturizer gently (as prescribed by physician); apply only a small amount (skin should not look greasy).

○ Do not scratch skin; if itching is bothersome, contact physician.

○ May take a prescription drug for severe itching.

• Instruct patient to avoid bruises or blisters on healed or healing skin:

    • Healed or healing skin is very sensitive to even slight trauma.

○ Avoid wearing tight-fitting clothes over the healed area (e.g., tight jeans, bras, girdles, shoes).

○ Wear loose-fitting clothes, such as jogging pants, sweatshirts, large tee shirts.

○ Wear rubber gloves when washing dishes if hands are burned.

○ Avoid hitting or bumping healed areas (e.g., contact sports).

    • Bruising may contribute to blister formation.

○ Wear white cotton clothes over healed areas.

○ Avoid direct exposure to sun; wear protective clothing and a sunscreen of SPF of 15 or above (call physician if reaction to sunscreen occurs).

    ○ Skin will be more sensitive to ultraviolet rays.

○ Wear protective clothing when weather is cold.

○ Avoid overexposure to cold.

    ○ Patient is at greater risk for frostbite in burn-injured areas due to altered circulation.

• Advise patient as to how skin will look in the process of healing:

○ Discoloration may include dark-pink, deep red, or greyish-red skin.

    • Discoloration occurs in the process of healing due to different changes in blood circulation. All changes are subject to individual variations.

Interventions	Rationale
○ If legs or feet were burned, color change is especially apparent after getting out of bed. ○ Scarring may occur that will give skin a "bumpy" or unsmooth appearance (Color Plate 18).	
• Explain purpose and use of a pressure garment (as applicable) (Color Plate 19): ○ Helps to minimize scarring. ○ Garment is made to individual measurements. ○ Smooths out skin and keeps muscles and skin growing in good functional positions. ○ Must be worn directly over the skin. ○ Must be worn 24 hours a day for about 10 to 13 months (physician will determine time); may remove mask and gloves at mealtimes; remove everything prior to bath or shower. ○ Hands, legs, and feet may look deep red to purple due to circulatory changes upon removal. ○ Call physician if garment feels too tight (due to weight gain) or if it rubs and causes patient to bleed; it may need to be remeasured.	• Hypertrophic scarring can be prevented through the use of a pressure garment. Many patients find it difficult to wear this garment. Patient may comply more with proper information.
• Instruct patient on care of pressure garment (as applicable): ○ Wash by hand in a mild pure soap. ○ Rinse well in lukewarm water. ○ Squeeze out excess water (do not wring out). ○ Lay flat to dry on a clean towel.	• Patient is given two garments. One garment must always be clean. Proper care maintains proper life of garment.
• Instruct patient as to level of activity (as prescribed by physician): ○ Gradually increase tolerance level for sports, work, school, and so on. ○ Slowly start back to usual activities.	• If patient was in hospital for extended period of time, fatigue will be common.

COLLABORATIVE

• Initiate appropriate referrals as necessary (e.g., home nursing, burn support groups).	• Most minor burns do not require referrals; however, recovered patients with moderate to major burns will usually require some followup.
• Arrange return visit to physician; or provide patient with physician's phone number, emphasizing importance of return visit.	• Followup visit to physician is necessary for adequate care.

Nursing Diagnosis: Knowledge Deficit, Wound Healing, and Burn Treatments (*Continued*)

Interventions

- Provide phone number for concerns or questions.
- Provide patient with a physician's prescription for topical agents and any additional dressing materials and medications.

Rationale

- Patient needs a resource person to contact should there be any problems.
- Many patients can receive payment assistance if it is written on a prescription. All medications and treatments are in writing to prevent any confusion.

Nursing Diagnosis: Self-Care Deficit: Dressings

May Be Related To:

- Pain and discomfort
- Cognitive impairment — knowledge deficit
- Physical limitations due to burns
- Psychologic limitations

Possibly Evidenced By: Inability to perform return demonstration of dressings; verbalizations.

Desired Patient Outcomes: Patient will be able to perform dressings satisfactorily.

Interventions

INDEPENDENT

- Assess patient for causative or contributing factors related to self-care deficit. Assess degree of deficit.

- Encourage patient to be involved in goal-setting to determine the care plan.
- Develop a care plan based on individual situation. Involve significant others as appropriate.
- Provide positive reinforcement for progress made toward goals.

Rationale

- Interventions will depend upon etiology of self-care deficit. Note individual variations. Some patients may not even want to look at wound; others may be adept at washing the wound but not at applying the dressing.
- Helps patient to acknowledge limitations and deal with them appropriately.
- Each situation may have a different causative or contributing factor.

- Increases self-confidence in patient and significant others.

COLLABORATIVE

- Initiate referrals to appropriate agencies (e.g., home nursing; burn support groups).

- Even if patient can perform dressing satisfactorily prior to discharge, at least one visit from a nurse is necessary to ensure compliance to regimen.

MEDICAL-SURGICAL OR PEDIATRIC SETTING

Most moderate burns require hospitalization. The patient will be placed in a medical-surgical or a pediatric unit, depending on his or her age. Although the nursing diagnoses may be similar for the patient with a moderate burn and the patient with a major burn, the care for the patient with a moderate burn does not encompass critical care aspects.

NURSING CARE PLAN: CARE OF THE PATIENT WITH MODERATE BURNS IN A HOSPITAL SETTING

Nursing Priorities:

1. Maintain hemodynamic stability.
2. Minimize and control bacterial contamination to promote healing.
3. Minimize pain and discomfort.
4. Provide emotional support to patient and significant other.
5. Maintain adequate nutrition to meet caloric and protein demands for proper healing.
6. Maintain joint mobility by providing ROM exercises and proper splinting (as applicable).
7. Provide assistance and referrals as necessary.

Nursing Diagnosis: Fluid Volume Deficit, Potential First 24 to 72 Hours

May Be Related to:

- Increased capillary permeability (causes a shift of plasma, proteins, and electrolytes from the vascular spaces to the interstitial spaces)
- Evaporative loss from wound surface
- Decreased fluid intake
  (These changes occur to a lesser degree with minor and moderate burns.)

Possibly Evidenced By: Decreased blood pressure, increased pulse rate, decreased urinary output, decreased capillary refill, increased urine specific gravity, elevated hematocrit, decreasing mental status, thirst, and dry mouth.

Desired Patient Outcomes: Patient will maintain an adequate state of hydration as evidenced by stable vital signs, adequate urine output, and normal laboratory values.

Interventions	Rationale
INDEPENDENT	
• Obtain admission weight and monitor daily weight.	• A slight weight gain can be expected during the first 72 hours, due to fluid replacement in a moderate injury. However, daily weight checks may not be indicated unless a pre-existing condition deems it necessary.

Nursing Diagnosis: Fluid Volume Deficit, Potential First 24 to 72 Hours (*Continued*)

Interventions	Rationale
• Monitor vital signs.	• Adequate vital signs indicate adequate fluid resuscitation, either orally or IV. Serves as a guide for hemodynamic status.
• Monitor intake and output (I&O); observe urine color.	• Adequate urinary output indicates adequate hydration. If urine color changes to red or reddish-brown, further tests are indicated to determine presence of myoglobin and thus deeper tissue damage.
• Encourage oral fluid intake.	• Balanced electrolyte solution (e.g., Gatorade) and fruit juices should be encouraged rather than free water. ○ Adequate circulating volume insures sufficient oxygenation of tissues and thus promotes wound healing.

COLLABORATIVE

• Insert and maintain large-bore peripheral IV tube with moderate injury.	• Fluid replacement prevents fluid and electrolyte imbalance that may be associated with a moderate injury.
• Administer crystalloid IV fluids (e.g., lactated Ringer's solution) during first 24 hours. Afterward, oral fluids may be adequate.	
• Monitor laboratory values (e.g., serum electrolytes, complete blood count).	• Laboratory values aid in determining hydration status and necessity for replacement of electrolytes.

Nursing Diagnosis: Tissue Perfusion, Alteration In

May Be Related To:

• Decreased peripheral circulating blood volume (due to the fluid shift and the increased hydrostatic pressure of local wound edema)
• Decreased circulating volume (the body attempts to compensate by decreasing the peripheral circulation to ensure adequate circulation to major organs)

Possibly Evidenced By: Skin that is cool, pale, and clammy with diminished or absent peripheral pulses; poor capillary refill; numbness and tingling sensation in extremity, together with increased pain; anxiety, restlessness.

Desired Patient Outcomes: Patient maintains adequate tissue perfusion as evidenced by adequate capillary refill, skin color, and temperature. Peripheral pulses are present and equal. No anxiety or restlessness from decreased cerebral perfusion.

Interventions	Rationale
INDEPENDENT	
• Elevate the affected areas.	• Allows for increased venous return and decreases dependent edema, which can compress blood vessels and inhibit adequate circulation.
• Assess peripheral perfusion hourly or as necessary. Note pulses, color, edema, sensation, motion, capillary refill.	• Assesses peripheral perfusion. Assesses need for escharotomy.
• Measure circumference of burned extremities. Keep patient warm.	• Serves as a guide to edema formation. Cold induces vasoconstriction, thus decreasing circulation.
• Encourage ROM exercises and use of affected areas in daily activities and self-care.	• Movement promotes fluid mobilization, thus decreasing edema and increasing circulation.

Nursing Diagnosis: Skin Integrity, Impairment Of: Actual

May Be Related To:

• Burn Wound

Desired Patient Outcomes: Patient will develop normal closure of wound. Normal body temperature is maintained.

Possibly Evidenced By: Disruption of skin surface and destruction of skin layers.

Interventions	Rationale
INDEPENDENT	
• Assess skin color and temperature and body temperature.	• Serve as indicators regarding loss of body heat.
• Assess wound for state of healing.	• Dressing techniques are varied to match specific need of wound.
• Perform dressing changes quickly but efficiently.	• Increased exposure of patient during dressing changes increases loss of body heat.
• Increase room temperature; provide blankets.	• These measures are suitable in maintaining body heat, provided patient's temperature is not elevated.

Refer to Chapter 4, p. 64, for additional interventions and rationale.

Nursing Diagnosis: Pain

Refer to Chapter 9, page 169, for etiology, manifestations, desired patient outcomes, interventions, and rationale.

Nursing Diagnosis: Infection, Potential For

May Be Related To:

- Loss of skin integrity.
- Decreased resistance to infection.

Possibly Evidenced By: Elevated temperature, positive wound cultures, changes in wound drainage and appearance.

Desired Patient Outcomes: Patient will not develop wound infection and sepsis.

Interventions	Rationale
• Maintain protective environment. Isolate linens, dressings, utensils, and bathroom.	• Initially, complete isolation within a specific unit is usually not indicated with a moderate injury unless severe infection develops. Isolation of linens, utensils, bathroom use, and so on, is usually sufficient to prevent cross-contamination. However, gown, gloves, and mask are usually necessary during dressing change. (Policy and procedure may vary; usually wound and skin precautions.)
• Maintain aseptic technique during dressing changes.	• Aseptic technique decreases transfer of organisms and thus incidence of infection.
• Assess burn wound with each dressing change. Note color, amount, odor, and consistency of drainage; appearance of wound; tenderness; color of eschar; cellulitis around margin of wound.	• Careful assessment provides early indicators to presence of infection and allows for prompt treatment.
• Shave hair extending 1 inch beyond margin of burn wounds. Do not shave eyebrows.	• Hair is a medium for bacterial growth.
• Monitor temperature, IV sites, urine, and laboratory values such as WBC.	• Reddened catheter sites and presence of purulent drainage indicates infection. Cloudy urine with increased sediment may indicate urinary tract infection. Increased WBC in blood or urine may indicate infection.

COLLABORATIVE

• Obtain cultures—wound, urine, sputum, and blood—as ordered and whenever necessary.	• Change in amount, color, odor, and consistency of wound drainage, sputum, or urine indicates a need for cultures. Tem-

Interventions	Rationale
	perature elevation above a certain range (e.g., greater than 102°F or 38.9°C) may warrant a blood culture. Results of cultures allow for early detection and prompt treatment.
• Perform hydrotherapy or wound cleansing as ordered (usually daily or twice daily according to needs of wound and patient).	• Hydrotherapy provides frequent cleansing of wounds and thus minimizes infection. Frequency of treatment depends on presence of drainage and on patient's tolerance. With a moderate injury, this procedure may be performed in a shower. (Refer to Hydrotherapy Procedure, Chapter 4, page 50.
• Debride any loose blister epithelium and necrotic tissue during hydrotherapy procedure.	• Removal of dead tissue decreases incidence of infection and promotes healing. If blisters appear infected, they are removed.
• Apply topical agents as ordered.	• Topical agents aid in minimizing infection. (Refer to Topical Agents, Chapter 4, page 44. These antimicrobial agents may be ordered specifically according to wound culture and sensitivity reports.
• Administer systemic antibiotics when appropriate.	• Systemic antibiotics are not commonly indicated with a moderate injury unless the patient develops a systemic infection. They are ordered according to blood culture reports.
• Administer tetanus toxoid prophylaxis.	• Prevents tetanus. Use Hypertet and toxoid if patient has never been immunized. Use DT in children less than 7 years old.

Nursing Diagnosis: Nutrition, Alteration In: Less Than Body Requirements

May Be Related To:

- Hypermetabolic state
- Protein-wasting from burn wound

Possibly Evidenced By: Weight loss, decreased plasma proteins, decreased albumin, decreased caloric intake.

Desired Patient Outcomes: Patient will maintain adequate nutritional intake, stable weight and maintenance of plasma proteins and albumin.

Interventions	Rationale

Refer to Chapter 9, page 172, for interventions and rationale.

Nursing Diagnosis: Mobility, Impaired Physical

(Refer to Chapter 9 for etiology, manifestations, desired patient outcomes, interventions and rationale.)

Nursing Diagnosis: Sleep Pattern Disturbance

May Be Related To:

- Pain and discomfort of burn wound.
- Hospital environment and routine.

Possibly Evidenced By: Verbalizations; irritability; restlessness; dark circles under eyes; frequent yawning; interrupted sleep.

Desired Patient Outcomes: Patient will experience improvement in sleep pattern, and an increased sense of well-being.

Interventions	Rationale
INDEPENDENT	
• Determine contributing factors and minimize same.	• Controlling anxiety and pain will provide a more restful sleep.
• Eliminate unnecessary noise and distractions.	• Provides for a quiet environment.
• Organize care to provide adequate periods of rest/sleep.	• Prevents patient from being disturbed.
COLLABORATIVE	
• Provide analgesics and/or sedation as ordered.	• With appropriate pain relief and sedation, patient will be more able to relax and sleep.

Nursing Diagnosis: Anxiety

May Be Related To:

- Threat to health status

(Refer to Chapter 7, page 98, for manifestations, desired patient outcomes, interventions, and rationale.)

Nursing Diagnosis: Fear

(Refer to Chapter 7, page 94, for etiology, manifestations, desired patient outcomes, interventions, and rationale.)

Nursing Diagnosis: Self-Concept, Alteration In

May Be Related To:

• Change in appearance

(Refer to Chapter 7, page 89, for etiology, manifestations, desired patient outcomes, interventions, and rationale.)

Nursing Diagnosis: Family Process, Alteration In

(Refer to Chapter 7, page 97, for etiology, manifestations, desired patient outcomes, interventions, and rationale.

Nursing Diagnosis: Social Isolation

(Refer to Chapter 7, page 90, for etiology, manifestations, desired patient outcomes, interventions, and rationale.)

Nursing Diagnosis: Coping, Ineffective Family

(Refer to Chapter 7, page 92, for etiology, manifestations, desired patient outcomes, interventions, and rationale.)

BIBLIOGRAPHY

Artz, CP, Moncrief, JA, and Pruit, BA: Burns: A Team Approach. Saunders, Philadelphia, 1979.

Boswich, JA (ed): The Art and Science of Burn Care. Aspen Publishers, Rockville, MD, 1987.

Brodzka, W, Thornhill, HL, and Howard, S: Burns: Causes and risk factors. Arch Phys Med Rehabil 66:746, 1985.

Carrougher, G and Marvin, J: Mechanical debridement. Journal of Burn Care and Rehabilitation 10(3):271, 1989.

Desai, MH: Epidemiology, assessment, and treatment of burn injuries. Emerg Care Q 1(3):51, 1985.

Heinrich, JJ, Brand, DA, and Cuono, CB: The role of topical treatment as a determinant of infection in outpatient burns. Journal of Burn Care Rehabilitation 9:3, 1988.

Hills, SW and Birmingham, JJ: The Fleschner Series in Critical Care Nursing: Burn Care. Fleschner Publishing, Bethany, Connecticut, 1981.

Hummel, RP (ed): Clinical Burn Therapy: A Management and Prevention Guide. John Wright—PSG, Boston, 1982.

Jacoby, F: Nursing Care of the Patient with Burns. CV Mosby, St Louis, 1976.

Mott, SR, James, SR, and Sperhac, AM: Nursing Care of Children and Families. Addison-Wesley, Redwood City, CA, 1990, pp 1164–1172.

Salisbury, R, Newman, NM, and Dingeldein, GP (eds): Manual of Burn Therapeutics. Little, Brown, & Co, Boston, 1983.

Warden, GD: Outpatient care of thermal injuries. Surg Clin North Am 67(1):147, 1987.

Chapter 9

LORNA L. SCHUMANN

CARE OF THE PATIENT WITH MAJOR BURNS

An estimated 2 million people are burned each year. Of these, 70,000 require hospitalization and 6000 to 9000 die.[1,2] Burns account for an annual loss of $13.6 billion due to income and property loss.[3] Major burns account for the largest portion of the costs of hospitalization and annual dollar loss.

Major burn injuries are classified by the American Burn Association (ABA) as those second-degree burns of greater than 25 percent total body surface area (TBSA) (greater than 20 percent TBSA in children) or all third-degree burns greater than 10 percent TBSA in both children and adults[4,5] (Refer to Chapter 2, page 23, for methods of estimating percentages of burns). Additional burn involvement also categorized as a major burn includes burns of the eyes, ears, face, hands, feet, or perineum; inhalation injuries; electrical injuries; burn injuries complicated by associated injuries, such as puncture wounds, head injuries, and fractures; and poor-risk patients such as insulin-dependent diabetics, the elderly, neonates, and so forth.

STATISTICS OF MAJOR BURNS

A data retrieval system has been developed by the National Burn Information Exchange (NBIE)[6] to process patient information on a national level and develop statistical data that can lead to improved patient care. Participants in the NBIE (approximately 35 percent of the nation's total designated burn beds) submit information forms on both burn survivors and burn mortalities. The NBIE information form is used to collect personal patient information and data related to medical history, concurrent injuries, percent of burn, type of burn, need for ventilatory support, type of topical burn agents used, wound care system, fluid therapy replacement, types of antibiotics used, complications, and discharge or mortality information.[7] Further information related to the data collection forms can be obtained by writing the National Burn Information Exchange in Ann Arbor, Michigan.

Data from these forms are then compiled at the Michigan State University computer center for annual distribution to participants. Morbidity and mortality data can be used by various units for comparison with individual patient outcomes. Figures 9–1 and 9–2 present data on burn patient survival statistics based on age groups, the percent of total area burned (see Fig. 9–1), and the percent of full-thickness area burned (see Fig. 9–2). In both instances patients over age 60 have the lowest survival rates and patients between age 5 and 34 have the highest survival rates.

Other statistics that influence survival rates and burn severity may include a positive past medical history. Past medical history is defined in this context as previous health problems that significantly affect mortality and morbidity of burn patients. Of the 21,440 patients in the NBIE data base, 5600 had a positive past medical history.[8] Frequently occurring problems included cardiovascular diseases (20 percent), pulmonary diseases (11 percent), central nervous system diseases (11 percent), emotional disorders (10 percent), and metabolic disorders (8 percent). Figure 9–3 shows the survival curves corresponding to patients with no past medical history as compared with those patients who had one, two, three, or more past medical health problems.

The effect of past medical health problems on patient survival is statistically significant. Each past medical problem that exists in a burned patient is comparable in terms of severity to a burn injury of 11 percent total body surface area.[9]

A retrospective study of 1271 patients at the University of Alabama Burn Center[10] was instigated to identify the primary causes of morbidity and mortality in burn patients. The period studied was 1971 to 1982. Using the aforementioned classification standards set by the ABA, 71.2 percent of the burns were classified as major burns. Patient ages ranged from 15 to 81, with the mean being 40.2 years. The mean age and mean percent burn of survivors was significantly lower than nonsurvivors (p = 0.0001). Complications

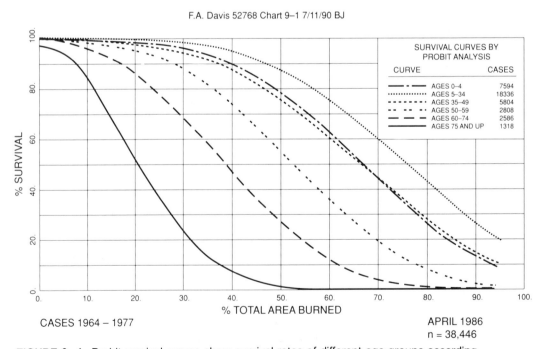

F.A. Davis 52768 Chart 9–1 7/11/90 BJ

SURVIVAL CURVES BY
PROBIT ANALYSIS

CURVE		CASES
— · —	AGES 0–4	7594
··········	AGES 5–34	18336
- - - - -	AGES 35–49	5804
- - · - - ·	AGES 50–59	2808
— — —	AGES 60–74	2586
————	AGES 75 AND UP	1318

% SURVIVAL

% TOTAL AREA BURNED

CASES 1964 – 1977

APRIL 1986
n = 38,446

FIGURE 9–1. Probit survival curves show survival rates of different age groups according to the percent of total area burned. (From Feller, I, and Jones, CA: The National Burn Information Exchange. Surg Clin North Am 67:167, 1987, with permission.)

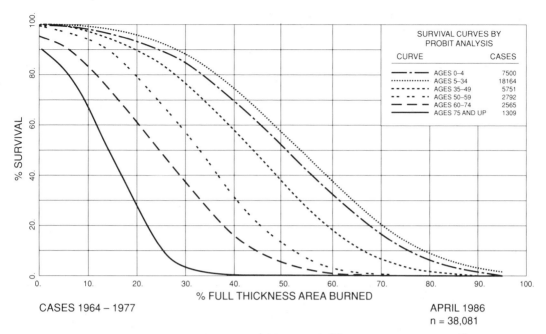

CASES 1964 – 1977

APRIL 1986
n = 38,081

FIGURE 9-2. Probit survival curves show survival rates of different age groups according to the percentage of full-thickness burn. (From Feller, I, and Jones, CA: The National Burn Information Exchange. Surg Clin North Am 67:167, 1987, with permission.)

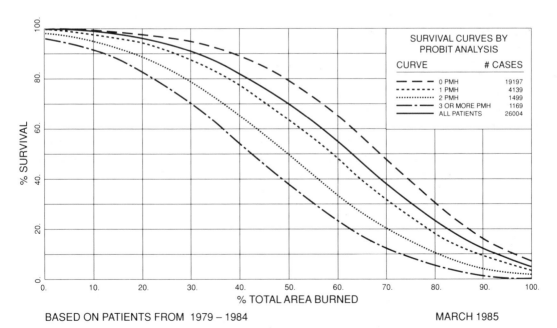

BASED ON PATIENTS FROM 1979 – 1984

MARCH 1985

FIGURE 9-3. Burned patient survival by frequency of past medical problems. Probit survival curves show better survival rates for groups with fewer past medical histories. (From Feller, I, and Jones, CA: The National Burn Information Exchange. Surg Clin North Am 67:167, 1987, with permission.)

of burn injury significantly associated with mortality included septicemia, myocardial infarction, respiratory insufficiency, pulmonary embolus, pneumonia, respiratory burn, bacteremia, renal failure, burn wound sepsis, gastrointestinal ulcer, hemolytic disorders, pneumothorax, stroke, and liver failure. Many of the patients had more than one of these diagnoses. Pre-existing conditions found to be significantly related to mortality were alcoholism; heart disease; circulatory disease; mental disorders; and diseases of the respiratory, endocrine, and digestive systems.[11]

PLACEMENT OF PATIENT

In general, patients with major burns are transported to a burn center in which special equipment, personnel, and facilities are available for optimum patient treatment (refer to Chapter 19, page 353). Burn patients require a great deal of wound care treatment, special monitoring, medical-surgical intervention, and a team approach that may not be feasible in many settings.

Many of the large metropolitan areas of the United States have elaborate burn care centers that function as emergency departments (ED), thus bypassing the regular ED. These centers may also contain their own operating room, recovery room, outpatient burn clinics, and rehabilitation facilities. When these facilities are functioning above 100 percent capacity, patients with lesser burns or those in the rehabilitation phase can be cared for on general surgical units with wound care managed by the burn service.

NURSING ASSESSMENT

Over the last two decades, the treatment of major burns has taken a new focus. Treatment modalities such as early wound excision and closure and the use of broad-spectrum antibiotics have greatly decreased the mortality figures. Sophisticated methods for providing nutritional support have been developed to meet the high caloric needs of burn patients. Because the needs of a major burn patient are tremendous, the nurse needs to assess the patient and his or her family holistically. The patient faces pain, suffering, loss, and scarring, both physically and emotionally. An additional area of concern is children in whom the burn is suspected to be caused by child abuse.

The nurse begins the process of patient assessment by determining the severity of the burn. The factors that influence determination of the severity of the burn are the percent of TBSA involved, the depth of the burn, the involvement of specialty areas (e.g., eyes, ears, hands), associated injuries, and poor-risk patients as defined earlier.

SYSTEMIC EFFECTS

Major burns can potentially affect all systems of the body. The direct damage to skin results in fluid and electrolyte loss and initiation of the burn stress response that leads to systemic effects. The following sections present the various body systems and the potential alterations that may result from a major burn.

Cardiovascular Effects

The pathophysiologic mechanisms associated with initial fluid shift, dehydration, and burn shock lead to decreased cardiac output. The decreased cardiac output is further complicated by hemoconcentration as a result of plasma loss. Burn shock follows the same pathway as other forms of hypovolemic shock characterized by decreased venous return, decreased ventricular filling pressures, decreased stroke volume, decreased cardiac output, decreased blood pressure, increased peripheral vascular resistance, and decreased tissue perfusion.[12-15] Compensatory mechanisms that increase the production of catecholamines in an attempt to increase cardiac output and blood pressure are activated. Sympathetic adrenergic stimulation leads to vasoconstriction of the blood vessels of the intestines, kidney, liver, stomach, spleen, lungs, and skin in an effort to maintain arterial pressure and venous return. The decreased blood flow to these vital areas can lead to loss of organ function, cellular hypoxia, and metabolic acidosis, if the patient is without adequate fluid resuscitation.[16-19]

The volume loss seen in major burn patients is multifocal. Fluid and plasma proteins are shifted from the vascular compartment into the interstitial spaces due to increased vascular permeability. Large amounts of sodium are translocated into skeletal muscle and other tissues. The sodium shift pulls water with it, further increasing hypovolemia and leading initially to hyperkalemia. However, due to the release of aldosterone, potassium is lost in the urine, and this leads to hypokalemia. In addition to other fluid volume losses, evaporative water loss through burn tissue can amount to 4 to 15 times normal. The estimated mean loss is 1.5 ml to 3.5 ml/kg per TBSA.[20]

NURSING CONSIDERATIONS

Cardiovascular assessment for the major burn victim includes monitoring those functions that reflect cardiac output, fluid volume status, and tissue perfusion. Routine monitoring includes:

- Monitoring of vital signs
- Monitoring input and output (maintain output at 30 to 70 ml/hour for adults and 1 ml/kg per hour for children)[21]
- Monitoring central venous pressures and/or pulmonary artery pressures
- Monitoring urine specific gravity
- Monitoring cardiac rhythm and rate
- Assessing peripheral pulses and compartment pressures
- Assessing capillary refill, skin warmth and color, note areas and degree of swelling
- Assessing escharotomy site for area, size (circumference), depth, and success of procedure
- Monitoring daily weights

Hematologic Effects

Severe hematologic changes can occur in major burns due to vascular changes and tissue damage. Pathophysiologic mechanisms in the early burn period (first 48 hours) lead to direct cellular damage and initiation of the inflammatory process. The release of vasoactive substances such as histamine causes increased vascular permeability associated with leakage of plasma and proteins into tissue.

Zawacki in 1974[22] identified three zones of tissue damage. These zones are analogous to the zones of tissue damage seen in myocardial infarction. The zone of greatest cellular damage is called the *zone of coagulation*. Cellular necrosis is prominent, and the normal inflammatory process of healing initiated by tissue damage is inhibited or blocked. The second zone or *zone of stasis* affects the vascular dermis and is character-ized by thrombosis. Leukocytes and platelets aggregate in the viable capillaries causing ischemia and thrombosis, which is further complicated by decreased blood flow due to vasoconstriction.[23] With optimum care, this area will usually recover circulation.

The final and least affected zone is the *hyperemic zone* which composes the burn borders. The normal inflammatory process for wound healing has been activated in this area and vascular integrity is maintained.

During the initial 48 hours postburn, fluid shifting leads to hypovolemia and, if not corrected, to hypovolemic shock. As mentioned previously, plasma moves from the vascular space into interstitial spaces due to increased capillary permeability, causing edema and blisters (Fig. 9–4). With fluid movement, sodium is also translocated into tissues, thus causing hyponatremia. Hyperkalemia is also a result of the fluid shift, due to fluid loss from the vascular space. The rapid fluid shift, in addition to evaporative losses, leads to hypovolemia.

Hematocrits in patients with burns greater than 40 percent TBSA may range from 50 to 70 percent during this phase.[24,25] Serial hematocrit studies can be useful in determin-ing adequate fluid volume restoration. The period of high hematocrits is then offset by red blood cell (RBC) destruction during the initial burn period. Progressive anemia due to cell mass loss of 3 to 9 percent occurs for the first 2 weeks postburn. The cell mass loss is due to tissue destruction and hemolysis from intense heat and to an unknown circulat-ing plasma factor that causes a significant reduction of half-life in the normal RBC.[26] Red blood cell loss is further aggravated by early surgical debridement of the wound to promote early wound closure. Frequent blood transfusions may be required to maintain a hematocrit above 30 percent.[27]

Other blood components damaged by the intense heat include platelets and white blood cells (WBCs). Platelet function and half-life are decreased. Platelet and leukocyte aggregation progresses to thrombosis, which is further complicated by increased blood viscosity and hypercoagulability. Early leukocytopenia tends to be a poor prognostic sign, indicating the body's inability to fight off an infection.[28]

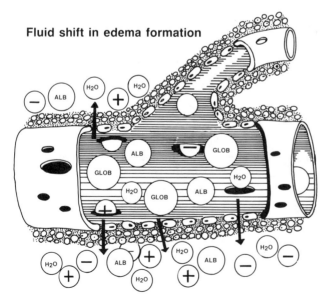

Fluid shift in edema formation

FIGURE 9–4. Fluid shift due to in-creased capillary permeability.

NURSING CONSIDERATIONS

Nursing assessment during the period of hemoconcentration and hemodilution is critical to patient survival and involves the following actions:

- Monitoring vital signs
- Monitoring urinary output, urine specific gravity, urine hemochromogens
- Monitoring laboratory values, especially complete blood count (CBC), electrolytes, wound cultures, ABGs, creatinine, and osmolarity
- Monitoring central venous pressures and/or pulmonary artery pressures

Metabolic Effects

(Refer also to Chapter 6, page 77.)

The metabolic demands seen in burn patients are very high. The body's defense mechanisms have been activated as a result of the injury. The increased secretion of catecholamines, cortisol, the renin-angiotensin system, antidiuretic hormone, and aldosterone to maintain homeostasis places the patient in a state of hypermetabolism.

The metabolic demands of the body are met early in the burn period by the breakdown of glycogen in the liver. The normal liver contains limited supplies of glycogen, which are depleted in 48 hours in the fasting state.[29] As a result of hypermetabolism, glycogen stores are depleted at a much faster rate. In the severe burn patient this high metabolic state may be maintained for months until wound closure is accomplished, thus requiring an aggressive nutritional supplement program. This hypermetabolic state is further accentuated by the presence of associated injuries and surgical intervention for debridement and wound closure. Table 9–1 lists causes for caloric losses in burn patients.

The extent of hypermetabolism is proportional to the severity of the burn.[30,31] Three factors that influence this high metabolic and catabolic rate are increased plasma catecholamine levels, evaporative heat and water loss from the burn, and elevated glucagon levels.[32] In addition to increasing metabolic consumption, heat production and oxygen

TABLE 9–1. Caloric Losses in Burn Patients

Cause	Potential Loss
Hypermetabolism	
Adult (Curreri)	(25 kcal) × (kg body weight) + (40 kcal) × (% burn)/day
Child (Polk)	(60 kcal) × (kg body weight) + (35 kcal) × (% burn)/day
Fluid Evaporation (580 kcal loss with each liter H_2O)	
20–40% burn	1–2 liters H_2O
40–60% burn	3–4 liters H_2O
60–90% burn	5–8 liters H_2O
Protein Loss (burn wound exudate)	Increases with the severity of the burn
Dressing Changes	Fluid and electrolytes
	Increased protein loss
Surgery	Blood, fluid, electrolytes
	Increased caloric loss
Increased Catabolism with Infection and Sepsis	Increased caloric loss
	Increased fluid evaporation
Decreased Effectiveness of Anabolic Process	Decreased protein utilization

consumption are also increased (refer to Chapter 6, page 77). Severe catabolism also begins in the early burn period. Catabolism is associated with a negative nitrogen balance, weight loss, and decreased wound healing.

The nutritional plan for burn patients is multifocal. Besides increasing caloric intake, an effort must be made to decrease energy expenditures, which is best accomplished by decreasing pain, stress, and shivering due to cold. Pain relievers and antianxiety medications can be administered to decrease the stress response. Warmth can be given by regulating room temperature and applying external sources of heat such as heat shields and heat lamps.

Infection is another major source of caloric expenditure. The use of topical antimicrobial agents has successfully decreased the rate of infection in burns less than 60 percent TBSA.[33] Adjunct therapy with systemic antibiotics prescribed on the basis of cultures and sensitivities has further decreased high metabolic rates. Monitoring wound cultures assists the burn team in early determination of wound sepsis and hence early treatment. Early excision and wound closure has been a major contributor in decreasing nutritional expenditure.[34]

In addition to reducing metabolic demands, nutritional supplementation is necessary. After caloric, protein, and nitrogen requirements are determined, a plan for replacement can be made. Nitrogen replacement should be calculated on the basis of caloric needs to provide a ratio of kilocalories-to-nitrogen of about 100:1 to 150:1.[35] Numerous formulas are available for estimating nutritional requirements. Some are based on the percent of burn and others on basal metabolic rate (BMR). Table 9–2 lists various formulas available for determining nutritional requirements of burn patients.[36]

Nutritional support for burn patients is best administered orally or enterally due to the increased susceptibility of the burn patient to infection when the parenteral route is used. This can be accomplished by using high-calorie, high-protein hospital diets, oral supplements, and tube-feeding formulas. If these are not adequate for patient needs or the enteral route is not available, peripheral intravenous supplements and total parenteral nutrition may be used.[37] Due to the poor nutritional intake and dietary habits of many Americans, supplemental enteral feedings have become the mainstay in burn therapy. Important considerations in planning a dietary routine for the patient are age, sex, body build, severity of the burn, medical history, eating habits, and likes and dislikes.

In general the recommended daily diet of a burn patient is seen in Table 9–3.

The use of a small silastic nasogastric feeding tube controlled by a mechanical pump allows for the delivery of continuous supplemental nutrition. This method is usually well tolerated by the patient. Major side effects with hyperosmolar supplements are vomiting and diarrhea. These can be controlled to some extent by using products with a lower osmolality. A wide variety of commercial products are available to meet individual patient needs.

Three main types of enteral products are available: (1) elemental, (2) polymeric, and (3) modular. The elemental products contain little or no fat, furnish needed amino acids and monosaccharides, and have a higher osmolality. Because of their high osmolality, diarrhea may be a problem. Polymeric products contain high molecular weight proteins, fats, and carbohydrates. Their lower osmolality decreases the problem of diarrhea. Modular formulas provide specific elements designed to meet the needs of patients with specific disease processes.

Tolerance to tube feedings should be assessed by starting the formula at half-strength at 50 ml/hour until there are no gastric residuals. Progression is then made to three-forths strength and then to full-strength at 50 ml/hour. Each step in the protocol is monitored by checking for gastric residuals. Normally a patient will remain at each step

**TABLE 9-2. Formulas for Estimating Nutritional Requirements
of Burned Patients***

	Date	Age Range	(% TBSA) Burned	NUTRITIONAL REQUIREMENT Calories	NUTRITIONAL REQUIREMENT Protein
1. Wilmore	1974	Adult	>40	2000-2200/m²/day	94 g/m²/day
2. Curreri	1974	Adult	Any	25 × (body weight in kg) 40 × (% TBSA burned)	
3. Muir & Barclay	1974	Adult	<20	35 kcal/kg/day	1.5 g/kg/day
			20-30	40 kcal/kg/day	2 g/kg/day
			30-40	50 kcal/kg/day	3 g/kg/day
			40-50	60 kcal/kg/day	5 g/kg/day
4. Davies & Liljedahl	1971	Child	Any	60 kcal/kg/day + 35 kcal/%BSA/day	3 g/kg/day + 1 g/%BSA/day
		Adult	Any	20 kcal/kg/day + 70 kcal/%BSA/day	1g/kg/day + 3 g/%BSA/day
5. Wilmore	1972	Child	<49	1350-1450/m²/day	
			>40	1950-2050/m²/day	
		Adolescent	<40	1200-1300/m²/day	
			>40	1675-1850/m²/day	
		Adult	<40	1100-1150/m²/day	
			>40	1550-1625/m²/day	
6. University of California, San Diego	1980	Any age	Any	1.4 (BMR × m² × 24 hour) + wt(growth + 0.6 BSAB)	Wt (RDA + 0.05BSAB)
7. Boston	1982	Child	<20 kg	BEE × 1.75	3 g/kg/day
		Adult	>20 kg	BEE × 2	1.5-2.5 g/kg/day

*Key: BSAB = body surface area burns; BEE = basal energy expenditure.
Adapted from Watchel, TL, et al: Nutritional support for burned patients. In Wachtel, TL, Kahn, K, and Frank, HA (eds): Current Topics in Burn Care. Aspen Publications, Rockville, MD, 1983, p. 109, with permission.

for about 24 hours before advancing the formula. Once the full-strength formula stage has successfully been attained, the amount of formula given per hour can be increased.[38]

NURSING CONSIDERATIONS

Frequent re-evaluation and revision of the patient's nutritional needs and nutritional program are made. Nutritional needs may be increased or decreased dependent on the patient's condition.

Metabolic-nutritional assessments made by the burn team are critical to meeting individual patient needs. They include the following actions:

- Assessing the patient's eating habits
- Monitoring calorie needs
- Monitoring bowel sounds at least every 4 hours
- Monitoring intake and output (I & O)
- Monitoring serum albumin levels and serum transferrin or iron binding capacity
- Monitoring calorie and protein intake
- Monitoring vitamin replacement
- Monitoring weight
- Assessing patient for diarrhea, constipation, abdominal cramping, or bloating

TABLE 9-3. Recommended Daily Diet for Burn Patients

Calories: Sufficient to meet metabolic needs
    Fat: 40% of calories
    Carbohydrates: 40% of calories
    Protein: 20% of calories
Protein: 2-4 g/kg body weight
Vitamins
    Vitamin C: 1.0-1.5 g/day
    Thiamine: 10-50 mg/day
    Multivitamin with folic acid: requirement depends on deficiencies
Minerals
    Iron: 600-1200 mg/day
    Zinc: 220 mg/day

Gastrointestinal Effects

Acute gastrointestinal (GI) problems that can develop after burn trauma include gastric dilatation, Curling's ulcer, paralytic ileus, and superior mesenteric artery syndrome.

Gastric dilatation is a fairly common problem due to fluid shifting, dehydration, immobility, and narcotic analgesia. It usually occurs in the first week postburn and should be suspected when the patient repeatedly vomits small quantities of food after each meal. Vomiting may also occur later in the burn period but is usually related to superior mesenteric artery syndrome. Gastric dilatation may lead to fecal impaction.[39] It may or may not be associated with paralytic ileus (nonmechanical obstruction of the bowel).[40] During the first few days postburn, when gastric motility is depressed and gastric dilatation is common in burns of greater than 20 percent TBSA, it is highly recommended that the patient be placed on nasogastric (NG) suction and remain NPO, or be fed through a feeding tube into the duodenum (Refer to Chapter 6, page 83, for further discussion).

Curling's ulcer (acute gastroduodenal ulcer) presents a major problem in burn patients because it causes bleeding (sometimes massive) in a patient who already has hematologic problems due to the burn. The major clinical presentation of the ulcer is bleeding observed either rectally (tarry stools) or in the patient's vomitus (bright red or "coffee ground" hematemesis). Curling's ulcer has been shown to occur in 75 percent of burn patients who are routinely checked via endoscopy,[41] yet not all of the patients present with positive symptomatology. The routine use of histamine blockers and antacids given prophylactically has done much to decrease the incidence of gastrointestinal ulceration.

The etiology of Curling's ulcer is not known, but it is thought to be associated with the stress response and gastric ischemia. The stress response encompasses factors such as sepsis, elevated cortisol levels, decreased GI blood flow due to shunting, elevated catecholamine levels, increased gastric mucosal permeability, and changes in the GI tract due to hypersecretion of acid.[42-44] (See Color Plate 20 for an example of a gastric ulcer in an electrical burn patient.)

Paralytic ileus is a form of intestinal obstruction associated with major burns. The patient presents with severe abdominal distention, gastric distress, absence of bowel tones, and vomiting. Incidence of paralytic ileus has decreased over the last 10 years due to the use of NG suction during the initial burn period and until bowel tones return. Sepsis may also be a cause of paralytic ileus. The burn team needs to consider the use of hyperalimentation during this period in order to provide adequate nutrition.

Superior mesenteric artery syndrome is a fairly rare gastric problem that occurs due to inadequate caloric support[45] and/or compression of the superior mesenteric artery.[46] Clinical presentation includes rapid weight loss, nausea, and vomiting after eating. Pathophysiologically, the third portion of the duodenum becomes dysfunctional due to decreased blood supply, which leads to partial or complete intestinal obstruction. Treatment encompasses the use of hyperalimentation and positioning the patient in the prone or right posterolateral position to relieve pressure on the superior mesenteric artery. The patient should be fed in the prone position.

NURSING CONSIDERATIONS

Frequent evaluation and assessments of the gastrointestinal system during the initial burn period are important for assessing bowel function and potential bleeding problems. These include the following actions:

- Assessing for mouth and abdominal injuries on admission
- Assessing proper placement of the NG or feeding tube, at least every 8 hours
- Monitoring bowel tones every 4 hours
- Guaiac stools and NG aspirate
- Monitoring for constipation or diarrhea or both
- Monitoring pH of gastric contents every 2 to 4 hours.

Renal Effects

Oliguric renal failure or acute renal insufficiency can occur in burn patients as a result of hypovolemia and accompanies reduced cardiac output. Up to 10 percent of fatally burned patients develop renal insufficiency.[47] Acute tubular necrosis in burn patients can be caused by tissue necrosis from cell destruction due to crushing injury, burn injury, incompatible blood transfusion, or x-ray contrast media. Other causes of renal damage include occlusion of the nephron and tubules due to build up of hemoglobin released from destroyed RBCs in the early stages of the burn and/or the accumulation of myoglobin from the destruction of muscle mass in electrical burns. The pathophysiologic mechanism of renal tubular necrosis due to hemolysis is the presence of hemochromogens in the urine that directly damage tubular cells.

> Grossly visible hemochromogens are present in up to 25 percent of patients with electrical injury, because plasma haptoglobin and other binding proteins are unable to handle the sudden load of hemoglobin, myoglobin, and protein degradation products released from large volumes of injured muscle.[48]

Other causes of renal damage are the potent antibiotics and/or pressor agents given to burn patients.

Adequate fluid resuscitation greatly decreases the incidence of renal dysfunction even in the most severely burned patients. Inadequate resuscitation leads to decreased renal plasma flow. In addition, glomerular filtration rate may be decreased in severe burns. Evaporative losses further compound the problem, because significant amounts of fluid can be lost. Hourly monitoring of urine output in the critical period is the best method of prevention of renal insufficiency. Ideally urine output in an adult should be maintained in the range of 0.5 to 1 ml/kg of body weight per hour, averaged over a 2-hour period. In addition to measuring output, the nurse also monitors the urine for the following values:

- Specific gravity, which is a reflection of the hydration state
- Glucose, which is a reflection of the stress response

- Protein, which is a reflection of renal tubular damage
- Ketones, which are a reflection of metabolism of fats and proteins, usually seen in the starvation state or when a patient is taking in insufficient calories
- pH, which is a reflection of acid-base balance
- The presence of hemochromogens, hemoglobin, and myoglobin in the urine

Elevated serum and urine glucose occur secondary to the stress-trauma response. Severe injury, surgical intervention, and critical illness cause an increase in glucose production in the liver (gluconeogenesis).[49,50] Insulin production remains normal or increased, but insulin utilization is decreased. The stress response also leads to an increase in other stress hormones such as glucagon, growth hormone, glucocorticoids, and catecholamines, which in turn elevates glucose levels even higher.[51] When the tubular maximum for glucose (TM_c) in the kidneys is exceeded, glucose spills over into the urine and is excreted. The normal serum renal threshold for glucose is considered to about 180 mg/dl. The high serum glucose seen in burn patients also leads to osmotic diuresis with the potential for losing large volumes of fluid.[52]

ELECTRICAL BURNS AND RENAL RESPONSES

Electrical burns present a special problem in the management of the renal system. Extensive internal tissue destruction caused by the passage of electrical current occurs without obvious external damage. It is therefore important to alter the burn resuscitation formula to calculate fluid volume replacement and monitor urinary output closely to titrate as indicated. Intravenous fluids are maintained at a rate sufficient to provide a urinary output of 70 to 100 ml/hr.[53] Renal damage may occur from damage due to severe shock, direct electrical current, and/or abnormal protein and muscle breakdown. Mannitol is administered to prevent acute tubular necrosis and the development of myoglobin casts.[54] Loop diuretics are *not* administered because they decrease the patient's total fluid volume.

Occasionally oliguric renal failure may be severe enough to require hemodialysis. Serum and urine creatinine and blood urea nitrogen (BUN) are reliable diagnostic measures of renal function. Although rarely done, hemodialysis may be necessary to remove excess body fluids, maintain acid-base and electrolyte balance, and remove waste products and toxins. In addition, plasmapheresis may be used in some cases for patients not responding to fluid therapy or for septic patients to decrease circulating cell antibodies.. Plasmapheresis can be used to draw off excess plasma with the replacement of packed red cells to combat anemia. Peritoneal dialysis is not recommended for burn patients due to the high incidence of infection.

NURSING CONSIDERATIONS

Other important nursing assessments are necessary to complete the evaluation for the renal system:

- Monitoring I & O
- Monitoring serum and urine electrolytes and osmolarity
- Monitoring specific gravity
- Monitoring the urine for spilling of protein, glucose, ketones, bilirubin, blood, and pH
- Monitoring serum creatinine and BUN.

Pulmonary Effects

(Refer also to Chapter 18.)

Pulmonary dysfunction can be a complication of burn injury (pneumonia or circumferential chest burns) or directly related to smoke inhalation (inhalation of carbon monoxide, toxic chemicals or both), and thermal injury (rare). They can be further grouped into two categories: those that occur in the first 48 hours postburn and those that occur later in the course of treatment. Pulmonary complications can be life-threatening and are one of the major causes of death in burn patients.[55,56]

PULMONARY DYSFUNCTION: FIRST 48 HOURS

Hyperventilation is a common element of major burns and is generally proportional to the severity of the injury. Oxygen consumption increases due to the hypermetabolic state and fear. Airway resistance increases in patients who suffer smoke inhalation injury. Lung sounds can be normal or abnormal with rales, rhonchi, and wheezes. In addition, it is not uncommon to see the PaO_2 drop below 80 mmHg in these patients.

Immediate complications include those that accompany inhalation of carbon monoxide, chemical toxins, and heat (rare).[57] A clinical presentation is described in Table 9–4.

Early diagnosis and treatment is crucial for survival. Ninety percent of the severely burned patients require ventilatory support of some kind (mask, cannula, or mechanical ventilation) during the course of treatment.[58] The nurse and respiratory therapist are responsible for providing oxygen support and monitoring respiratory function. Adjunct therapy includes the use of antibiotics, steroids (controversial), bronchodilators, intermittent positive pressure breathing (IPPB) treatments, hyperbaric oxygenation, and mechanical ventilation support. Endotracheal suctioning and tracheal lavage may be necessary for clearing the airway of mucus and carbonaceous materials. An escharotomy may be necessary to relieve tightness caused by circumferential burns of the chest and neck. Maintenance of pulmonary toilet (turn, cough, and deep breathe; postural drainage) will assist the patient to mobilize and expel pulmonary secretions.

LATER PULMONARY DYSFUNCTION

Those complications that occur in the second group (more than 48 hour postburn) include pneumonia, pulmonary embolism, atelectasis, pneumothorax, pulmonary

---

TABLE 9–4. Signs and Symptoms of Pulmonary Complications

History
    Burn occurred in a confined area
Burns of specific body areas
    Face
    Neck
    Nose
    Mouth
    Ears
    Hands (in children)
Singed nasal hair
Carbonaceous material in the nose and mouth
Hoarseness
Productive cough with carbonaceous material
Blistering on lips, mouth, or oral mucosa

Data from Gaston, SF and Schumann, LL: Inhalation injury: Smoke inhalation. AJN 80:94, 1980.

edema, and adult respiratory distress syndrome (ARDS).[59] They occur secondary to infection, hypovolemic shock, immobility, and/or overhydration. They are not as easily treated as smoke inhalation.

Mechanical ventilation may be required to provide adequate oxygenation and acid-base balance. Careful monitoring of arterial blood gases (ABGs) is essential to pulmonary assessment because warning signs like cyanosis and stridor are late signs. Subtle changes in clinical signs and symptoms may be overlooked due to the fact that hyperventilation, tachycardia, pain, anxiety, and restlessness are common to all burn patients. In severe burns arterial blood gas monitoring and continuous blood pressure monitoring are facilitated by the use of an arterial line. In addition, the nurse also needs to monitor the patient's fluid balance and nutritional balance to prevent overhydration and to maintain adequate proteins and calories. Colloids may be administered to maintain adequate albumin levels for prevention of edema. Treatment regimens with IPPB and bronchodilators are essential adjuncts to oxygen therapy. The use of antibiotics is indicated after culture and sensitivity are determined. (Refer to Chapter 18, page 333, for a more detailed explanation.)

NURSING CONSIDERATIONS

Nursing assessments related to the respiratory system monitor the patient's need for and response to therapy that promotes effective gas exchange. These assessments include the following:

- Assessing for signs and symptoms of inhalation injury on admission
- Assessing carboxyhemoglobin level on admission and until the level returns to normal
- Monitoring breath sounds at least every 4 hours
- Monitoring breathing pattern (labored, tachypnea, and so on)
- Monitoring ABGs, CBC, and electrolytes
- Monitoring sputum: color, amount, odor, consistency
- Assessing the patient for signs and symptoms of respiratory distress
- Monitoring serial chest x-rays
- Monitoring I & O
- Assessing the patient for fatigue related to the effort to breathe
- Monitoring pulmonary function tests, when appropriate
- Monitoring effect of rigorous pulmonary toilet
- Monitoring pulmonary artery pressures and cardiac output when appropriate
- Monitoring the effect of suctioning and endotracheal lavage

Immunologic Effects

(Refer also to Chapter 2, page 20.)

The skin is a person's first line of defense. Loss of skin integrity due to a burn creates a loss of this defense mechanism. Approximately 75 percent of the deaths related to major thermal burns are directly related to infection.[60] The burn wound offers a large area for entry of bacteria and an ideal media for bacterial growth. Severe infection can easily develop, despite intensive local and systemic intravenous treatment with high-potency broad-spectrum antibiotics. Sensitivity to infection is also increased by obstruction of blood flow and defects in the immune response following a full-thickness burn.

Common microorganisms seen in burn patients include *Pseudomonas aeruginosa*, *Staphylococcus aureus*, and *Streptococcus* species. Other microorganisms common to wounds and to septic shock are *Escherichia coli*, *Klebsiella*, *Enterobacter*, and *Serratia*.

Viral and fungal infections may also occur in burn patients as their resistance to infection decreases. Colonization of the burn wound may begin as early as 24 hours postburn, but most often begins after the fifth day postburn.[61]

Burn trauma leads to cellular release of vasoactive substances such as histamine which further leads to transient vasoconstriction (5 to 10 minutes) followed by vasodilation. With the loss of vascular integrity comes the accumulation of plasma proteins and fluid in the extravascular space. In addition to the trapping of neutrophils in capillary beds, this prevents adequate mobilization of host defense mechanisms. The function of neutrophils is also depressed, leading to the inability to phagocytize bacteria and enzymatically dissolve bacteria.

The host defense mechanism can be divided into three classifications: (1) the external defense mechanism of an intact integument and mucosal barrier, which is lost in the injury; (2) the internal defense mechanisms of the nonspecific inflammatory system; and (3) the specific immune system.[62,63]

NONSPECIFIC IMMUNE RESPONSES

The *nonspecific inflammatory system* is also composed of the skin and mucosal barrier. Within a few hours postburn, the wound fills with exudate composed of plasma proteins, blood cells, and fibrin strands. Polymorphonuclear leukocytes (PMNs) and macrophages move into the area and begin the process of removing cellular debris and injured tissue fragments. They also act by engulfing and destroying invading microorganisms. The initial chemotaxic response decreases during the second week postburn, thus allowing for increased bacterial growth. In addition to depressed phagocytic activity, the ability to kill bacteria is also depressed. Depression of the reticuloendothelial system has also been noted following burn injury.[64]

SPECIFIC IMMUNE RESPONSES

The *specific immune system* responses involve the thymus-derived lymphocytes (T cells) and the bursa-equivalent lymphocytes (B cells) and their products. The immune system recognizes and destroys specific antigens. T lymphocytes, B lymphocytes, and macrophages work together to control the immune response and destroy antigens. Burn injury depresses the specific immune system and increases the patient's susceptibility to infection.

NURSING CONSIDERATIONS

Monitoring of bacterial counts is essential to the management of the burn wound and the prevention of sepsis. Quantitative bacterial colonization can be determined by wound biopsy. A punch biopsy of the full-thickness eschar is excised and sent for determination of number and types of organisms. This method is more satisfactory than monitoring of surface cultures because of the poor correlation between surface cultures and deep wound cultures.[65] Bacterial counts of 10^4 per gram of tissue are treated for sepsis.

Nursing assessment related to the immune system includes:

- Monitoring for signs and symptoms of infection or sepsis
- Monitoring wound cultures
- Monitoring the metabolic response to burn injury
- Monitoring the CBC and differential
- Monitoring patient's response to intravenous antibiotics and subeschar clysis
- Monitoring the response to topical antibiotics

- Monitoring wound healing
- Monitoring nutritional intake
- Monitoring of serial photographs of the wound surface

Neurologic Effects

Upon admission, most burn victims are awake, alert, and oriented. If this is not the case, then one or more of the following may be suspected: head injury, drug or alcohol abuse, or carbon monoxide poisoning. Also, fluid and electrolyte imbalances are precursors to neurologic complications. Changes in levels of consciousness, such as increasing restlessness may be an early sign of fluid volume deficit and hypovolemia. Seizures may occur in hypervolemia (water intoxication), in hyponatremia, or as a result of associated injuries. Treatment of the underlying cause and administration of anticonvulsant medication(s) are appropriate therapy to resolve the problem.

Electrical injuries also cause direct nerve damage because electrical current travels down the neuromuscular bundles and blood vessels. If the point of electrical contact is the skull, then direct cerebral damage may occur. Spinal cord injury (SCI) may occur secondary to electrical injury and myotonic contraction of the spinal cord. SCI is the most common permanent sequela seen as a result of electrical injuries. It occurs when the electrical current moves from arm to arm or from arm to leg.[66] Even if no visible burn is sustained, the patient with an electrical injury should be treated as if he or she has a SCI (log roll, bed flat, correct body alignment) until the injury has been ruled out by radiologic examination of the spine.

Neurologic damage can be classified into two groups: those of early onset that appear shortly after the injury and those of late onset that may be caused by thrombosis of the associated nutrient vessels or spinal cord vessels.[67] The early-onset group shows neurologic deficits, shortly after the injury, which commonly affect the motor neurons. The deficits appear to resolve over time, but complete resolution is uncommon. Patients who develop deficits late frequently have more severe deficits such as quadriplegia, hemiplegia, or localized nerve deficits. Recovery is variable, but resolution of the deficits is rarely as good as with those patients who have early onset of neurologic deficits.

NURSING CONSIDERATIONS

Nursing assessment of the neurologic system is important to monitor response to therapy or changes in condition. Such assessment includes the following actions:

- Monitoring the level of consciousness (Glascow Coma Scale)
- Monitoring mental status
- Monitoring motor strength and reflexes
- Monitoring pupillary response
- Monitoring the effects of physical and occupational therapy
- Monitoring muscle functioning
- Monitoring effects of anticonvulsants
- Monitoring for signs and symptoms of sepsis
- Implementing SCI precautions (i.e., Philadelphia collar, flat in bed, log roll) until negative spinal series confirmed

Musculoskeletal Effects

Musculoskeletal complications can be multifocal, stemming from associated injuries or as a result of the burn wound healing process. Patients may present with fractures associated with burn injuries. Fractures of long bones from falls or auto accidents are not uncommon (see Color Plates 21 and 22). Cast application over the burn area is contraindicated because of the increased medium for bacterial growth provided by the warm, moist environment under the cast. Open reduction of fractures may sometimes be attempted but carries with it the high incidence of infection due to burn wound contamination and potential for septicemia.

TRACTION

Skeletal traction is the preferred method of treatment for long-bone fractures. Traction holds the reduced bones in proper alignment for healing and relief of pain and pressure on peripheral nerves. It allows for the application of topical antimicrobials and the visualization of the wound. In 1979 Pruitt[68] described the use of skeletal traction in 17 burn patients. One of these patients developed a bone infection.

Proper care of pin sites with the application of gauze-soaked antimicrobial agents (betadine is commonly used) decreases the incidence of bone infection. Pin care is performed every 8 hours and after tubbings.

EXPOSED MUSCLE OR BONE

Exposed bone or muscle due to electrical injury or deep burn injury may lead to complications of osteomyelitis and infection and/or necrosis of muscle. Some burn centers advocate the application of topical antimicrobials as essential to prevention of infection. Sulfamylon is recommended for deep burn wounds. Other burn centers cover the exposed nerve and tendon with sterile normal saline gauze, taking great caution not to allow drying, while treating the surrounding burn areas with topical antimicrobials.

HYPERTROPHIC SCARRING AND CONTRACTURES

Another area of concern related to musculoskeletal complications is the development of hypertrophic tissue and contractions. Contractures result from the proliferation of scar tissue in deep burns. Normal tissue is pulled into the scar area. Scar tissue is easily injured due to the lack of adequate blood flow. Willis, Larson, and Abston in 1973,[69] determined that collagen forms in two distinct ways:

1. Whirlpools of collagen evolve into nodular swirls
2. Fibers evolve in parallel form in the direction of stress. Parallel fibers are much less likely to develop contractures. Thus therapy aims at the development of parallel fibers by maintaining exercise, splinting, therapeutic positioning, early mobilization, traction, and the use of pressure garments and Ace wraps.

Because the normal position of comfort is the flexed state, flexion contractures are the most common. This makes proper positioning essential to the prevention of contractures. Another factor that promotes contracture formation is delayed healing, especially in areas of joint movement. This leads to the proliferation of red vascular granulation tissue, which increases contracture formation. Dependent edema in burned extremities further adds to contracture formation.

Therapeutic positioning involves avoidance of positions of comfort (flexion), frequent repositioning to avoid pressure areas, and use of therapeutic adjuncts to maintain proper alignment. Splints are used to prevent or correct contractures. They are custommade from thermoplastic materials to provide optimum therapy and comfort.

NURSING CONSIDERATIONS

Nursing assessment of the musculoskeletal system is critical to detect complications early and promote maximum rehabilitation. It involves:

- Monitoring neurovascular assessment: pulses, reflexes, paresthesia, color, warmth
- Monitoring the circumference of extremities
- Monitoring patient positioning to maintain elevation of burned extremities and prevent contractures
- Monitoring pain response in relation to the exercise program
- Monitoring the effects of the exercise program
- Assessing the patient's ability to perform range of motion and activities of daily living
- Assessing daily the effectiveness of the splint program and monitoring for evidence of pressure areas secondary to poor fit.

Psychologic Effects

(Refer also to Chapter 7.)

To accomplish psychologic adjustment of patients suffering from major burns requires a multidisciplinary approach. An individualized program is developed to meet each person's problems. Many factors enter into the existing state of events. These include personal characteristics; beliefs; feelings of fear, anxiety, and pain; psychologic trauma associated with the accident (e.g., loss of loved ones in the fire); severity of the burn; disfigurement; loss of independence and function; separation from family and friends; feelings of powerlessness; and loss of normal coping mechanisms. Individuals respond differently to burn injuries. Their preburn psychologic adaptation mechanisms in response to stress are often a clue to the response they will exhibit in the burn unit. Those who were well adjusted prior to the burn tend to continue to be well adjusted afterward.

The psychologic problems can be divided into three periods—acute, intermediate, and rehabilitation. The acute period is characterized by the waxing and waning of confusion, memory loss, insomnia, lethargy, combativeness, and fear of death. Common causes of psychologic dysfunction during this period include electrolyte imbalance, hypoxia, cerebral edema, medications, and infectious processes. The intermediate period is characterized by pain, depression, regression, nightmares, and behavior problems. The patient may also exhibit loss of bowel and bladder function. The final period is the rehabilitation period, which is characterized by readjustment, depression, regression, fears of deformity and mutilation, and (in men) concerns about impotence.

The burn team needs to develop a good rapport and a trusting relationship with the patient and his or her family. Providing flexible visiting hours and taking time to listen to patient and family concerns go a long way toward this end.

Many patients develop defense mechanisms of repression, denial, and suppression to deal with the pain and grief they are suffering. One of the goals of the burn team is to help patients deal with their feelings without removing their protective defense mechanisms.

As the patient improves, maladaptive defense mechanisms and behaviors can be modified with the use of behavior modification techniques. An individual plan is developed for each patient. Often psychologic wounds do not heal as fast as physical wounds, and therefore may require long-term therapy.

Nursing assessment of psychologic adaptation and adjustment allows early identification of problems and interventions to assist the patient when needed. It includes:

- Monitoring the patient's and families progression through the grieving process
- Assessing the patient's response to pain and treating appropriately
- Monitoring the patient's response to relaxation therapy and biofeedback training
- Assessing the patient's willingness to talk about feelings and concerns.
- Assessing the patient's readiness to discuss sexual concerns.

Septic Shock

The pathophysiologic mechanisms of septic shock are complex. It develops rapidly and progresses to death in a matter of hours, unless vigorous treatment is initiated.

Burn victims are exposed to a variety of sites of bacterial invasion. Besides the burn wound itself, other sites include those of indwelling urinary catheters, IV catheters, and surgical wounds from associated injuries.

The symptoms of septic shock can be classified into those related to warm shock (early stage) and cold shock (late stage). The early clinical characteristics of septic shock include chills, fever, nausea, vomiting, oliguria, diarrhea, and change in mental status.

WARM SHOCK

Warm shock reflects a hyperdynamic state characterized by tachycardia due to beta-adrenergic stimulation. Alpha-adrenergic stimulation leads to vasoconstriction of certain blood vessels of the lungs, splanchnic bed, skin, and kidneys. In the presence of adequate fluid volume, cardiac output and cardiac index are increased. The skin remains warm and dry. Tachypnea and respiratory alkalosis are present. While marked hypotension may be present, prognosis is generally good. Failure to respond to therapy leads to cold shock.

COLD SHOCK

Cold shock reflects a hypodynamic state due to increased capillary permeability or loss of extracellular fluid volume. Tachycardia persists and is accompanied by decreased cardiac output, cardiac index, and systemic vascular resistance. Hypotension, altered level of consciousness, metabolic acidosis, and lactic acidemia are present. The increased capillary permeability leads to pulmonary interstitial edema. The decreased cardiac output leads to ischemia of the gastrointestinal tract and decreased renal blood flow.

As with other forms of shock, septic shock is characterized by hypotension and inadequate tissue perfusion. The inadequate tissue perfusion in this case is associated with massive vasodilation related to gram-negative (*Pseudomonas, Klebsiella, Enterobacter, E. coli*, and *Serratia*) or gram-positive bacteremia (*Pneumococcus, Streptococcus, Staphylococcus*, and *Actinomyces*). Other sources of septic shock include viruses, fungi (common in long-term major burns), *Chlamydia*, and *Protozoa*. Invasion by bacteria leads to a threefold reaction: release of chemical substances from damaged tissues, release of exotoxins from live bacteria, and release of endotoxins from dead bacteria. The massive vasodilation seen in septic shock patients is due in part to the release of endotoxins into the circulation. It appears likely that endotoxins also influence the endogenous opiate system, enhancing vasodilation and decreasing cardiac contractility. In addition to endotoxin release, other substances such as bradykinin and myocardial depressant factor (MDF) exert further forces that lead to decompensation of the cardio-vascular system and ischemia to major organ systems.

Chemical substances released from damaged tissues include histamine and packets of chemicals contained in lysosomes. Histamine release leads to increased capillary permeability. Lysosomal enzymes release powerful substances such as acid phosphatase, ribonuclease, beta-glucuronidase, cathepsin D, and arylsulfatase which, in addition to causing local damage, also release or activate vasoactive polypeptides.[70] Bradykinin and MDF are two such vasoactive substances that play a prominent role in septic shock. Bradykinin is a potent vasodilator that also acts to increase capillary permeability. MDF is liberated from the ischemic pancreas, depresses myocardial contractility (up to 50 percent), and causes splanchnic vasoconstriction. The combination effect of these chemi-cal substances is increased capillary permeability, depressed myocardial contractility, vasodilation, decreased perfusion, and multisystem failure.

The standard treatment plan for the patient in septic shock requires the nurse to pay particular attention to adequate oxygenation, careful monitoring of the vital signs, careful monitoring of fluid and electrolyte and acid-base balance, assisting with obtain-ing blood and wound cultures, monitoring laboratory values, administering antibiotics, assessing mental status, and frequent monitoring of hemodynamic values and arrhythmia status. Vasopressive agents will also be administered to provide cardiovascular support. The use of naloxone to control the hypotension caused by endotoxins is currently under investigation.

NURSING CONSIDERATIONS

Nursing assessment for the septic shock patient is critical to patient survival. It includes:

- Monitoring wound status
- Monitoring fluid and electrolytes
- Monitoring blood, wound, and urine cultures
- Monitoring vital signs
- Monitoring hemodynamic status: pulmonary artery pressures and cardiac output
- Monitoring the effects of vasopressive agents and naloxone
- Monitoring the effects of antibiotics
- Monitoring the level of consciousness
- Monitoring ABGs, WBC, differential, and glucose.

Fluid Resuscitation

Burn injury leads to capillary damage, which promotes the development of abnormal capillary permeability. Generalized increased capillary permeability occurs in burns greater than 25 percent TBSA.[71] The greatest loss of plasma occurs during the first 12 hours and then tapers down during the second 12 hours postburn with continuing extensive leak for the first one to three days.[72,73] Optimal fluid volume replacement during this period is essential to cardiac output, renal perfusion, and tissue perfusion. During the initial resuscitation period, an escharotomy may be necessary as fluid accu-mulates under the eschar and inhibits vascular perfusion, respiratory movement or both.

Children, patients with electrical burns, smoke inhalation patients, and burn patients who are alcoholics require more fluids than the standard formulas provide. Elderly patients require smaller fluid volumes than do other adults, thus the lower end of the fluid range would be the more accurate estimate of fluid needs for this age group. The nurse monitors the effectiveness of fluid resuscitation by the following criteria:

1. Urine output of 20 to 50 ml/hour or 1 ml/kg body weight per hour in children and 30 to 70 ml/hour in adults[74]
2. Central venous pressure (CVP) less than 12 mmHg
3. Clear sensorium
4. Absence of ileus or nausea
5. High-normal pulse rate 100 to 120 in children and 80 to 100 in adults

Numerous fluid resuscitation formulas are in use in various burn units. Currently, the Parkland formula developed by Baxter is the most widely used in the United States.[75] Table 9–5 lists some of the major formulas used in burn resuscitation. Each of the formulas provides adequate sodium replacement. In general, fluid replacement is based on the patient's kilograms of body weight and the percent of TBSA burn. Because the greatest plasma loss occurs in the first 24 hours postburn, the greatest replacement also needs to occur during that period. It is important to remember that any formula is only a guideline for fluid replacement and requires continuous monitoring of the patient's status (vital signs, urine output, electrolyte balance, and hemodynamic pressures) for optimum resuscitation.

After calculating the fluid volume necessary for the first 24 hours, half of that volume is given during the first 8 hours and the remainder over the next 16 hours. For example, a 70-kg patient with a 60 percent burn would require 4 ml × 70 kg × 60 percent burn = 17 liters for the first 24 hours with half of that volume delivered in the first 8 hours.[76,77] To deliver the first 8-hour volume, it may be necessary to make up the time lost before the infusion was started; therefore, the burn team calculates from the time of injury and replaces accordingly.[78]

Replacement of colloidal fluids appears not to be beneficial in the initial postburn period.[79,80] When capillary permeability has returned to normal, usually after the first 24 hours, administration of colloids (albumin or plasma) is recommended.[81] The Parkland formula recommends administering 0.3 to 0.5 ml/kg per percent burn over the first 8 hours of the second 24 hours. In addition, D_5W replaces Ringer's lactate solution during the second 24 hours to maintain an adequate urine output.[82]

TABLE 9–5. Burn Resuscitation Formulas*

Name	Baxter's Parkland Formula	Evans Formula	Brooke Formula	Monafo's Hypertonic Formula
First 24 Hours				
Crystalloid	Ringer's lactate	Normal saline	Ringer's lactate	Hypertonic lactated saline
Amount of Fluid (ml/kg/% burn)	3–5 ml	1.0 ml	1.5 ml	Variable, to maintain urinary output 70 ml/hr
Colloid	0	+	+	0
Glucose in Water	0	2 liters	2 liters	0
Second 24 Hours				
Crystalloid	0	Normal saline	Ringer's lactate	Hypertonic saline
Glucose in Water for Adequate Urine Output	2 liters	2 liters	Variable	0
Colloid	+	+	+	0

*Key: + = contained in formula; 0 = not contained in formula.

NURSING CONSIDERATIONS

Nursing assessment during the fluid resuscitation period helps minimize organ system complications by identifying complications early. Such assessment includes:

- Monitoring vital signs and hemodynamic parameters, pulmonary artery pressures, and cardiac output at least hourly
- Monitoring electrolytes and CBC, reporting abnormalities
- Monitoring urine output reporting levels less than 20 ml/hour in children and 30 ml/hour in adults
- Monitoring the patency of the urinary catheter
- Monitoring I & O hourly and reporting abnormalities
- Obtaining admission weight and monitoring the patient's weight daily at approximately the same time of day with the same amount of clothing
- Monitoring dressings and burn sites to assess for bleeding

Pain Control

PHARMACOLOGIC THERAPY

Pain control presents a major problem in the care of a burn patient. The amount of pain suffered by a burn patient is inversely proportional to the amount of third- and fourth-degree burns the patient has.[83] Partial-thickness burns, donor sites, and the edges of third-degree burns are associated with a large amount of pain because of exposed nerve endings. The burn patient has both chronic pain and periods of intense pain associated with wound care therapy and surgical procedures. Intravenous analgesia with morphine sulfate during the critical period is essential. Some units use other analgesics such as methadone or fentanyl on a regular basis, rather than morphine. Patient-controlled analgesia (PCA) has been beneficial in reducing the intensity of pain and decreasing the amount of medication necessary for pain relief. It also provides the patient with some means of control over his or her environment. Intravenous administration of analgesics in the initial period is important due to the unreliable absorption rate from intramuscular sites in burn patients.

Sedatives and tranquilizers may help allay the anxiety associated with a severe burn. Anxiety may exaggerate the pain experiences. In 1961 Lynn and Eysenck[84] found that the higher the anxiety level, the greater the pain response. Other factors such as fatigue, stress, cultural factors, learned behavior, and depression also affect the patient's perception of pain. A well-rounded pain program that uses both pharmacologic and nonpharmacologic measures and gives the patient more control of the environment is the optimum plan.

A common method used to evaluate a patient's pain level is called the visual analogue scale.[85] Patients are asked to identify their pain level along a continuous unnumbered 10 cm line. Figure 9–5 shows a typical visual analogue scale. At one end of the scale is "no pain" and at the other extreme is "pain as bad as it could possibly be." A few patients have difficulty visualizing pain on a continuous line, but the majority have no difficulty. This method has the advantages of being sensitive and reliable without the control of numbers or pain descriptors.[86]

NONPHARMACOLOGIC THERAPY

In addition to pharmacologic agents, stress reduction methods such as visualization (imagery), hypnosis, and relaxation techniques are helpful in combating pain and anxiety. Other nonpharmacologic measures for pain relief include the use of transcutaneous electrical nerve stimulation (TENS), acupuncture, acupressure, biofeedback therapy,

Visual Analogue Scale

no pain _____ pain as bad as it
could possibly be

Trofino: Nursing Care of the
Burn-Injured Patient

FIGURE 9–5. Visual Analog pain rating scale.

and auditory stimulation such as comedy, music, and distraction. Other methods for assisting with comfort and decreasing pain levels include elevation of burned extremities and position patient for comfort while maintaining proper body alignment to prevent contractures.

NURSING CONSIDERATIONS

Frequent evaluation of the burn patient's pain level is important for pain control. Nursing assessment for pain control includes:

- Monitoring the patient's pain response
- Monitoring effectiveness of pain medications
- Monitoring effectiveness of nonpharmacologic therapy.

Rehabilitation

New advances in burn care have greatly increased the patient's survival rate. With more patients surviving, rehabilitation has become an even more important aspect of total patient care. The rehabilitative phase of care for the patient with a major burn can encompass many years. The planning of the rehabilitation of the patient ideally begins shortly after admission.

Rehabilitation impinges upon many areas of burn care. It encompasses mobility, function, and wound healing, and psychosocial changes. Restoration or maintenance of mobility and function is a top priority in patient care. Control of scarring and contractures correlates with mobility and function. Plastic surgery (refer to Chapters 4, 20, and 21) may be an ongoing process for many years. Psychosocial changes occur due to the very devastating effect of the burn and the recovery process (refer to Chapter 7).

The care of the patient in relation to rehabilitation encompasses many members of the burn team, most notably physicians, nurses, occupational therapists, physical therapists, psychologists, psychiatrists, social workers, vocational rehabilitation counselors, home health nurses and aides, and, as appropriate, play therapists and school teachers. The roles of each of these burn team members varies throughout the course of the patient's recovery according to the patient's needs while in the hospital and at home (refer to Chapter 8). The rehabilitative care of the patient also differs according to his or her age (refer to Chapters 14 and 15); any special considerations (refer to Chapters 13, 16, 17, and 18); and specific burned areas (refer to Chapters 10, 11, and 12).

NURSING CONSIDERATIONS

Nursing assessment of rehabilitation involves the following:

- Frequent evaluation of patient's mobility level
- Frequent evaluation of patient's psychosocial level
- Monitoring of wound healing (scarring, contractures)

PATIENT HISTORY

Accurate assessment and evaluation of burn patients involves obtaining a complete health history and doing a complete physical examination. This procedure frequently follows a routine course provided by a standard nursing assessment form. Health care workers should make every effort to consolidate their data-gathering process because patients frequently complain that many people have asked them the same questions.

In obtaining a patient's history, it is advantageous to provide a quiet, comfortable atmosphere. The history-taking process provides the nurse with both objective and subjective data related to the patient's anxiety level and psychologic status. It also provides a foundation for the development of the patient's individualized nursing care plan. If the patient is unable to provide subjective data, the examiner obtains information from those at the scene of the accident (e.g., fire fighters, observers, paramedics) and from family members.

Obtaining the following data will provide hospital personnel with an accurate profile of the burn patient from which to classify the extent of injury and provide optimal care. It is important to obtain an accurate history of the exact mechanism of burn injury and associated injuries. Early in the history-taking process, the exact location of pain at both wound sites and sites of associated injuries is determined.

If the burn is from flames, the nurse notes whether it occurred in a closed space and whether the victim was exposed to smoke or if an explosion occurred. It is also important to note the type of burning materials such as nylon (carpets), acrylics, wood, polyvinylchloride (cable insulation, wall and floor coverings), polyurethane (upholstery), and polystyrene (foam materials). Some of these substances produce systemic toxicity; others are pulmonary irritants.

If the burn was caused by an electrical source, it is important to determine the voltage involved, the duration of exposure, and whether the victim was grounded. As electrical burns are often associated with falls, the cause of associated injury is determined (e.g., fall from a tree or ladder (refer to Chapter 3, page 34).

With chemical burns, it is important to note the type of chemical and the length of exposure to the substance. Also important is the presence or absence of noxious fumes (refer to Chapter 3, page 31).

It should be determined if the burn history coincides with the type of burn itself. Abuse is suspected in cases of cigarette burns, burns of the buttocks, extensive scalding burns, and circumferential burns of the feet and buttocks, especially those with clear demarcation lines.

In addition to the aforementioned data that relate specifically to the burn, the nurse obtains a medical history as well, regarding allergies (e.g., food, drugs, tape, iodine); immunizations (including date of last tetanus vaccine); past medical-surgical problems; previous hospitalizations; family health history; social history related to the use of drugs, alcohol, and tobacco; dietary history and preferences; sleep pattern; and history of bowel and/or bladder problems. As a final step in the history-taking process, the nurse determines if the patient has any health problems not previously elicited by reviewing physical systems.

PHYSICAL ASSESSMENT

The initial physical examination is similar to that performed for any trauma patient. The process is begun by focusing on the ABCs (airway, breathing, circulation). The patient is observed for a patent airway (especially if smoke inhalation is suspected), and assessed for the adequacy of ventilation, blood pressure, and pulses. High-flow oxygen is initiated if smoke inhalation injury is suspected. The next step in assessment is to focus on the four components of the physical assessment, which include inspection, palpation, percussion, and auscultation.

Inspection

GENERAL

The nurse observes the general appearance of the patient. The patient is assessed as a whole to determine the acuity of his or her condition. Any distinguishing characteristics such as difficulty speaking or hoarseness due to laryngeal edema are noted. The nurse assesses age, sex, body build, race, nutritional status, motor activity, mental status, edema, blisters, signs of distress, and general areas of burn.

Severity and extent of the burn is determined by percent, depth, and location of the wounds. The nurse also notes any high-risk specialty areas that are burned and assesses for any associated life-threatening injuries. At the time of the general assessment, the nurse also obtains baseline vital signs.

LOCALIZED INSPECTION (HEAD-TO-TOE)

Face, Head, and Neck. The patient's face is evaluated for expression and symmetry. The oral and nasal cavities are observed for sooty material, flame burns, bloody or sooty sputum, singed nasal hairs, dry red mucous membranes, conjunctivitis, rhinorrhea, and facial edema. The neck is observed for circumferential burns and the patient is monitored for dyspnea or stridor or both.

Mental Status. The patient's speech is observed for clarity of thinking, orientation, memory, cognitive skills, and expression of thought. These data can frequently be obtained during the history-taking process.

Respiratory System. In assessing the respiratory system it is helpful to observe chest movements from both the patient's side and from the end of the bed. The nurse observes the respiratory pattern, thoracic configuration (e.g., barrel chest), adequacy of lung expansion (symmetry and depth), appearance of dyspnea, cyanosis (peripheral and central), and use of accessory muscles to breath. *Take special note of circumferential burns of the chest.*

Neurologic System. The standard routine for assessment of neurologic status is determination of the Glascow Coma Scale value. Coma is defined as a score of 7 or less. The nurse assesses the patient's motor response, verbal response, and eye opening response. Additional assessments include pupil size and equality in response to light. Motor strength also is evaluated.

Cardiovascular System. The precordium is assessed for apical impulse, retractions, and heaves or lifts.

Gastrointestinal System. The abdomen is observed for distention, bleeding, symmetry, and scars.

Musculoskeletal System. The patient's extremities are observed for size, symmetry (noting any deformities), contour, edema, and movement. Circumferential burns are especially noted.

Palpation

The patient's chest and abdomen are palpated for any areas of tenderness. Possible fractures of the extremities also are palpated, noting any areas of tenderness. The wound is palpated to determine elastic versus leathery eschar. Finally, peripheral pulses are palpated to determine adequate blood flow.

Percussion

Percussion is infrequently used in routine nursing assessment but is helpful in determining liver or splenic enlargement. Percussion is also used to determine bladder fullness.

Auscultation of Major Systems

Auscultation of the major organ systems is one of the most important assessments the nurse will do. Frequently it is the nurse who identifies significant early changes and intervenes to make corrections. The nurse routinely (every 4 hours) auscultates the heart, lungs, and abdomen.

The lungs are auscultated for the presence of wheezes, rales, rhonchi, and pleural friction rub. Also, the nurse assesses for diminished breath sounds and any evidence of stridor. It is important to listen to lung sounds both anteriorly and posteriorly. A pleural friction rub, if present, is best heard anteriorly in the lower lateral chest below the xiphoid process.

The cardiovascular system is assessed by auscultating heart sounds at the apex, along the left sternal border and over the pulmonic and aortic valves (second intercostal space to the left and right of the sternum). The nurse monitors heart sounds for pericardial friction rub, murmurs, S_3, S_4, and clicks.

Auscultation of the abdomen precedes palpation and percussion due to the effect in increasing bowel sounds. The abdomen is also auscultated for the presence of bowel sounds and the presence of abdominal bruits. It is recommended that the examiner listen for at least 5 minutes before concluding that bowel sounds are absent.

DIAGNOSTIC STUDIES

Diagnostic Test	Rationale
Complete Blood Count	To identify pre-existing anemia; to monitor hemoconcentration during the initial fluid shift; to determine appropriate fluid volume replacement during the phases of hemoconcentration and hemodilution, as well as postsurgically.
Urinalysis	To assess for the presence of glucose, ketones, albumin, hemoglobin, and myoglobin (hemochromogens).
Spot Urinalysis at Bedside	To assess glucose, ketones, pH, protein, bilirubin, and blood; to assess specific gravity for determination of hydration status.
Serum Creatinine and BUN	To assess renal function during the emergent phase when renal damage is a potential complication due to tissue damage and fluid shifting. The BUN is also elevated in severe dehydration and increased protein metabolism. To assess renal function for patients receiving nephrotoxic antibiotics.

Cultures: Wound, Urine, Sputum, Blood	To assess for sites of infection; to obtain baseline information; to determine appropriate therapy for specific infecting organism; to prevent severe infections.
Chest x-rays	To obtain baseline films; to assess for pneumonia, smoke inhalation, adult respiratory distress syndrome, atelectasis, or other pulmonary disease process; to assess pulmonary status in conjunction with other pulmonary parameters.
Serum Albumin	To assess nutritional status; to assess protein loss through tissue damage.
Serum Electrolytes and Osmolarity	To determine electrolyte changes caused by the fluid shifts or surgical intervention or both; to assess electrolyte changes due to burn complications such as diabetes, infection, and heart disease.
Arterial Blood Gases	To assess for adequate oxygenation; to obtain baseline parameters; to monitor for acid-base balance.
Oxyhemoglobin	To rule out smoke inhalation; to determine type of respiratory equipment needed to ventilate the smoke inhalation patient.
Xenon Lung Scan	To determine areas of poor perfusion or poor ventilation on patients with smoke inhalation.
Bronchoscopy	To locate sites of bleeding in the tracheobronchial airway; to remove foreign matter such as soot, damaged tissue, and mucus particles; to visualize area and cause of obstruction, to assess degree of laryngeal inflammation and edema.
ECG	To help identify dysrhythmias; to evaluate effects of cardiac medications; to assess the effects of fluid shift on the cardiac status; to obtain baseline data.
Serum Glucose	To monitor stress response and pseudo-diabetes. Insulin therapy may be necessary in some patients.

NURSING CARE PLAN: CARE OF THE PATIENT WITH MAJOR BURNS

Nursing Priorities

1. Maintain a patent airway; intubation may be necessary
2. Identify and manage associated life-threatening injuries, such as blocked airway, massive hemorrhage, and cardiac dysrhythmias

3. Maintain a homeostatic balance in fluids and electrolytes
4. Minimize pain and suffering due to treatments
5. Minimize and control bacterial contamination to promote healing
6. Maintain adequate nutrition to meet caloric and nitrogen demands for proper healing
7. Maintain joint mobility by providing range-of-motion (ROM) exercises and proper splinting

8. Assist the patient to deal with the fear, grief, and loss associated with disfigurement of major burns
9. Maintain a holistic approach to nursing care by meeting the needs of the patient physically, emotionally, culturally, spiritually, and psychologically
10. Initiate discharge planning at admission, modify as necessary, to prepare the patient to return to activities of daily living (ADLs)

Nursing Diagnosis: Airway Clearance, Ineffective

May Be Related To:

- Smoke inhalation injury (from inhalation of heat, toxic and/or noxious gases); inhalation injury can lead to symptoms of hypoxemia, orolaryngeal, tracheal, and pulmonary irritation and swelling
- Edema following burns of the face or neck

Possibly Evidenced By: Facial burns with singed nasal hairs, hoarseness, croup, carbonaceous sputum, difficulty breathing, tight chest, swollen and blackened mucous membranes, wheezing, cyanosis (late sign or may be masked by high levels of carbon monoxide), increasing cough, swollen face and neck, and circumoral and circumnasal edema. Chest examination may be normal or may show decreased breath sounds, rales, and rhonchi.

Desired Patient Outcomes: The patient will maintain adequate levels of oxygenation (PaO_2 80 to 100 mmHg.) and unlabored respirations; lung sounds will be present and clear in all lobes.

Interventions	Rationale
INDEPENDENT	
• Observe for signs and symptoms of airway dysfunction by:	• Airway obstruction or dysfunction leads to inadequate oxygenation of vital tissues.
○ Auscultating lungs at least every 4 hours.	
○ Monitoring character, rate, and depth of respirations.	
○ Observing for cyanosis, hoarseness, increasing anxiety, increasing cough, stridor, wheezing.	
• Suction as necessary.	• Assists in maintaining a clear airway.
• Monitor ABGs.	• Assists in modification of treatment according to condition (e.g., decrease or increase FIO_2 based on PaO_2, increase rate to blow off more O_2).
• Encourage patient to turn, cough, deep-breathe, and/or use incentive spirometer every 2 to 4 hours.	• Promotes lung expansion. Assists in ventilation, in mobilizing secretions.

Interventions	Rationale
• Elevate head of bed.	• Decreases swelling of face and neck.
• Monitor I & O.	• Assists in modification of fluid therapy. Adequate hydration aids in liquefying secretions. Overhydration leads to pulmonary edema.
• Monitor pulmonary artery and CVP pressures as indicated.	• Hemodynamic monitoring is helpful in assessing cardiovascular status.

COLLABORATIVE

• Administer humidified oxygen.	• Prevents hypoxemia and acidosis.
• Administer chest physiotherapy.	• Promotes drainage of secretions.
• Administer mycolytic agents as prescribed.	• Assists in liquefying secretions.

Nursing Diagnosis: Gas Exchange, Impaired

May Be Related To:

• Smoke inhalation injury and heat-damaged tracheal-bronchial tissue

Possibly Evidenced By: Increased cough with increased sputum, labored breathing, dypsnea, decreased lung sounds, rales and/or rhonchi, decreased PaO_2, restlessness, confusion, tachycardia, and, in severe cases cyanosis, flaring nares, retractions.

Desired Patient Outcomes: The patient will maintain adequate gas exchange as evidenced by:

○ Clear lung sounds
○ Respiratory pattern regular and unlabored
○ PaO_2 80 to 100 mmHg.
○ $PaCO_2$ 35 to 45 mmHg.
○ Effective mobilization of secretions

Interventions	Rationale
INDEPENDENT	
• Monitor lung sounds and character, rate, and depth of respirations. Monitor ability to cough.	• Assesses changes in pulmonary function so that therapy can be modified. Indicates signs of stress, hypoxia, and increasing respiratory effort.
• Monitor ABGs.	• Assesses levels of oxygen to monitor hypoxia, hypercarbia, and acidosis. Guides oxygen therapy.
• Encourage patient to turn, cough, deep-breathe, and use incentive spirometer every 2 to 4 hours.	• Mobilizes secretions and promotes lung expansion.
• Monitor vital signs.	• Establishes baseline data from which to assess changes in cardiopulmonary status. Indicates signs of respiratory distress.

Nursing Diagnosis: Impaired (*Continued*)

Interventions	Rationale
• Note amount, color, and consistency of pulmonary secretions (note presence of carbonaceous sputum).	• Infectious agents will change the color, consistency, and amount of sputum. Carbonaceous sputum is diagnostic for smoke inhalation.

COLLABORATIVE

Interventions	Rationale
• Administer humidified oxygen.	• Promotes oxygenation to maintain adequate PaO_2.
• Administer bronchodilators and antibiotics, as prescribed.	• Respiratory pharmacologic agents used to: ○ Decrease bronchospasms and mucosal edema ○ Control infection
• Obtain sputum cultures.	• Monitors microbial growth and assists physician in selecting appropriate antibiotic therapy.
• Assist in providing/maintaining endotracheal intubation/mechanical ventilation.	• May be necessary to ensure adequate ventilation and oxygenation.

Nursing Diagnosis: Tissue Perfusion, Alteration In

May Be Related To:

- Decreased circulating blood volume from the fluid shift and the tourniquet effect of circumferential burns.
- Blood loss with decreased cardiac output and decreased tissue perfusion (associated with problems of lactic acidosis and the potential for renal shutdown)
- Release of myocardial depressant factor

Possibly Evidenced By: Increased heart rate; thready pulse; skin that is cool, pale, and clammy; diminished or absent peripheral pulses; decreased urine output; anxiety, restlessness, and lethargy; decreased pulmonary artery and CVP pressures; metabolic acidosis with increasing respiratory rate; and stupor or coma, if severe.

Desired Patient Outcomes: The patient will maintain adequate cardiac output and optimal tissue perfusion as evidenced by presence of peripheral pulses and adequate circulation, sensation, and motion (CSM).

Interventions	Rationale

INDEPENDENT

Interventions	Rationale
• Elevate the burned extremity above the level of the heart.	• Enhances return of fluid to the heart and decreases edema formation.
• Assess peripheral perfusion hourly (pulses, color, swelling, sensation, motion, capillary refill).	• Assesses need for escharotomy. Assesses peripheral perfusion.

Interventions	**Rationale**
• Measure circumference of burned extremities.	• Assists in identifying edema formation.
• Monitor cardiac output if pulmonary artery catheter is in place.	• Indicator of fluid volume deficit and cardiac function to determine replacement needs.
• Monitor cardiac rhythm.	• Assists in identifying and treating arrhythmias.
• Monitor laboratory data (platelets, prothrombin time, partial thromboplastin time, bleeding time). Observe for increasing bleeding tendencies, hemorrhage, as well as increased clotting time.	• May be an early indicator of bleeding problems such as disseminated intravascular coagulation (DIC). An atypical DIC may occur in the first 10 days postburn despite adequate fluid resuscitation.
• Monitor urine output.	• Assesses adequacy of circulation and maintenance of renal perfusion.

COLLABORATIVE

• Assist with intracompartmental pressures.	• Determines the need for escharotomy. Prepare for escharotomy if pressure is consistently greater than 25 mmHg.[29]
• Assist with escharotomy.	• Removal of eschar, which allows for edema expansion and permits peripheral perfusion.
• Monitor escharotomy site for bleeding, and assess the extremity for CSM and pain relief.	• Assesses blood loss. Monitors increasing edema.
• Administer blood products, as ordered.	• May be necessary to replace cells lost by tissue destruction.
• Administer albumin/plasma, as ordered.	• Administration of protein volume expanders may be necessary to return edema fluids to the vascular system and promote diuresis.

Nursing Diagnosis: Fluid Volume Deficit, Potential

May Be Related To:

- A rapid shift of plasma and plasma proteins into the interstitial spaces due to increased capillary permeability and vasodilation (sodium and chloride also shift into the muscle and tissues)
- Evaporative losses from the wound surface
- Untreated fluid shifts can result in hypovolemic shock; metabolic acidosis results from the decreased circulation and poor peripheral perfusion
- Decreased fluid intake

Possibly Evidenced By: Decreased blood pressure, increased pulse, decreased urinary output, decreased central venous pressure, decreased pulmonary artery pressures, decreased urine specific gravity, elevated hematocrit, weight loss, and decreasing mental status.

Desired Patient Outcomes: The patient will maintain adequate fluid and electrolyte balance. Tissue perfusion will be maintained and hypovolemia prevented.

Nursing Diagnosis: Fluid Volume Deficit, Potential (*Continued*)

Interventions	Rationale
INDEPENDENT	
• Obtain admission weight and monitor weight daily.	• Assess weight gains and losses common to fluid shifting. Measures fluid loss.
• Record all I & O, hourly. Record hourly specific gravity.	• Serves as a guide for fluid loss and replacement.
• Report urine output of less than 3 ml/hour.	• Assesses adequacy of circulation and maintenance of renal perfusion.
• Monitor the patency of the urinary catheter.	• Necessary to prevent clots and casts from blocking the catheter. Maintains accuracy of output.
• Monitor vital signs and hemodynamic parameters, at least hourly.	• Serves as a guide for fluid replacement and hemodynamic status.
• Monitor electrolytes, CBC.	• Serves as a guide for electrolyte replacement. Serves as a guide for blood product replacement.
• Monitor dressings and burn sites to assess for bleeding.	• Assesses blood loss and need for action in controlling blood loss.
• Maintain IV patency.	• Maintains a site for replacement therapy and IV medications.
COLLABORATIVE	
• Administer IV fluids and electrolyte replacements as prescribed.	• Fluid resuscitation in burn therapy begins immediately and is based on the severity of the burn and the formula used by each hospital.
• Elevate the head of the bed as prescribed.	• Promotes lung expansion and ventilation and perfusion of lung fields.
• Assist in the placement of hemodynamic monitoring lines (CVP, pulmonary artery catheter).	• Serves as a guide for fluid replacement. Assesses cardiac output and fluid volume.
• Administer blood and blood products as prescribed.	• Blood replacement may be necessary due to hemolysis of cells from the burn and postsurgically after debridement. Other blood products may be needed due to burn tissue destruction.
• Administer fluid challenges/mannitol for myoglobinuria.	• Routinely given to patients who develop myoglobin in their urine due to tissue destruction. The goal is to maintain urine output above 100 ml/hour and prevent acute tubular necrosis.

Nursing Diagnosis: Fluid Volume Excess, Potential

May Be Related To:

- Iatrogenic causes of overhydration during fluid resuscitation
- Surgical stress response
- Excess fluid and/or sodium intake

Possibly Evidenced By: Edema, weight gain, intake greater than output, shortness of breath, dyspnea, orthopnea, rales, rhonchi, restlessness, anxiety, elevated pulmonary artery and central venous pressures, infiltrates on chest x-ray, low urine specific gravity, jugular vein distention, development of a third heart sound, dilutional changes in electrolytes, and decreased hematocrit and hemoglobin.

Desired Patient Outcomes: The patient will maintain optimum fluid and electrolyte balance. Tissue perfusion will be maintained and hypervolemia prevented.

Interventions	Rationale
INDEPENDENT	
• Obtain admission weight and monitor weight daily at the same time of day with the same amount of clothing.	• Assess weight gains common to fluid shifting and fluid retention.
• Record I & O hourly in the critical period. Record hourly specific gravity.	• Serves as a guide for fluid therapy.
• Monitor vital signs and hemodynamic parameters, at least hourly, and report abnormal results. Titrate fluid replacement according to hemodynamic pressures.	• Serves as a guide for fluid replacement and hemodynamic status.
• Monitor electrolytes, CBC, and other diagnostic tests, and report abnormal results.	• Serves as a guide for electrolyte replacement. Serves as a guide for blood product replacement.
• Monitor for physical assessment changes at least every 4 hours. Monitor breath sounds and heart sounds. Monitor for fluid overload, edema especially in dependent body areas. Assess for neck vein distention. Monitor peripheral pulses. Monitor mental status.	• Routine physical assessments assist the nurse identifying early changes of fluid overload.
• Limit the amount of time in the Hubbard tank to no more than 20 minutes.	• Longer periods of time in the Hubbard tank allow electrolyte leeching and fluid absorption.
COLLABORATIVE	
• Assist in the placement of hemodynamic monitoring lines (CVP, pulmonary artery catheter).	• Serves as a guide for fluid replacement. Assesses cardiac output and fluid volume.
• Elevate the head of the bed, as prescribed.	• Promotes lung expansion and ventilation and perfusion of lung fields.

Nursing Diagnosis: Fluid Volume Excess, Potential (*Continued*)

- Administer IV fluids and electrolyte replacements as prescribed. Restrict sodium and fluid intake, as necessary.

- Administer diuretic and/or mannitol, as needed.

- Fluid resuscitation in burn patients needs to be closely monitored to maintain optimum fluid and electrolyte balance.
- Removes excess fluid from body and flushes debris from the kidneys.

Nursing Diagnosis: Altered Urinary Elimination Pattern

May Be Related To:

- Decreased circulating blood volume secondary to third spacing prior to fluid resuscitation.
- Oliguria secondary to myoglobinuria and acute tubular necrosis

Possibly Evidenced By: Decreased urinary output; brown-black urine; blood in urine.

Desired Patient Outcomes: Patient will maintain adequate urinary output as manifested by a urine output of 0.5 to 1.0 ml/kg per hour[34] (if hemachromogens present, a minimum output of 0.1 ml/kg/ per hour).

Interventions

Rationale

INDEPENDENT

- Measure urine hourly, noting color, amount, blood, glucose, protein, and myoglobin.
- Palpate bladder.
- Observe for blood at the meatus.

- Determines renal functioning and adequacy of fluid resuscitation.

- Determines distention.
- Blood at the meatus may be a sign of a urethral tear.

COLLABORATIVE

- Insert Foley catheter, as ordered, in patients with 20 percent or more burns. Send a urine specimen to the laboratory for a urinalysis test.

- Patients with this extent of burns receive fluid resuscitation, and urine output must be accurately measured. Specimen serves as baseline. In the patient with electrical burns, urine output should be 100 ml/hour.[35] If myoglobin still present with increased fluid administration, give 25 g of mannitol immediately, and 12.5 g should be added to each subsequent liter of fluid.[36] In the child, mannitol dosage is reduced appropriately.

Nursing Diagnosis: Bowel Elimination, Alteration In: Constipation

May Be Related To:

- Alterations in circulatory supply to the bowel resulting in a paralytic ileus
- Internal injury secondary to trauma, falls, and so on

Possibly Evidenced By: Decreased bowel sounds, vomiting, abdominal distention, decreased frequency of bowel movements, nausea, abdominal pain and tenderness.

Desired Patient Outcomes: Patient will maintain adequate gastric functioning and bowel elimination.

Interventions	Rationale
INDEPENDENT	

• Assess GI status by:
  ○ Auscultating for bowel sounds
  ○ Palpating for abdominal distention, tenderness, and pain
	• Decreased bowel sounds are a sign of impending ileus or intestinal trauma. With multiple trauma, abdominal injury can occur such as liver laceration; splenic rupture, laceration, or contusion; small bowel perforation; or pancreatic contusion.

• Maintain patient NPO if multiple trauma, until abdominal injury can be ruled out.	• Prevents further damage.
• Measure amount, color, heme content, and pH of vomit or NG aspirate.	• Determines GI functioning and possible internal bleeding.
COLLABORATIVE	
• Assist with or insert NG tube as ordered in patients with greater than 25 percent burns;[38] place to low intermittent or low continuous suction (vented NG tube).	• Allows for gastric decompression. Do not nasally insert an NG tube in a patient with a suspected basilar skull fracture: the tube can go through a dural tear into the brain.
• Secure NG tube; if facial burns, tie as for endotracheal tube.	• Prevents dislodgment.
• Administer antacids as ordered to maintain gastric pH less than 5.	• Prevents ulceration of gastric mucosa. Determines GI functioning and possible internal bleeding.

Nursing Diagnosis: Pain

May Be Related To:

- Exposure of nerve endings in partial-thickness burns
- Donor site procurement

Possibly Evidenced By: Verbalization of pain, withdrawal, whimpering, crying, screaming, facial grimaces, clenched teeth, tight lips, and knotted

Nursing Diagnosis:
Pain (*Continued*)

brow. Patient may rub the painful area and may resist moving the affected area.

evidenced by stated relief, nonverbal cues, and vital signs.

Desired Patient Outcomes: The patient's pain is minimized or controlled as

Interventions	Rationale
INDEPENDENT	
• Assess and record the nature, location, quality, intensity, and duration of pain.	• Monitors individual responses to pain. Monitors response to therapy and changes in pain response.
• Assess level of pain through verbalization, facial expression, and body positioning. Rate pain or have patient rate pain on a visual analogue scale.	• Pain is a subjective sensation of hurt and is best determined by the patient. Changes in location, character, and intensity of pain may indicate developing complications.
• Accept individual responses to pain.	• Pain perception or expression are influenced by multiple factors such as cultural or ethnic background, coping mechanisms, past experience, and other unknown individual differences.

• Observe for psychophysiologic responses to pain:
  ○ Increases in blood pressure, pulse, and respiratory rate
  ○ Increased restlessness and irritability
  ○ Increased muscle tension
  ○ Facial grimaces
  ○ Guarding
	• Pain responses are variable and dependent on cultural and psychologic influence. Physical and mental parameters change in response to pain.

• Offer pain medication a half hour before pain-provoking treatments.	• Analgesics given prior to exercise and treatments assist patient to perform at a higher level of function.
• Evaluate effectiveness of analgesics.	• Need to monitor for oversedation versus undermedication.
• Offer diversional activities: music, radio, television, books, games.	• Diversional activities assist in helping the patient focus on things other than burn pain.
• Properly position patient. Elevate extremities above the level of the heart.	• Increases comfort. Elevation of burned extremities decreases edema and pain from swelling.
• Use relaxation techniques to increase comfort.	• Increases comfort by increasing patient control and ability to deal with pain.
• Explain procedures and their importance (e.g., ROM, tubbings, dressing changes).	• Educating patients about what to expect assists in decreasing anxiety and fear of the unknown.
• Perform dressing changes efficiently. Have supplies ready.	• Prevents air hitting open wounds, thereby decreasing pain.

Interventions	Rationale
• Attempt to allay fear and anxiety by allowing time to verbalize concerns.	• Provides patients with more control. Assists patients to begin dealing with concerns.
• Maintain comfortable environment (30 to 33°C, bed cradle, quiet environment).	• With skin surface loss, the body is unable to self-regulate to environmental temperature changes. Pressure from bed linens may cause pain.

COLLABORATIVE

• Administer analgesics and sedatives, as prescribed.	• Need to control pain and promote sleep without oversedating the patient.
• Administer IV morphine sulfate during the critical period. Other medications such as methadone or fentanyl may also be used.	• Intramuscular injections are not absorbed well in burn patients because of edema and poor tissue perfusion.
• Cover wound with biologic dressings and grafts.	• Biologic dressings decrease nerve exposure and thus decrease pain.
• Instruct patients in the use of self-administered analgesics.	• Such methods increase patient's control over situation.

Nursing Diagnosis: Infection, Potential For

May Be Related To:

• Loss of skin integrity
• Decreased resistance to infection in addition, multiple dressing changes and tubbings increase fluid loss and provide increased opportunity for contamination

Possibly Evidenced By: Elevated temperature; positive wound cultures; changes in wound status (odor, redness, tenderness, swelling, and amount of drainage); and signs and symptoms of sepsis.

Desired Patient Outcomes: The patient will not develop wound infection and sepsis.

Interventions	Rationale
INDEPENDENT	
• Shave hair to at least 1 inch around burn areas (excluding eyebrows).	• Hair is a medium for bacterial growth.
• Strict isolation during tubbing and dressing changes.	• Decreases bacterial contamination.
• Monitor vital signs at least hourly in the critical period.	• Early detection of signs and symptoms of infection lead to prompt treatment.
• Monitor WBC count.	• Increased WBCs may indicate an infectious process. Silvadene may suppress WBCs.

Nursing Diagnosis: Infection, Potential For (*Continued*)

Interventions	Rationale
• Monitor wound cultures.	• Wound biopsies are routinely done and surfaces cultured to determine type of organisms and cell counts.
• Monitor wound for changes in drainage: odor, redness, tenderness, swelling, and amount of drainage.	• Assists in identification of infectious processes.
• Monitor indwelling catheters—IV, Foley, and other invasive lines. Date and time insertions, line changes, and so on.	• Early detection of infectious processes leads to early treatment.
• Maintain strict aseptic technique during wound management.	• Decreases chance of infection and reduces exposure to pathogens.
• Monitor effect of topical agents.	• If the topical agent in use is not controlling the bacterial count, then a different agent should be tried.
• Implement isolation techniques.	• Decreases chance of contamination and infection.
• Instruct visitors in appropriate burn unit protocols.	• Proper hand-washing techniques plus use of gloves, gown, and mask decrease contamination.

COLLABORATIVE

• Administer antibiotics and topical agents, as prescribed.	• Useful in eliminating or controlling infectious processes.
• Collect wound cultures, as ordered.	• Assists in identifying and treating infectious processes.
• Administer subeschar clysis with antibiotics.	• Adjunct to topical agents for treatment of burn wound sepsis.

Nursing Diagnosis: Nutrition, Alteration In: Less Than Body Requirements

May Be Related To:

• Hypermetabolic rate
• Inability to ingest and digest food
• Severe protein wasting from the burn wound

Possibly Evidenced By: Weight loss, decreased plasma proteins, decreased albumin, decreased caloric intake to meet high nutritional needs, negative nitrogen balance, and decreased muscle mass.

Desired Patient Outcomes: The patient will maintain 90 percent of preburn weight as well as maintaining plasma proteins and a positive nitrogen balance.

Interventions	Rationale

INDEPENDENT

- Monitor caloric and protein intake. Monitor I & O.

- Assess the patient's eating habits. Determine family eating patterns, food allergies, and cultural eating habits.

- Provide high-protein powdered milk drinks.
- Monitor daily weights.

- Assess muscle tone.

- Consult with a dietician in planning patient's diet.

- Encourage family and friends to bring in patient's favorite foods.
- Assess bowel sounds; check for abdominal distention. Observe for signs and symptoms of gastrointestinal disorders.
- Monitor glucose levels.

- Maintain oral hygiene.

- Reinforce good eating habits.

- Avoid painful procedures during feeding times.

- Caloric and protein requirements need to be met in order to maintain a positive nitrogen balance and provide calories for healing.
- Providing the patient with food that he or she likes assists in encouraging the patient to eat more. Intake of 4000 to 5000 kilocalories per day may be necessary to promote healing of major burns.
- Adds calories and protein to the diet without being filling.
- Assesses fluid volume changes and weight loss due to inadequate caloric intake.
- Assesses muscle loss due to inadequate caloric intake and immobility.
- Dietary planning includes obtaining patient likes and dislikes and meeting daily requirements.
- Encourages patient to eat more.

- Gastrointestinal problems occur due to severe injuries and high-level stress.

- Pseudodiabetes may become a problem in major burns.
- Good oral hygiene provides for:
  - Healthy gums and teeth
  - Improved appetite
  - Decreased source of infection
- Positive reinforcement encourages good eating habits. Allows patients to feel good about their efforts.
- Severe pain decreases the desire to eat.

COLLABORATIVE

- Administer antacids and histamine blockers, as prescribed.

- Administer vitamin and mineral supplements, as prescribed.

- Guaiac NG drainage and stools.

- Prevention and treatment for ulcer formation. Histamine blockers inhibit gastric acid secretion.
- Replaces losses and promotes healing. Vitamin C promotes healing. Vitamin needs are increased due to increased losses and increased metabolic demand.
- Detects gastric and intestinal bleeding.

Nursing Diagnosis: Nutrition, Alteration In: Less Than Body Requirements (*Continued*)

Interventions	Rationale
• Administer total parenteral nutrition (TPN) and/or enteral feedings, as prescribed.	• Supplements or replaces oral intake to increase caloric and protein intake. TPN administration is not used unless other nutritional replacement methods are inadequate due to the high risk of sepsis.

Nursing Diagnosis: Mobility, Impaired Physical

May Be Related To:

- Inhibited movement because of intense pain
- Development of hypertrophic tissue and contractures

Possibly Evidenced By: Limited range of motion, contractures, guarding, posturing, and rigidity of movement.

Desired Patient Outcomes: The patient will be returned to optimal physical function through prevention of contractures and hypertrophic tissue and adherence to rehabilitation protocol.

Interventions	Rationale
INDEPENDENT	
• Provide active and passive ROM, every 1 to 2 hours, while patient is awake.	• Assists in prevention of loss of movement and development of contractures.
• Elevate burned extremities above the level of the heart.	• Decreases edema and increases venous return.
• Maintain proper body alignment using splints.	• Prevents or limits contracture formation. Maintains joint function.
• Medicate the patient with analgesics, as needed, prior to exercise and ambulation.	• Decreased pain facilitates mobility.
• Assess joint mobility every 4 hours and during dressing changes.	• Consistent evaluation of joint mobility promotes early treatment measures.
• Initiate the rehabilitation process on admission.	• Prevents loss of joint function. Promotes a regular program of care that enlists patient participation.
• Promote occupational therapy activities and diversional activities that assist in exercise. Coordinate ADLs, therapy, hydrotherapy, and nursing care.	• Promotes exercise and maintains joint function with activities other than the routine exercise program. Combining activities produces improved results by enhancing effects of each and providing for longer rest periods between grouped activities.

Interventions	Rationale

COLLABORATIVE

- Use the circoelectric bed, per physician's order; use frequent turning and low-pressure beds.
- Apply splints, per order.

- Assist with escharotomy or fasciotomy.

Refer to nursing diagnosis Tissue Perfusion, Alteration in, on page 164, of this care plan.

- Facilitates wound care. Decreases the incidence of pressure sores.

- Prevents or limits contracture formation.
- Improves circulation to edematous extremities.

Nursing Diagnosis: Fear

May Be Related To:

- Fear of hospitalization
- Fear of disfiguration, disability, or death
- Fear of separation from friends and family

Possibly Evidenced By: Verbalization of fear, noncommunication, clenched teeth, wringing of hands, and increased diaphoresis.

Desired Patient Outcomes: The patient will be able to:

- Verbalize fears and concerns, identify sources of fear.
- Communicate positive feelings about self and body image.
- Express hope and confidence in recovery.
- Identify and use support systems.
- Integrate at least one fear-reducing coping mechanism in daily behavior.

Interventions	Rationale

INDEPENDENT

- Encourage the patient and family to verbalize fears and concerns. Set aside one-on-one time.
- Establish a trusting relationship with the patient, family, and friends.
- Prepare the patient for the appearance of the wound.

- Explain procedures and progress to the patient and family.
- Contact ancillary services to assist patients and their family members deal with concerns.
- As much as possible, allow for flexible visiting hours.
- Allow patients to progress at their own pace through the grief stages.

- Offers emotional support. Allows the patient the opportunity to express and begin dealing with concerns.
- Enhances trust and patient cooperation in the plan of care.
- Allows patient the opportunity to realistically deal with the healing process and the future appearance of the scar tissue.
- Assists in overcoming problems associated with fear of the unknown.
- Provides a wide variety of personnel to assist in dealing with all types of problems and concerns.
- Promotes patient-family interaction in dealing with the grief process.
- Patients deal better with grief when they proceed at their own pace.

Nursing Diagnosis: Fear
(*Continued*)

Interventions	Rationale
• Set limits on maladaptive behavior.	• Assists patients in dealing with problems realistically. Assists patients to develop positive coping mechanisms.
• Provide positive reinforcement for progress.	• Promotes progression toward independence and self-care. Improves self-image.
• Assist the patient in learning relaxation techniques, hypnosis, visualization, and diversional and/or guided imagery techniques.	• Promotes relaxation and diversion from the current problems.
• Encourage socialization with other burn patients.	• Provides opportunities for burn patients to see other burn wounds. Acceptance by other burn patients improves self-esteem.
• Encourage a visit from a burn survivor from a burn recovery organization.	• Visitation provides moral support and realistic information.

COLLABORATIVE

• Administer analgesics, sedatives, and hypnotics as needed to allay fear and anxiety.	• Certain pharmacologic agents act to relieve anxiety and provide relaxation.

Nursing Diagnosis: Knowledge Deficit, Wound Healing and Burn Treatments

May Be Related To:

• Lack of knowledge of the healing process
• Lack of knowledge about the development of scar tissue and the need to prevent it by exercise and the use of splints and pressure garments
• Lack of knowledge about nutritional needs

Possibly Evidenced By: Inability to answer questions related to care of wound and outpatient regimen.

Desired Patient Outcomes: The patient is able to:

• Verbalize understanding of nutritional requirements.
• Verbalize understanding of outpatient regimen.
• Demonstrate ability and knowledge to care for healing areas.
• Verbalize and demonstrate exercises and application of splints.
• Demonstrate knowledge of development of scar tissue and prevention of contractures.

Interventions	Rationale
INDEPENDENT	
• Explain procedures and tests.	• Decreases patient's anxiety while increasing patient's knowledge about progression of care in burn treatment.

Interventions	**Rationale**
• Explain reasons for frequent assessments.	• Allows patient the opportunity to know what to expect. Decreases anxiety about the unknown. Promotes patient cooperation.
• Explain reasons for tubbing and dressing changes.	• Promotes patient cooperation.
• Explain reasons for using splints and performing ROM exercises. Demonstrate correct use of splints and proper ROM.	• Allows patient the opportunity to know what to expect. Promotes patient cooperation. Maintains joint function.
• Begin discharge planning on admission.	• Facilitates patient-family participation in the treatment program.
• Teach the patient the stages of wound healing processes.	• Facilitates patient participation. Improves patient compliance after discharge.
• Reinforce explanations of the necessity to wear splints and pressure garments at home.	• Knowledge that wearing these items will improve wound healing and decrease scar tissue formation encourages patient compliance.
• Stress the importance of maintaining an exercise program at home.	• Assist in maintaining and regaining joint function.
• Provide information about local support groups for burn victims.	• Provides patients and families opportunities to seek additional resources for help after discharge.

Nursing Diagnosis: Anxiety

(Refer to Chapter 7, page 98, for etiology, manifestations, desired patient outcomes, interventions, and rationale.

Nursing Diagnosis: Fear

(Refer to Chapter 7, page 94, for etiology, manifestations, desired patient outcomes, interventions, and rationale.)

Nursing Diagnosis: Self-Concept, Alteration In

(Refer to Chapter 7, page 89, for etiology, manifestations, desired patient outcomes, interventions, and rationale.)

Nursing Diagnosis: Family Process, Alteration In

(Refer to Chapter 7, page 97, for etiology, manifestations, desired patient outcomes, interventions, and rationale.)

Nursing Diagnosis: Social Isolation

(Refer to Chapter 7, page 90, for etiology, manifestations, desired patient outcomes, interventions, and rationale.)

Nursing Diagnosis: Coping, Ineffective Individual and Family

(Refer to Chapter 7, page 92, for etiology, manifestations, desired patient outcomes, interventions, and rationale.)

Nursing Diagnosis: Post-Trauma Response

(Refer to Chapter 7, page 93, for etiology, manifestations, desired patient outcomes, interventions, and rationale.)

Nursing Diagnosis: Grieving: Anticipatory/Dysfunctional

(Refer to Chapter 7, page 94, for etiology, manifestations, desired patient outcomes, interventions, and rationale.)

Nursing Diagnosis: Adjustment, Impaired

(Refer to Chapter 7, page 95, for etiology, manifestations, desired patient outcomes, interventions, and rationale.)

Nursing Diagnosis: Powerlessness

(Refer to Chapter 7, page 96, for etiology, manifestations, desired patient outcomes, interventions, and rationale.)

REFERENCES

1. Pruitt, BA: Other complications of burn injury. In Artz, CP, Moncrief, JA, and Pruitt, BA (eds): Burns: A Team Approach. WB Saunders, Philadelphia, 1979, p 523.
2. Berkowitz, RL: Burns. In Krupp, MA, Schroeder, SA, and Tierney, LM (eds): Current Medical Diagnosis and Treatment, 1987. Appleton and Lange, Norwalk, CT, 1987, p 991.
3. Silverstein, P and Lack, BO: Epidemiology and prevention. In Boswick, JA (ed): The Art and Science of Burn Care. Aspen Publishers, Rockville, MD, 1987, p 11.
4. Fitzgerald, RT: Prehospital care of burned patients. Critical Care Quarterly 1:13, 1978.
5. Archambeault-Jones, C and Feller, I: Burn nursing is nursing. In Wachtel, TL, Kahn, V, and Frank, HA (eds): Current Topics in Burn Care. Aspen Publishers, Rockville, MD, 1983, p 187.
6. Feller, I and Jones, CA: The National Burn Information Exchange. Surg Clin North Am 67:167, 1987.
7. Ibid, p 169.
8. Ibid, p 176.
9. Ibid, p 176.
10. Dimick, AR, et al: Ten-year profile of 1,271 burn patients. Journal of Burn Care and Rehabilitation 6:341, 1985.
11. Ibid, p 341.
12. Fitzgerald, RT, p 13.
13. Dains, JE: Integumentary system. In Thompson, JM, et al (eds): Clinical Nursing. CV Mosby, St Louis, 1986, p 623.
14. Rogers, CL: Monitoring techniques in the acute phase of burn injury. In Wagner, MM: Care of the Burn-Injured Patient: A Multidisciplinary Involvement. PSG Publishing, Littleton, MA, 1981, p 73.
15. Moncrief, JA: The body's response to heat. In Artz, CP, Moncrief, JA, and Pruitt, BA (eds): Burns: A Team Approach. WB Saunders, Philadelphia, 1979, p 23.
16. Dains, JE, p 623.
17. Rogers, CL, p 73.
18. Moncrief, JA, p 23.
19. Baxter, CR: Pathophysiology and treatment of burns and cold injury. In Rhoads, JE and Hardy, JD: Textbook of Surgery ed 5. Lippincott, Philadelphia, 1977, p 198.
20. Leape, L: Tissue changes in burned and unburned skin of rhesus monkeys. J Trauma 10:488, 1970.
21. Berkowitz, RL, p 993.
22. Zawacki, BE: Reversal of capillary stasis and prevention of necrosis in burns. Ann Surg 180:98, 1974.
23. Braen, G and Jelenko C: Thermal injuries. In Rosen, P, et al: Emergency Medicine: Concepts and Clinical Practice. CV Mosby, St Louis, 1983.
24. Loebl, EC, Baxter, CR, and Curreri, PW: The mechanism of erythrocyte destruction in the early postburn period. Ann Surg 178:681, 1973.
25. Kenner, CV: Burn injury. In Kenner, CV, Guzzetta, CE, and Dossey, BM (eds): Critical Care Nursing: Body-Mind-Spirit. Little, Brown & Co, Boston, 1981, p 817.
26. Loebl, Baxter, and Curreri, p 681.
27. Moncrief, JA, p 23.
28. Baxter, CR, p 198.
29. Curreri, PW: Metabolic and nutritional aspects of thermal injury. Burns 2:16, 1975.
30. Ibid, p 16.
31. Bradburn, GB: Direct measurements of total metabolism of a burned patient. Arch Surg 105:410, 1972.
32. Trunkey, DD, et al: Burns and other thermal injuries. In Dunphy, JE and Way, LW (eds): Current Surgical Diagnosis and Treatment, ed 3. Lange Medical Publishers, Los Altos, CA, 1977, p 226.
33. Wilmore, DW: Nutrition and metabolism following thermal injury. Clin Plast Surg 1:603, 1974.
34. Wilmore, DW, et al: Alterations in hypothalamic function following thermal injury. J Trauma 15:697, 1975.
35. Luterman, A, Adams, M, and Curreri, PW: Nutritional management of the burn patient. Critical Care Quarterly 7:34, 1984.
36. Wachtel, TL, et al: Nutritional support for burned patients. In Wachtel, TL, Kahn, V, and Frank, HA (eds): Current Topics in Burn Care. Aspen Publications, Rockville, MD, 1983, p 107.

37. Ibid, p 114.
38. Ibid, p 113.
39. Trunkey, DD, et al, p 226.
40. Kenner, CV, p 817.
41. Trunkey, DD, et al, p 226.
42. O'Neill, JA, et al: Effect of thermal burns on gastric mucous production. Surg Gynecol Obstet 131:29, 1970.
43. McAlhany, JC, et al: Histochemical study of gastric mucosubstances after thermal injury: Correlation with endoscopic evidence of acute gastroduodenal disease. J Trauma 15:609, 1975.
44. McAlhany, JC, Czaja, AJ, and Rosenthal, A: Acute gastroduodenal disease after burns. In Artz, CP, Moncrief, JA, and Pruitt, BA (eds): Burns: A Team Approach. WB Saunders, Philadelphia, 1979, p 512.
45. Reckler, JM, et al: Superior mesenteric artery syndrome as a consequence of burn injury. J Trauma 12:972, 1972.
46. Robson, MC, Krizek, TJ, and Wray, RC: Care of the thermally injured patient. In Zuidema, GD, Rutherford, RB, and Ballinger, WF (eds): The Management of Trauma, ed 3. WB Saunders, Philadelphia, 1979.
47. Monafo, WW and Freedman, BM: Electrical and lightning injury. In Boswick, JA (ed): The Art and Science of Burn Care. Aspen Publishers, Rockville, MD, 1987, p 241.
48. Ibid, p 244.
49. Wilmore, DW: Metabolic changes after thermal injury. In Boswick, JA (ed): The Art and Science of Burn Care. Aspen Publishers, Rockville, MD, 1987, p 137.
50. Wolfe, RR, Desai, MH, and Herdon, DN: Metabolic response to excision therapy. In Boswick, JA (ed): The Art and Science of Burn Care. Aspen Publishers, Rockville, MD, 1987, p 145.
51. Wilmore, DW, p 140.
52. Ganong, WF: Review of Medical Physiology, ed 13. Appleton and Lange, Norwalk, CT, 1987, p 229.
53. Artz, CP: Electrical injury. In Artz, CP, Moncrief, JA, and Pruitt, BA (eds): Burns: A Team Approach. WB Saunders, Philadelphia, 1979, p 351.
54. Ibid, p 351.
55. Petroff, PA and Pruitt, BA: Pulmonary disease in the burn patient. In Artz, CP, Moncrief, JA, and Pruitt, BA (eds): Burns: A Team Approach. WB Saunders, Philadelphia, 1979, p 95.
56. Archambeault-Jones, CA and Feller, I: Burn care. In Kinney, MR, et al: AACN's Clinical Reference for Critical-Care Nursing. McGraw-Hill, New York, 1981, p 741.
57. Gaston, SF and Schumann, LL: Inhalation injury: Smoke inhalation. AJN 80:94, 1980.
58. Archambeault-Jones, CA, p 741.
59. Petroff, PA, p 95.
60. Van Dijk, WC, et al: Neutrophil function, some opsonic activity and delayed hypersensitivity in surgical patients. Surg 92:21, 1982.
61. Moran, K and Munster, AM: Alterations of the host defense mechanism in burned patients. Surg Clin North Am 67:47, 1987.
62. Ibid, p 47.
63. Arturson, MG: The pathophysiology of severe thermal injury. Journal of Burn Care and Rehabilitation 6:129, 1985.
64. Schmidt, K, et al: Phagocytic activity of granulocytes and alveolar macrophages after burn injury measured by chemiluminescence. Burns 10:79, 1983.
65. Kenner, CV, p 817.
66. Monafo, WW and Freedman, BM, p 242.
67. Kenner, CV, p 826.
68. Pruitt, BA, p 523.
69. Willis, B, Larson, D, and Abston, A: Positioning and splinting the burned patient. Heart Lung 2:696, 1973.
70. Archambeault-Jones, CA, p 741.
71. Berkowitz, RL, p 991.
72. Ibid, p 992.
73. Ayres, SM, Schlichtig, R, and Sterling, MJ: Care of the critically ill, ed 3. Year Book Medical Publishers, Chicago, 1988, p 358.
74. Berkowitz, RL, p 993.
75. Ibid, p 993.
76. Wachtel, TL and Fortune, JB: Fluid resuscitation for burn shock. In Wachtel, TL, Kahn, VC, and Frank, HA (eds): Current Topics in Burn Care. Aspen Publishers, Rockville, MD, 1987, p 41.

77. Demling, RH: Fluid resuscitation. In Boswick, JA (ed): The Art and Science of Burn Care. Aspen Publishers, Rockville, MD, 1987, p 189.
78. Dimola, MA, Acres, CA, and Winkler, JB: Burns. In Kinney, MR, Packa, DR, and Dunbar, SB (eds): AACN's Clinical Reference for Critical-Care Nursing, ed 2. McGraw-Hill, New York, 1988, p 1414.
79. Nicosia, JE and Petro, JA: Manual of Burn Care. Raven Press, New York, 1983.
80. Pruitt, BA, Mason, AD, and Moncrief, JA: Hemodynamic changes in the early postburn patient: The influence of fluid administration and of a vasodilator. J Trauma 11:36, 1971.
81. Berkowitz, RL, p 993.
82. Wachtel, TL, p 41.
83. Rauscher, LA and Ochs, GM: Prehospital care of the seriously burned patient. In Wachtel, TL, Kahn, V, and Frank, HA (eds): Current Topics in Burn Care. Aspen Publishers, Rockville, MD, 1987, p 1.
84. Lynn, R and Eysenck, H: Tolerance for pain, extraversion and neuroticism. Percept Mot Skills 12:161, 1961.
85. Huskisson, EC: Measurement of pain. Lancet 2:1127, 1976.
86. Berry, J and Huskisson, EC: A report on pain measurement. Clinical Trials 9:13, 1972.

CARE OF SPECIFIC ANATOMIC BURNS

Chapter 10

DENISE A. SADOWSKI, RN, MSN

BURNS OF THE EYES AND EARS

Burn injuries to the face are considered to be one of the most traumatic and devastating insults to the human body (Color Plate 23). More specifically, burn injuries to the eyes and ears present a major treatment dilemma because of the intricate makeup of these individual body parts (Color Plates 24 and 25).

The immediate goal of treatment for acute burn injury to the eyes and ears is to prevent further damage and complications. Patients with burns to these areas should have a complete assessment done in a precise, systematic manner. It is imperative that the initial evaluation be thorough so that appropriate treatment interventions and therapeutic management can be implemented. The long-term sequelae can be devastating if proper care is not initiated.

EYE BURNS

Burn injury directly to the eyes can occur from flames (heat injury); chemicals; ultraviolet, infrared, gamma, and x-rays; laser; contact; or late sequelae from electrical injury. Heat injury and chemicals account for most of the burn injuries occurring in or near the eyes. Damage to the eyes can include the eyelid, conjunctiva, and cornea as well as deeper tissues. The injury can be severe enough to cause significant infections, eyelid contractures, corneal ulceration, and even permanent loss of vision.

Burn Injuries

Burn injuries usually occur to the eyelids because of the secondary reflex lid closure and Bells' phenomenon. They can be classified as minimal, moderate, and major. Minimal injury includes a superficial partial-thickness burn that heals in approximately 1 week. These burns are usually moist and tender with blisters.[1] Moderate injury consists of a deeper partial-thickness burn that usually heals on its own without surgical intervention. Edema and pain will be present. The edema present during the early postburn period is of benefit to the patient because it protects the globe from becoming dry. The eye is able to remain moist and further damage is usually prevented.

Major eyelid injury involves deep partial- and full-thickness burns that require skin grafting. The skin over the lid is hard and leatherlike and will not swell. These full-thickness injuries to the lid can be associated with deeper tissue involvement, including corneal damage. The major cause of corneal damage is rapid contracture and ectropion formation. This incomplete closure of the lids causes drying out of the cornea and possible ulcer formation. Lubrication or artificial tears need to be instilled into the eyes very hour and p.r.n. (as necessary) to help prevent the corneas from drying out and prevent corneal ulceration and infection. The nurse visually inspects the eyes frequently for exposure of the globe and to take appropriate action if it does become exposed.

The use of tarsorrhaphy, the method of suturing the lids together to protect the corneas, is not common practice in burn care today.[2] More complications than benefits are associated with tarsorrhaphies. The suture can pull through, leaving unsightly notches in the tarsal plate and free lid margin. The tarsorrhaphies can also pull apart when contractures begin and the globes are no longer protected. Reconstruction of the lids can be difficult with the use of tarsorrhaphies because it compromises the amount of skin that can be placed on the lid. It is difficult to place a graft on a lid that is sutured to its partner. In lids that are nonviable, the tarsorrhaphies can be lost because the nonvital tissue sloughs away, leaving the globe exposed. The use of tarsorrhaphies, therefore, is not advocated early in the burn course and is not an adequate protection for the globe in the later period of burn healing.

Caring for burns of the eyelids involves early and thorough cleansing with mild soap and debridement of the necrotic tissue. Cotton-tipped applicators soaked with saline are helpful in cleaning the inner and outer canthus of the eye. This removes foreign material and crusts from the eye. This should be done three times a day and p.r.n. in order to prevent further damage and infection. A mild, ophthalmic antibiotic ointment can be applied over the lids. The patient should be examined by an ophthalmologist, who will stain the eye with fluorescein and perform a slit-light examination to determine if there is any damage to the cornea and conjunctiva. An analgesic agent should be administered as needed to provide some pain relief.

Chemical Injuries

Chemical injuries to the eye may occur from acids. These are usually self-limiting unless there is prolonged contact. They may also occur from alkaline substances, which cause more extensive damage and a higher incidence of residual ocular impairment. This damage may include a vascularized, opacified cornea, corneal ulceration, keratinization of the conjunctiva, and secondary glaucoma and cataracts. Chemical burns to the eyes can damage all of the cornea and a conjunctival epithelium and represent an urgent ocular emergency. (refer to Chapter 3, page 31).

The amount of injury depends on the strength and concentration of the chemical, duration of contact, and its toxicity. Alkaline solutions tend to cause more disasterous eye burns because of their ability to penetrate rapidly into the eye and bind to the external ocular tissue, thereby resisting removal during irrigation. The extent of injury to the cornea and conjunctiva, as well as the eyelid, will influence the results for maintenance of vision.

These patients will initially complain of severe pain as soon as the chemical enters the eye. The pain increases and intraocular pressure dramatically rises. This increase of pressure occurs from the shrinkage of collagen in the fibrous coats of the eye and the release of prostaglandins.

Immediate care for chemical eye burns is irrigation with copious amounts of water or normal saline for at least 20 to 30 minutes to dilute the chemical and wash it out to decrease any potential harmful effects. Foreign particles and contact lenses are removed from the eyes prior to irrigation. Occasionally a neutralizing solution may be used if it can be identified and is available.

Many devices exist to adequately irrigate the eyes. One of the easiest and simplest to use is intravenous (IV) tubing connected to a bag of normal saline. The end of the tubing is placed across the bridge of the nose and pointed directly at the inner canthus of the eye. This allows the solution to run across the eye and flush the chemical out. The flush should not be directed from the outer canthus inward because the chemical has the tendency to penetrate the eye deeper versus being flushed out, and may splash to the other eye. This irrigation may need to continue for 4 to 6 hours after injury depending on the chemical involved and the amount of injury suspected. An ophthalmic antibiotic ointment should be instilled into the eye every 4 to 6 hours following irrigation. Some physicians also may use steroid preparations.

It is important that eversion of the upper eyelid is accomplished and that eyelids are kept open with retractors or manually. This is necessary to ensure the chemical has been flushed adequately from all surfaces.

Contact Burns

Contact burns of the eyes are rare but can occur from hot flying objects (i.e., molten metal or glass, match heads, cooking oil) or direct corneal contact (i.e., lighted head of a cigarette or cigar and electric curling irons). The severity of the injury depends on the duration of contact, intensity of the heat source, and area of contact in the eye. Fortunately, these injuries are usually not severe because of the rapid blink reflex that protects the cornea from exposure to sources of heat.

With contact burns of the eyes, the patient will immediately begin to complain of pain, tearing, blurred vision, and photophobia. Water or saline can be used to irrigate the eye to decrease the heat present. The patient should be instructed not to rub the eye, in order to prevent further damage to the corneal epithelium. A topical ophthalmic antibiotic should be instilled three to four times a day, and the eye should be patched to prevent straining. These contact burns are usually easily treated and vision sequelae is rare.

Electrical Burns

Eye damage from electrical burns is often not manifested for several months after the initial injury. Usually the eyes do not present with any abnormal findings at the time of the acute burn. Cataracts are the most common form of eye injury that occurs, and it may take up to 3 years following the injury before one appears. The incidence of cataract formation is usually higher in patients who had the entry site on the head or neck. Followup care after the acute injury should include periodic visits to the ophthalmologist to screen for any potential visual deficits.

Nursing Considerations

All patients who sustain a burn injury to the eye are prone to difficulties in interacting with the environment because of potential or actual visual disturbances. During the care of a patient who had sustained an eye burn, it is important for the nurse to realize there might be some alterations in vision. Nurses will identify themselves as they approach the patient so as not to startle or cause anxiety for the patient. With massive edema of the eyelids or difficulty opening the eye because of pain, knowing who is around and what the nurse or other health team member is going to do helps decrease anxiety.The patient and/or family are instructed about the occurrence of eyelid edema, how and why it develops, and an average length of time it may last, depending on the severity of the injury and the potential long-term effects.

Mechanisms need to be discussed with the patient if possible in how the nurse and other health team members will communicate with the patient during this stressful experience. Tactile stimulation for word meanings, emotional support and comfort, soft voice tones so as not to frighten the patient, and describing where objects are in the patient's environment are some ways to help alleviate anxieties and increase communication with the patient. It is important to remember that the patient still needs to remain oriented to the environment. Ingenious ways of doing this help make the burn injury less stressful for the patient and better enable the patient to handle the situation.

Patient History

A detailed and thorough history of the burn injury should be obtained from the patient, if possible, or a family member and rescue workers to assist in ascertaining the severity of the injury. A comprehensive and complete history allows for appropriate interventions to be performed.

The exact account of the burn injury, the time it occurred, and any associated injuries or complaints by the patient should be ascertained in order to assist with appropriate care. This is important because specific interventions (i.e., fluid resuscitation) may relate to the time and severity of the injury. Any precipitating factors leading up to the injury or problems that occurred after the injury was sustained can also be helpful in providing care. The specific type of burn injury—flame, chemical, or contact—needs to be known, as well as the duration of contact with the heat source.

It is important to ascertain the care given at the scene of the accident and during transport to determine if appropriate interventions were performed and in deciding future interventions. If the patient wore contact lenses, be sure they were removed. Determine if any other foreign particles were removed from the eyes and what they were. Also assess if the eyes were irrigated, what type of solution was used, and how long the irrigation lasted. Finally, determine whether an IV infusion was started and what type of solution and medications, if any, were given.

The patient's pain level also needs to be determined because it can reflect severity of the injury. Ask the patient where the pain is (unilateral versus bilateral eyes), the quality of the pain (e.g., burning, throbbing, sharp), aggravating or alleviating factors, and the intensity of the pain. A 1-to-10 scale for adults and a face chart for a child is helpful in assessing the intensity of the pain.

Vision may be lost partially or totally from the injury. The nurse determines if the patient is experiencing any photophobia, visual acuity disturbances, and/or pruritus of the eyes.

Pertinent background information is helpful to know in caring for the patient on a long-term basis. Determine the patient's age, any known allergies, pertinent family history, past medical history (especially eye ailments like cataracts or glaucoma), and any medications the patient is currently taking, including ophthalmic drops and ointments.

Once the subjective data are gathered, a more thorough physical inspection can be done. The physical signs that are detected on examination help in evaluating the burned eyes and assists with appropriate therapeutic interventions.

Singed eyelashes and eyebrows often indicate more extensive ocular burn damage. Eyelids should be inspected for position, edema, redness, lacerations, abrasions, excessive bleeding and ability to close. The conjunctiva and sclera are examined for color, edema, lacerations, abrasions, and any foreign objects. The corneas are inspected for opacity and markings, which can have an effect on vision. Pupils are assessed for size (e.g., those that are usually semidilated and fixed may signify a chemical injury), shape, reaction to light, and equality. Assess the patient's visual acuity for any blurriness and ability to focus. An ophthalmologist examines the eyes for edema of corneal epithelium, clouding of the lens, and any cells floating in the anterior chamber of the eyes. Due to the rapid swelling of the lids, it is critical to obtain an immediate ophthalmology consultation.

All of these physical assessment techniques and skills constitute an integral part in determining the severity of burn injury to the eyes. Thorough and comprehensive histories and physical examinations lead to prompt and appropriate therapeutic interventions.

EAR BURNS

Burn injury to the external ear is not an uncommon consequence with burns occurring on the face and neck. Because of its exposed anatomic position, poor vascularity, lack of subcutaneous tissue, and the superficial location of the cartilage, burns of the ear are often deeper than other areas of the body.[3] As a result, burns of the ear require early attention and thorough treatment.

Burn Injury

Burns to the ear can occur by direct thermal injury, usually resulting in deep partial-thickness or full-thickness involvement. The deep partial-thickness burn may not directly expose the cartilage but, because of contracture of the overlying eschar and edema formation, a decrease in vascularity can result in necrosis of the underlying cartilage.[4,5] With full-thickness injury, there is a lack of blood supply to the cartilage, leading to necrosis of the tissue.

The area is treated with an antimicrobial agent (silver sulfadiazine or mafenide acetate) or wet normal saline soaks. The eschar should not be debrided but rather allowed to separate spontaneously. Hypersensitivity can develop to the antimicrobial agents, especially mafenide acetate, and pseudochrondritis — or inflammation of the ear — can develop.[6,7] Because of this, mafenide acetate is not being used as widely for ear burns as in the past.

Chondritis

Burns to the ears can result in an infection known as chondritis. Although not very common, it is a serious problem because it can destroy the unburned as well as the burned cartilage, thereby altering the shape of the ear.

The development of chondritis is usually insidious and occurs 2 to 6 weeks postinjury. It may occur after the ear appears to be healed. *Pseudomonas aeruginosa* is the predominant organism, with *Staphylococcus aureus* the next most common organism found on the infected ear.[8]

The patient begins to complain of dull pain and tenderness in the affected ear. The pain increases in severity and the ear becomes red, edematous, and warm. The inflammation is initially localized in the helix or antihelix areas but spreads rapidly to involve the entire ear. Purulent drainage can occur and the ear may begin to protrude from the head because of the massive edema.

Once chondritis has developed, the goals are to minimize the spread of infection and to prevent further cartilage damage, severe ear deformity, and loss of the ear. The abscess should be incised and drained, and dead cartilage removed.[9] Wet normal saline soaks can be applied over the ears. Pressure caused by thick dressings or pillows should be avoided. Systemic antibiotics may also be indicated. The treatment of chondritis is not always satisfactory in minimizing cartilage damage or ear deformity. The earlier this infection is recognized and treated, the greater the chance for successful results.

Caring for the patient who has sustained ear burns involves meticulous and thorough cleansing of the entire ear with soap and water three times a day. A cotton-tipped applicator is helpful in getting into the small areas of the ear. This helps to remove antimicrobial agents previously applied so that they do not cake onto the ear, interfering with eschar separation. Cotton-tipped applicators also help to debride some of the loose eschar that is separating. This dead tissue should not remain on the ear because of the potential to cause infection. An antimicrobial agent or saline soaks with a soft, light protective dressing is then applied.

The patient should be positioned so that no pressure is on the ear from dressings or pillows. A gauze sponge between the ear and the scalp may help protect the exposed cartilage from rubbing against the sheets. A 2-inch margin of hair behind the ear may have to be shaved to prevent hair from interfering with the burn.

Nursing Considerations

Because of the massive edema that can occur with ear burns as a result of the initial injury or infection, the patient may experience some hearing deficit. The patient or family, or both, needs to be educated to the potential or actual problem, and ways must be developed to communicate with the patient. The patient needs to understand how and why the edema is occurring to begin coping with the loss. Different forms of tactile stimulation can be developed to mean different things to the patient, especially if hearing loss is severe. This can also be a way of providing emotional support and comfort. A communication system needs to be developed so the patient does not lose contact with the environment if hearing loss occurs. It is important to remember that the patient may experience anxiety over the temporary hearing impairment, and interventions need to be developed to alleviate this stress.

Patient History

A detailed and thorough history of the burn injury should be obtained from the patient, if possible, or from family members and rescue workers to ascertain the severity of the injury. A comprehensive and complete history allows for appropriate interventions to be performed.

The exact account of the burn injury to the ears, the time it occurred, and any associated injuries or complaints by the patient should be determined in order to assist with appropriate care. Any precipitating factors leading up to the injury or problems that occurred after the injury was sustained can also be helpful in providing care. The specific type of injury to the ears (e.g., flame, chemical), and the duration of contact with the source needs to be known because it can relate to the severity of the injury.

It is important to ascertain the care given at the scene of the accident and during transport in determining if appropriate interventions were performed and in deciding future interventions. The nurse determines how the burning process was stopped and what type of ointments, if any, and dressings were applied. If the patient wore hearing aids, they should have been removed. It should be determined what, if any, foreign particles were removed from the ears. Finally, the nurse determines if an IV infusion was started and what type of solutions and/or medications were given.

The patient's pain level also needs to be determined because it can reflect the severity of the injury. The patient is asked the exact location of the pain, the quality of the pain (such as burning, dull, sharp, throbbing), aggravating or alleviating factors,and the intensity of the pain. A 1-to-10 scale for adults and a face chart for children may help them assess pain intensity.

Hearing may be distorted partially or totally from the injury. The nurse determines if the patient is experiencing any difficulty hearing, or any buzzing or ringing in the ears. Ongoing assessments determine if the abnormalities are improving, stabilizing, or progressing.

Pertinent background information is also important to obtain, including the patient's age, known allergies, pertinent family history, past medical history (especially any hearing impairments), current use of hearing aids, and any medications currently taken, including ear drops or ointments.

Once the subjective data are gathered, a more thorough physical inspection can be done. The physical signs that are detected on examination help in evaluating the burned ears and assists with appropriate therapeutic interventions.

The auricles should be examined for any type of deformities, lesions, pain, or drainage. The drainage should be assessed for the type, amount, and color (if the drainage is bright red, internal bleeding may be suspected). Also, the auricles are assessed for tenderness, inflammation, and redness, as these can be signs of infection. The ear canal and drum are inspected for any discharge, edema, foreign bodies, redness, fluid, lesions, or drainage. The drainage is assessed for type, amount, and color. Bleeding can signify serious damage and must be attended to at once. If the patient has hearing loss, the degree of loss and whether it is unilateral or bilateral should be assessed.

All of these physical assessment techniques and skills are an integral part in determining the severity of thermal injury to the ears.Thorough and comprehensive histories and physical examinations lead to prompt and appropriate therapeutic interventions.

NURSING CARE PLAN: BURNS OF THE EYES AND EARS

Nursing Priorities

1. Manage eye or ear injury.
2. Minimize pain and discomfort
3. Minimize infection and prevent complications

4. Provide emotional support to patient and significant others (Refer to Chapter 7 page 89.)
5. Initiate discharge teaching

Nursing Diagnosis: Sensory-Perceptual Alteration In Vision

May Be Related To:

- Eye burns resulting from flames, chemicals, or direct contact with hot objects
- Ulceration or eyelid contractures as a result of burn injury

- Dressings applied over eyes to protect corneas

Nursing Diagnosis: Sensory-Perceptual Alteration In Vision (*Continued*)

Possibly Evidenced by: Blurriness; tearing or discomfort of eyes; actual visual impairment.

Desired Patient Outcomes: The patient will experience normal preburn vision as evidenced by no complaints of blurriness, tearing or discomfort in the eyes at time of discharge.

Interventions	Rationale
INDEPENDENT	
• For chemical injury, irrigate with copious amounts of water or saline for at least 20 to 30 minutes.	• Assists with neutralizing and removing the chemical from the eye, and prevents further damage.
• Arrange for an ophthalmic examination.	• Permits immediate and appropriate treatment. Helps prevent further complications.
• Assess involved eye or eyes every 2 hours and p.r.n. for blurriness, pain, conjunctivitis, and/or corneal drying, tearing, drainage, edema, tenderness, redness, and reaction to light.	• Determines changes as they are occurring, allowing for appropriate therapeutic interventions to be performed.
• Explain injury process at time of admission or soon after, and warn patient of partial or total vision loss.	• Prepares patient for potential outcomes, to decrease anxiety.
• Clean inner and outer canthus with saline-soaked cotton-tipped applicators every 4 hours and p.r.n.	• Promotes better vision and prevents buildup of exudate and crusts. Maintains cleanliness and helps prevent infection.
• Assist patient with activities of daily living (ADLs). Arrange personal articles, trays, and the like, to accentuate functional vision. Orient to room. Be consistent in arrangement of these items.	• Helps patient maintain basic hygiene skills and self-esteem. Helps meet safety needs.
• Anticipate patient's needs and decrease environmental barriers. Position furniture and items out of travel path. Place call bell within easy reach.	• Prevents physical injury to patient resulting from a cluttered environment.
• Provide appropriate diversional activities as tolerated (i.e., radio, talking books).	• Promotes relaxation and prevents boredom.
• Provides safety measures as appropriate (i.e., side rails, assistance with ambulation).	• Prevents physical injury to patient.
• Explain all procedures to patient prior to initiation.	• Minimizes fear in patient. Because vision is impaired, patient needs to comprehend what will occur.
• Announce yourself each time you approach patient or room.	• Minimizes fear and decreases anxiety.

Interventions	Rationale

COLLABORATIVE

- Assist ophthalmologist with examination, which involves staining the eye with fluorescein and performing a slit-light examination.
- Assist in removal of foreign particles or contact lenses from involved eye(s).
- Apply antimicrobial ointments to eyes and perform dressing changes as ordered.
- Instill artificial tears every hour and p.r.n.
- Use external shielding devices or eye patches as needed.

Rationale:

- Excessive edema of the eyelid may make examination difficult. Young children usually need to be assisted or restrained as necessary.
- Prompt removal of objects from eyes prevents further damage.
- Decreases chance of tissue irritation and infection and provides protection for the eyes.
- Helps to keep the eyes moist and prevents ulceration and infection.
- Prevents drying of the eyes. Assists in protecting from infection.

Nursing Diagnosis: Sensory-Perceptual Alteration In Hearing

May Be Related To:

- Burns to the ear resulting in direct burn injury and/or edema
- Infection resulting from complication of burns to the ears
- Dressings applied over the ears
- Ototoxic drug therapy

Possibly Evidenced By: Loss of hearing; pain; edema; tenderness; necrosis.

Desired Patient Outcomes: The patient will experience normal preburn hearing as evidenced by no complaint of tenderness, tinnitus, or discomfort in ears at the time of discharge.

Interventions	Rationale

INDEPENDENT

- Arrange for an otic examination.

- Assess helix and antihelix of the involved ear every 2 hours and p.r.n. for edema, redness, drainage, tenderness, pain, and hearing loss.
- Explain injury process at time of admission or soon after, and warn patient of partial or total hearing loss.
- Gently but thoroughly clean the outer ear with cotton-tipped applicators. Check ear canal every 2 hours and p.r.n. for exudate.

Rationale:

- Allow appropriate treatment without delay. Helps to prevent further complications.
- Determines changes as they are occurring, allowing for appropriate therapeutic interventions to be performed.

- Prepares patient and significant others for potential outcomes, and decreases anxiety.
- Decreases further drainage into the ear. Helps to prevent infection.

Nursing Diagnosis: Sensory-Perceptual Alteration In Hearing (*Continued*)

Interventions

- Carefully remove loose exudate and crusts from outer ear. Avoid debriding crusts still firmly attached to ear.
- Position the patient so no pressure from dressings or pillows is applied to the ear. If tracheostomy tape is tied around the face to hold endotracheal or nasogastric tube in place, check ears every 2 hours and prn to be sure tape is not rubbing on the ears.
- Place a gauze sponge behind the ear (between the ear and scalp).

- Shave a 2-inch margin of hair surrounding the ear.

- Provide patient comfort and assist with activities as needed.

- Coordinate with patient a communication mechanism, especially if hearing loss is severe.
- If mafenide acetate is being used, observe for signs of hypersensitivity that can mimic chondritis.

Rationale

- Removal of loose crusts helps to prevent infection. Removal of firmly attached crusts may cause further damage.
- Prevents pain, contractures, and impairment of blood supply to the ear.

- Protects the cartilage. Also prevents contractures and/or webbing. The ear can become adhered to the head if adjacent burned surfaces are not separated.
- Prevents infection and maceration from hair shaft. Prevents crusts from forming on hair. Aids in maintaining cleanliness near site.
- Ear burns can cause severe pain, especially when infected. By providing comfort as well as assisting with basic ADLs, anxiety will decrease and rest will be provided.
- Assists with orientation to the environment and minimizes fear and anxiety in patient.
- With prolonged use of mafenide acetate, the chance of hypersensitivity and complications for the patient is increased.

COLLABORATIVE

- Assist physician with the examination.

- Assist in removal of foreign objects and hearing aids.
- Apply antimicrobial ointment to outer ear, and change dressings as ordered.

- Apply saline soaks and a soft, light, protective dressing to exposed cartilage.

- Pain can make the examination difficult. Most young children dislike ear examinations and may require assistance in remaining still.
- Prompt removal of objects prevents further trauma to the ear.
- Decreases chance of tissue irritation and infection and provides protection for the ears.
- Exposed cartilage will be very painful. Soaks prevent further trauma, infection, and pain.

Nursing Diagnosis: Pain

May Be Related To:

• Itching or pruritus in eyes and ears caused directly by the injury, a sensitivity reaction to a specific agent (i.e., an antimicrobial agent), or the healing process
• Pain associated with direct injury, dressing changes, surgical intervention and routine care activities (refer to Chapter 9 page 169, Pain)

Possibly Evidenced By: Verbalizations; rubbing/scratching affected areas.

Desired Patient Outcomes: The patient's discomfort is minimized or controlled as evidenced by stated relief, nonverbal cues, vital signs, and no further skin breakdown.

Interventions	Rationale
INDEPENDENT	
• Supply substitute methods of dabbing the itchy area or applying cool, wet cloth over the ears or eyes.	• Prevents rubbing the burn areas and causing tissue breakdown. Scratching areas already inflamed further irritates and damages the skin.
• Keep areas clean and apply dressings per physician order or unit's protocol.	• Decreases the chance of tissue irritation and infection and keeps the area clean to help decrease the feeling of the need to scratch.
• Provide education to the patient as appropriate regarding the dangers of scratching injured or delicate tissue.	• Understanding concepts encourages adherence to specific treatment interventions.
COLLABORATIVE	
• Administer antipruritic medication per physician order before discomfort becomes severe.	• To provide comfort and decrease the urge to scratch the involved areas.
• Apply lotion to healed areas several times per day.	• Lubrication prevents dryness and, therefore, pruritus.

Nursing Diagnosis: Tissue Perfusion, Alterations in (also refer to Chapter 9 page 164)

May Be Related To:

• The use of mafenide acetate on burned ears, which can cause toxicity due to systemic absorption
• Capillary damage secondary to burn injury
• Excessive pressure on ears from pillows or sheets

Possibly Evidenced By: Metabolic acidosis, anxiety, restlessness, increased respiratory rate.

Desired Patient Outcomes: The patient will experience optimal tissue perfusion, normal acid-base balance, and no further tissue breakdown

Nursing Diagnosis: Tissue Perfusion, Alteration In (*Continued*)

Interventions	Rationale
INDEPENDENT	
• Remove all old mafenide acetate during wound care before applying a new layer of cream.	• Having large amounts of the agent on the burn area can cause toxicity because of the systemic absorption.
• Monitor patient for pain during and after application of mafenide acetate.	• Severe pain may occur from a hypersensitivity reaction to the agent.
• Assess ear burns during dressing changes and prn for edema, redness, inflammation, and tenderness.	• Hypersensitivity to the agent may develop, causing a pseudochrondritis.
• Avoid using pillows under head; instead, use a foam ring.	• Prevents pressure on the ears and impairment of blood circulation, leading to breakdown and necrosis.
• Position patient so no pressure from dressing is on the ears.	• Helps to protect the cartilage from rubbing against the head.

Nursing Diagnosis: Infection, Potential for (refer to Chapter 9).

Nursing Diagnosis: Fear (refer to Chapter 9 page 175, Fear).

Nursing Diagnosis: Knowledge Deficit, Wound Healing and Burn Treatment (refer to Chapter 9 page 176, Knowledge, Deficit).

Nursing Diagnosis: Home Maintenance Management, Impaired

May Be Related To:

• Lack of knowledge
• Burn injury
• Inadequate support systems

Possibly Evidenced By: Expressed or demonstrated difficulty in changing dressings; anxious patient and family members.

Desired Patient Outcomes: Patient is maintained at home with minimal or no difficulties; complications are minimized and avoided.

Interventions	Rationale

INDEPENDENT

- Assess patient and significant others for level of cognitive, psychologic, and physical functioning.
- Encourage questions from patient, family, and significant others.

- Instruct patient and family how to care for burned eyes and ears and have them demonstrate appropriate care.
- Provide a list of care that should be done on a daily basis.

- Arrange referrals as needed.
- Arrange a predischarge planning conference 2 to 3 days before discharge.

- Provides baseline data for teaching.

- Increases understanding of discharge care and assists the family with appropriate interventions.
- Demonstration of care helps the staff know whether or not the patient and family understand what was taught.
- Decreases the anxiety concerning what should be done — especially if the care involves many tasks.
- Provides outside assistance if needed.
- Determines that all care taught and demonstrated is correctly understood and clarifies any other questions the patient or family may have.

Nursing Diagnosis: Mobility, Impaired Physical

May Be Related To:

- Loss of vision

   (Refer to Chapter 9, page 174, for other etiologies, manifestations, desired outcomes, and interventions.)

Nursing Diagnosis: Social Isolation

May Be Related To:

- Impaired vision secondary to burns of the eyes
- Impaired hearing secondary to burns of the ears

Possibly Evidenced by: Inability to participate in desired activities; inability to participate in preinjury activities.

Desired Patient Outcomes: Patient can participate in activities at level of preinjury or at level acceptable to the patient.

Interventions	Rationale

INDEPENDENT

- Assess factors that may increase the patient's sense of isolation.

- Care is best directed to the patient's needs for interaction.

Nursing Diagnosis: Social Isolation (*Continued*)

Interventions	Rationale
• Identify support systems available to the patient. Refer to Chapter 7, page 90, for other interventions.	• These will assist the patient in achieving an optimum level of independence.

Nursing Diagnosis: Coping, Ineffective, Family/Individual

(Refer to Chapter 7, page 92, for etiology, manifestations, desired patient outcomes, and interventions.)

Nursing Diagnosis: Post-Trauma Response

(Refer to Chapter 7, page 93, for etiology, manifestations, desired patient outcomes, and interventions.)

Nursing Diagnosis: Grieving, Anticipatory

(Refer to Chapter 7, page 94, for etiology, manifestations, desired patient outcomes, and interventions.)

Nursing Diagnosis: Adjustment, Impaired

May Be Related To:

• Inadequate support systems for loss of sensory functions
• Assault to self-esteem

(Refer to Chapter 7, page 95, for other etiologies, manifestations, desired patient outcomes, and interventions.)

Nursing Diagnosis: Powerlessness

May Be Related To:

• Loss of vision
• Loss of hearing

(Refer to Chapter 7, page 96, for other etiologies, manifestations, desired patient outcomes, and interventions.)

Nursing Diagnosis: Anxiety

May Be Related To:

• Unknown outcome regarding vision
• Unknown outcome regarding hearing

(Refer to Chapter 7, page 98, for other etiologies, manifestations, desired patient outcomes, and interventions.)

Nursing Diagnosis: Family Process, Alteration In

(Refer to Chapter 7, page 97, for etiology, manifestations, desired patient outcomes, and interventions.)

Nursing Diagnosis: Self-Concept, Disturbance In

(Refer to Chapter 7, page 89, for etiology, manifestations, desired patient outcomes, and interventions.)

Nursing Diagnosis: Parenting, Alterations In

May Be Related To:

• Loss of vision
• Loss of hearing

(Refer to Chapter 7, page 105, for other etiologies, manifestations, desired patient outcomes, and interventions.)

REFERENCES

1. Frank, DH, Wachtel, T, and Frank, HA: The early treatment and reconstruction of eyelid burns. Trauma 23(10):874, 1983.
2. Peterson, HD: Eyelids. In Boswick, JA (ed): The Art and Science of Burn Care. Aspen Publishers, Rockville, MD 1987, p 341.
3. Purdue, GF and Hunt, JL: Chondritis of the burned ear: A preventable complication. Am J Surg 152:257, 1986.
4. Dowling, JA, Foley, FD, and Moncrief, JA: Chondritis in the burned ear. Plast Reconstruct Surg 42(2):115, 1968.
5. Goel, TK, Law, EJ, and MacMillan, BG: Management of the acutely burned ear. Burns 9:218, 1983.
6. Kroll, SS and Gerow, RJ: Sulfamylon allergy stimulating chondritis. Plast Reconstruct Surg 80(2):298, 1987.
7. Perry, AW, et al: Mafenide induced pseudochondritis. Journal of Burn Care and Rehabilitation 9(2):145, 1988.
8. Stewart, RC and Beason, ES: Chondritis of the ear: A method of treatment. J Trauma 19(9):686, 1979.
9. Engrau, LH: Acute care and reconstruction of head and neck burns. In Boswick, JA (ed): The Art and Sience of Burn Care. Aspen Publishers, Rockville, MD, 1987, p 336.

BIBLIOGRAPHY

Achauer, BM: Management of the Burned Patient. Appleton and Lange, Los Altos, California, 1987.
Bars, HA: Otologic aspects of ear burns. Am J Otol 2(3):235, 1981.
Bates, B: A Guide to Physical Examination. JB Lippincott, Philadelphia, 1974.
Boswick, JA: The Art and Science of Burn Care. Aspen Publishers, Rockville, MD, 1987.
Campbell, C: Nursing Diagnosis and Intervention in Nursing Practice. John Wiley & Sons, New York, 1978.
Carvajal, HF and Parks, DH: Burns in Children: Pediatric Burn Management. Year Book Medical Publishers, Chicago, 1988.
Cotlar, SW: Reconstruction of the burned ear using a temporary fascial flap. Plast Reconstruct Surg 71(1):45, 1983.
Dowling, JA, Foley, FD, and Moncrief, JA: Chondritis in the burned ear. Plast Reconstruct Surg 42(2):115, 1968.
Frank, DH, Wachtel, T, and Frank, HA: The early treatment and reconstruction of the eyelid burns. J Trauma 23(10):874, 1983.
Goel, TK, Law, EJ, and Macmillan, BG: Management of the acutely burned ear. Burns 9:218, 1983.
Grant, DA: Saving the burned ear. Texas Med 63:58, 1967.
Grant, DA, Finley, ML, and Coers, CR: Early management of the burned ear. Plast Reconstruct Surg 44(2):161, 1969.
Greminger, RF, Elliot, RA, and Rapperport, A: Antibiotic iontophoresis for the management of burned ear chondritis. Plast Reconstruct Surg 66(3):356, 1980.
Helvig, B: Trauma to the integument: Burns. In Howell, E, Widra, L, and Hill, MG (eds): Comprehensive Trauma Nursing Theory and Practice. Scott, Foresman and Co., Glenview, IL, 1988, p 378.
Hummel, RP: Clinical Burn Therapy: A Management and Prevention Guide. John Wright PSG, Boston, 1982.
Klein, RM, Bersen, RL, and Seidenberg, B: Firework burns of choroid and retina. Am J Ophthalmol 97(5):643, 1984.
Kroll, SS and Gerow, FJ: Sulfamylon allergy simulating chondritis. Plast Reconstruct Surg 80(2):298, 1987.
Mannis, MJ, Miller, RB, and Krachmer, JH: Contact thermal burns of the cornea from electric curling irons. Am J Ophthlamol 98(3):336, 1984.
Martin, R. Yonkers, AJ, and Yarlington, CT: Pericondritis of the ear. Laryngoscope 86:664, 1976.

Perry, AW, et al: Mafenide induced "psuedochondritis." Journal of Burn Care and Rehabilitation 9(2):145, 1988.

Pfister, RR: Chemical corneal burns. Int Ophthalmol Clin 24(2):157, 1984.

Pfister, RR: The effects of chemical injury on the ocular surface. Ophthalmology 90(6):601, 1983.

Purdue, GF and Hunt, JL: Chondritis of the burned ear: A preventable complication. Am J Surg 152:257, 1986.

Salisbury, RE, Newman, NM, and Dineldein, GP: Manual of Burn Therapeutics: An Interdisciplinary Approach. Little, Brown, & Co, Boston, 1983.

Stanley, JA: Strong alkali burns of the eye. N Engl J Med 273(23):1265, 1965.

Stewart, RC and Beason, ES: Chondritis of the ear: A method of treatment. J Trauma 19(9):686, 1979.

Wagner, MM: care of the Burn-Injured Patient. PSG Publishing, Littleton, Massachusetts, 1981.

Warpeha, RL: Resurfacing the burned face. Clin Plast Surg 8(2):255, 1981.

Chapter 11

DOREEN J. KONOP

PERINEAL BURNS

Although any burn is a potentially serious injury, the location of the burn is very important in assessing the severity and in planning and implementing the care for the patient. Burns to the perineum or genital area are more serious not only because of their delicate location, but also because they may pose particular problems related to treatment and wound healing. Perineal burns may result in scarring and functional impairments and, at the very least, increase a patient's anxieties because of the changes in body image as well as the pain and discomfort that is experienced. It is important that perineal burns be evaluated and treated by a physician and nursing staff who are trained and qualified in burn care. Thus, admittance to a burn unit is appropriate and necessary.

PATIENT HISTORY

The nurse obtains a history of the burn injury and notes the type, extent, and depth of the burn. Perineal burns are most often seen in patients whose injuries cover an extensive body surface area or are secondary to abuse. Flame injuries, contact burns, and scalds account for the majority of burns to the perineum, although they can result from chemical or electrical sources as well. Very often these burns may be the result of abuse and must be assessed, investigated, and reported.

The causative agent should be noted. If the burn resulted from a chemical injury, the chemical, duration of contact, and first aid care provided are determined. The local poison control center is contacted for more information on the particular chemical agent. If it is an electrical injury, the voltage and amperage of current and the duration of contact are determined. The patient's cardiac status is a priority for assessment.

Also obtained is pertinent historic information including the patient's age, past medical history, recent surgeries, allergies, alcohol consumption, tobacco use, social drug use, and present medications. Any emergency or prehospital care provided to the patient, including initial wound care, IV fluid administration, and medications, constitutes important information in planning immediate care.

A thorough history regarding perineal burns in children and adults is warranted. Circumstances and events surrounding the burn injury must be investigated and reported as indicated. Abuse is frequently a cause of perineal burns.

Note the level of pain. Perineal burns are often very painful due to their sensitive location on the body. The pain level will vary depending on the depth of the burn injury and the percent of body surface burned. Superficial and partial-thickness burns are extremely sensitive to tactile stimuli. Thus, any wound manipulation will cause significant pain and discomfort to the patient. Although tactile sensation is usually not present in full-thickness burns, most wounds will include some areas of partial-thickness injury, and therefore are painful also.

Anxiety and fear are usually experienced by all patients with burn injuries, especially when they involve the genital or perineal area. Although not always verbalized, many concerns exist among these patients regarding sexuality, function, and appearance.

PHYSICAL ASSESSMENT

Inspection

The appearance of the wound depends on the type and depth of burn (Color Plates 26 and 27). (Refer to Chapter 2, page 21, and Chapter 3, page 28.) The site or location of perineal burns differ in men and women due to anatomic differences. Perineal burns in the woman most often involve the area of the inner thighs and pubis. Rarely is the vulva affected because it is shielded and protected and is generally spared from direct burn trauma. However, the labia may become swollen and tender due to generalized edema formation. In males, the genitalia are exposed, less protected, and therefore more vulnerable to burn injuries (Color Plate 28). However, adjacent areas such as the groin or thighs are often found to be more severely injured. Gross edema formation of the penis and scrotum can be seen initially with most perineal burns. This edema resolves very slowly and is a great source of discomfort for the male patient.

Unfortunately, perineal burns are also seen in injuries sustained as a result of abuse, neglect, or assault. Children may be victims of abuse in instances precipitated by unsuccessful toilet training, incontinence, or careless bathing practices. Children who suffer immersion scalds will likely have burns to the buttocks and feet as well as the perineum. It is the nurse's and physician's responsibility to report any suspicion of abuse.

Recent attention has also been focused on spouse abuse, whereby domestic violence results in physical injury to husband or wife. These injuries may take the form of intentional scalds to various areas of the body, including genitalia. The documented incidence of this type of assault is misleading, mainly due to the reluctance of the victim to discuss the circumstances of the occurrence.

Finally, the elderly population has also been identified as being at risk of burn injuries related to abuse. Elderly abuse often takes the form of bathtub scalds or immersion accidents where the individual may have been left unattended or unsupervised during the time of the bath. This can result in severe burns to the perineum, buttocks, back, and legs. Lack of mobility and lack of independence, along with bowel or bladder control problems, help to make the elderly patient extremely vulnerable to abuse or neglect.

Urine Output

Urine output is a good indication of renal blood flow and adequacy of fluid replacement. Output will be low if the patient is hypovolemic. In perineal burns, edema formation of the genitals may cause obstruction of the urethra. A Foley catheter, necessary to maintain patency and to monitor the patient's intake and output status, should be inserted as soon as possible postburn.

ROUTINE CARE

General treatment of perineal burns essentially consists of local wound care, using an open technique if possible. Unlike other types of burns, aggressive surgical excision and grafting is not initially recommended. Rather, a conservative approach is more widely practiced because of the sensitive location of such burns and more importantly, because of the unique characteristics of the skin covering the genital and perineal area. The skin is naturally redundant, with many folds and creases. Despite burn trauma to the skin, many of the dermal appendages may actually be spared, thus allowing the wound to heal. It is important, then, to avoid traumatizing or destroying any remaining skin cells that are capable of re-epithelialization. For these reasons, the management of perineal burns focuses on promotion of healing and prevention of infection, using nonsurgical wound care practices. Topical antimicrobial creams and/or biologic dressings may be used.

If surgical excision and grafting are necessary, hygiene, immobilization, and positioning are extremely important for successful graft "take." Bedrest is indicated with legs abducted. A Foley catheter is used for urinary drainage and can also serve as a type of stent with penile burns.

NURSING CONSIDERATIONS

Several special considerations are related to the general care of perineal burns. Careful attention to cleanliness is necessary because of the risk of contamination and infection from contact with feces. Contact with urine is harmful because its inherent acidity causes excoriation and further trauma to the tissues. It is important to wash the burn wounds gently but thoroughly after bowel movements or urination. Frequent reapplication of topical creams will also be required. Although it is advantageous to use an open technique, dressings are usually necessary when caring for perineal burns in infants and children. The dressings should be minimal and nonconstricting and can be held in place with diapers if needed. Excessive pressure should be avoided.

Gross edema formation occurs initially in the genital and perineal area. Placement of a Foley catheter soon after the injury is necessary to ensure unobstructed urine flow. A suprapubic catheter may also be used. Also, bowel movements may be extremely painful for the patient with perineal burns. The nurse must monitor the patient's elimination status closely, as severe constipation or fecal impactions can result from the patient's reluctance to have a bowel movement.

Finally, a perineal burn is a physically and emotionally traumatic injury. Pain, embarrassment, and anxiety are important issues that the nurse should consider when formulating a plan of care. The nurse must act with sensitivity, not only in educating the patient but in maintaining his or her privacy and dignity. A patient's questions and concerns regarding sexual function and appearance need to be addressed openly and honestly. Because patient's may be reluctant to ask questions, other sources, such as counseling, need to be made available to the patient. The developmental stage of the patient helps guide the referral to appropriate resource persons.

NURSING CARE PLAN: PERINEAL BURNS

Nursing Priorities

1. Promote wound healing
2. Maintain elimination status (bowel/bladder)
3. Minimize and control pain
4. Minimize or prevent complications
5. Meet psychosocial needs of patient
6. Provide appropriate patient education

Nursing Diagnosis: Skin Integrity, Impairment Of: Actual

(Also refer to Chapter 4, page 64, Skin Integrity, impairment of)

May Be Related To:

- Perineal burn wound
- Graft site

Possibly Evidenced by: Disruption of skin surface and destruction of skin layers.

Desired Patient Outcomes: The patient will experience closure of burn wounds and complete "take" of grafts, which will allow for maximum elimination status and sexual functions.

Interventions	Rationale
INDEPENDENT	
• Perform all wound care procedures using sterile technique. Use protective isolation practices as necessary.	• Burn patients have a decreased resistance to infection. Aseptic technique and protective isolation helps to reduce the introduction of infectious organisms and prevents cross-contamination.
• Shave pubic hair, as well as other hair on or near burned areas, as often as needed during healing.	• Hair contains bacteria and is a good medium for bacterial growth. Removing hair helps to limit possible contamination of burn wound.
• If young child, not toilet-trained: ○ Cleanse and redress wounds frequently ○ Impregnate gauze pads with topical agent, place directly on wounds, and apply diaper to help secure dressings into place	• Wounds must be kept free of fecal and urinary materials to prevent further trauma or infection, or both.
• If adult with fecal or urinary incontinence: ○ Utilize Foley or condom catheters as necessary ○ Other methods as necessary: fecal incontinent pouches, special low-residue diets	• Cleanliness of wounds must be maintained as much as possible; otherwise, further trauma or infection, or both, may occur.

Nursing Diagnosis: Skin Integrity, Impairment Of: Actual
(*Continued*)

Interventions	Rationale
○ Secure dressings with adult diapers as described earlier	
○ Rectal Foley catheter to gravity drainage may be indicated for management of fecal incontinence.	
• Wash wounds twice daily, or as necessary, with appropriate antibacterial soap. Gently debride any loose skin or eschar from genitalia.	• Loose, necrotic tissue and exudate from burns must be cleansed in order to protect wounds from infection and to promote healing. A very conservative approach is necessary in debriding burns on the penis or scrotum. The skin on these areas is very loose and wrinkled. Spontaneous healing of these wounds often occurs because tiny areas or islands of epithelial tissue remain viable despite deep burn injury.
• Cleanse perineal area gently but thoroughly after bowel movements and urination.	• Fecal contamination or frequent exposure of burn wounds to urine may cause skin irritation, infection, or delayed wound healing.
• Observe and assess burn wounds daily noting progression of wound healing.	• Wound healing must be assessed, documented, and communicated to physician in order to monitor appropriateness of care.
• Assess burn wounds for signs of infection: pus, foul odor, or unexpected redness and edema. Monitor vital signs for temperature trends, and notify physician if temperature elevates to 38.5°C or above.	• Early recognition of infection allows for prompt treatment.
• Perform Foley catheter care twice a day. Observe urine for presence of sediment, mucus, or blood.	• A significant number of urinary tract infections occur in patients with extensive perineal burns and indwelling Foley catheters.

COLLABORATIVE

Interventions	Rationale
• Obtain wound cultures and sensitivities as per burn unit routine or if purulent drainage is present on burn. Obtain blood and urine culture if patient's temperature is above 38.5°C.	• Cultures will determine the type of organism as well as sensitivities for appropriate antibiotic therapy.
• Apply topical antimicrobial agent per physician order. Use open technique in burn wound care if possible; use bed cradle, and position legs spread apart.	• Antimicrobial agents will decrease surface colonization on burn wound. Open technique allows for constant observation of burn wound; eliminates bulky,

Interventions	Rationale
	uncomfortable and difficult dressings; and facilitates cleansing and reapplication of topical agents. Also, organisms thrive in dark, moist environments; using a bed cradle and spreading legs helps to avoid this.

Nursing Diagnosis: Pain

(Also refer to Chapter 9, page 169 "Pain")

May Be Related To:

• Exposure of nerve endings

Possibly Evidenced By: Verbalizations, anorexia, crying, screaming, facial grimaces, clenched teeth, knotted brow, immobilization of area, insomnia, and restlessness.

Desired Patient Outcomes: The patient will experience reduction in level of pain, as evidenced by verbalizations, nonverbal cues, vital signs, and use of rating scale.

Interventions	Rationale
INDEPENDENT	
• When scrotal edema is present, elevate scrotum with folded towels, sheepskin, or fluffed gauze when patient is in bed, and provide scrotal support when patient is out of bed.	• Elevation will aid in decreasing edema and associated pain. Scrotal support will decrease the perineal discomfort associated with standing, walking, or sitting.
• Ensure proper position of Foley catheter and drainage tubing. Tape or secure catheter to patient's leg to prevent excessive tension and contracture formation.	• Improper positioning or excess tension on Foley catheter can cause trauma and significant discomfort to the patient.
COLLABORATIVE	
• Use air bed or fluidized bed. Provide foam cushions when patient is sitting.	• Air or water bed may lessen discomfort associated with prolonged periods of bedrest for patients with perineal burns. Foam pads or pillows will cushion seats and make sitting more comfortable for the patient.

Nursing Diagnosis: Self-Concept, Disturbance In.

(Refer to Chapter 7, page 89.)

Nursing Diagnosis:
Sexual Dysfunction

May Be Related To:

- Perineal burns—discomfort and pain
- Physical disfigurement due to perineal burns and scar formation.
- Psychologic impact of burn injury

Possibly Evidenced By: Verbalizations of problem and actual or perceived limitations imposed by burn wound and/or therapy.

Desired Patient Outcomes: The patient will identify reasons for sexual dysfunction and identify appropriate remedies and alternative, satisfying/acceptable sexual practices.

Interventions	Rationale
INDEPENDENT	
• Encourage expression of feelings about perceived sexual dysfunction; have patient describe in own words.	• Development of appropriate interventions is based upon initial identification.
• Encourage patient and significant others to verbalize feelings regarding the perineal burns.	• Identifies feelings, fears, and misconceptions so that they may be dealt with constructively.
• Reinforce information given by physician.	• Many grafting procedures may be necessary to regain function.
• Assess patient's sexual relationship prior to trauma and appropriately suggest counseling and alternative methods.	• Interventions will be more successful if a satisfying sexual relationship was previously developed.
• Encourage use of lubricants as necessary.	• Healed skin will be more sensitive, dry, and itchy.
• Provide appropriate information regarding wound healing.	• Allows patient to understand realistically how long it will take for the wound to heal and expectations for grafting.

Nursing Diagnosis: Fear

May Be Related To:

- Fear of disfigurement
- Threat to self-concept
- Knowledge deficit

Possibly Evidenced By: Nervousness, uncooperative behavior, withdrawn or isolated behavior, verbalizations, sweating and wringing of hands.

Desired Patient Outcomes: The patient will experience reduction of fear manifested by discussion and verbalization of issues and concerns.

Interventions	Rationale
INDEPENDENT	
• Provide thorough explanations to patient and family regarding burn care. Patient should be informed of all tests,	• Patient education is necessary to help allay fears and anxieties and to increase patient compliance with treatments.

Interventions	**Rationale**
procedures, or activities prior to their performance.	
• Assess patients level of understanding. Elicit information that would indicate patient's comprehension of material.	• Patient may require reinforcement of previously taught material.
• Encourage patient to verbalize physical and emotional feelings. Allow issues of sexuality and body image to be freely discussed.	• A perineal burn is a great source of apprehension because it threatens a patient's perceived sexuality, self-esteem, and self-image.

COLLABORATIVE

• Assist patient, if necessary, in discussing personal concerns with physician. Encourage patient to ask questions.	• Nurse must act as a patient advocate in helping to facilitate effective communication.
• Use support systems such as social service, pastoral care, or psychiatric consultants to provide counseling and emotional support.	• Comprehensive care of the burn patient requires attention to emotional needs as well as physical needs.

Nursing Diagnosis:
Knowledge Deficit

(Refer to Chapter 9, page 176, Knowledge Deficit)

Nursing Diagnosis: Infection, Potential For

May Be Related To:

• Increased contamination from bacteria in perineal area

redness, tenderness, swelling, and amount of drainage).

Possibly Evidenced By:

Elevated temperature; positive wound cultures; changes in wound status (odor,

Desired Patient Outcomes:

The patient will remain free from infection

Interventions	**Rationale**
INDEPENDENT	
• Wash wounds gently but thoroughly after bowel movements and urination.	• Helps decrease contamination.
• Ensure all dressings are nonconstricting. Avoid excessive pressure.	• Prevents trauma to healing and injured tissues.

Nursing Diagnosis: Infection, Potential For (*Continued*)

Interventions	Rationale
• Protect the patient's need for privacy and modesty during treatments.	• Embarrassment and modesty are common reactions; it may be difficult for the patient to express these.

(Refer to Chapter 4 for other etiologies, manifestations, desired patient outcomes, interventions.)

Nursing Diagnosis: Social Isolation

(Refer to Chapter 7, page 90 for etiology, manifestations, desired patient outcomes, and interventions.)

Nursing Diagnosis: Coping, Ineffective Family/Individual

(Refer to Chapter 7, page 92 for etiology, manifestations, desired patient outcomes, and interventions.)

Nursing Diagnosis: Post-Trauma Response

(Refer to Chapter 7, page 93 for etiology, manifestations, desired patient outcomes, and interventions.)

Nursing Diagnosis: Grieving

(Refer to Chapter 7, page 94 for etiology, manifestations, desired patient outcomes, and interventions.)

Nursing Diagnosis: Adjustment, Impaired

(Refer to Chapter 7, page 95 for etiology, manifestations, desired patient outcomes, and interventions.)

Nursing Diagnosis: Powerlessness

(Refer to Chapter 7, page 96 for etiology, manifestations, desired patient outcomes, and interventions.)

Nursing Diagnosis: Anxiety

May Be Related To:

- Uncertainty regarding future sexual functioning
- Uncertainty regarding future elimination patterns

(Refer to Chapter 7, page 98 for etiologies, manifestations, desired patient outcomes, and interventions.)

Nursing Diagnosis: Family Process, Alteration In

(Refer to Chapter 7, page 97 for etiology, manifestations, desired patient outcomes, and interventions.)

Nursing Diagnosis: Parenting, Alteration In

(Refer to Chapter 7, page 105 for etiology, manifestations, desired patient outcomes, and interventions.)

BIBLIOGRAPHY

Doenges, M, et al. Nursing Care Plans, ed 2. FA Davis, Philadelphia, 1989.

Feller, I and Grabb, WC: Reconstruction and Rehabilitation of the Burned Patient. Chapter 78. National Institute for Burn Medicine, Ann Arbor, Michigan, 1979.

Furnas, DW and McCrow, JB: Resurfacing the genital area. Clin Plast Surg 7(2): 235, 1980.

McDougall, WS et al: The thermally injured perineum. J Urol 121(3):320 1979.

Sawhney, CP: Management of burn contractures of the perineum. Plast Reconstruct Surg 72(6):837, 1983.

Weimer, C, Goldfarb, IW, and Slater, H: Multidisciplinary approach to working with burn victims of child abuse. Journal of Burn Care and Rehabilitation 9(1):79 1988.

Chapter 12

MADELEINE T. MARTIN

BURNS OF THE HANDS AND FEET

Burns of the hands and feet are both similar to and different from burns of other parts of the body. Similarities include assessment criteria, emergency treatment measures, and possible sources of tissue damage such as electricity, chemicals, and flames. Differences are related primarily to the unique and important anatomic structure of the hands and feet, the functional importance of both, and their sensory role—particularly of the hands.

Except for the palms and soles, anatomically the hands and feet have relatively thin dermal and epidermal layers protecting a complex structure of bones, joints, muscles, nerves, and vascular bed. Thus, tissue damage more easily exposes these structures, increasing the severity of injury and having long-term implications for rehabilitation and maintenance of function.

Both hands and feet have great functional importance for patients. Injury to the foot affects mobility. The hand, a highly specialized organ, is important for both delicate and sensitive maneuvers, as well as for tasks requiring gripping power and strength. Even small injuries render the patient dependent on others for many self-care tasks. The potential also exists for a forced occupation change if the person suffers long-term loss of fine and gross hand movements.

As sensory organs, the hands are particularly important. Burn injury affects this sensation in varying ways throughout the course of recovery. During the acute phase, pain severity may have physiologic and psychosocial implications. In the later and posthealing phases, scar tissue has been found to be less sensitive, affecting a patient's responses to environmental stimuli.

PATIENT HISTORY

Initially, a history is obtained of the events surrounding the injury. As for any emergency, the first priority is to ensure that there are no life-threatening injuries. The history of the accident will assist in determining the cause of the burn (i.e., thermal, electrical, chemical, or frostbite), as well as length of contact with the skin.

212

The past medical history should be obtained to determine other management issues such as diabetes, hypertension, and so forth. Patient age also contributes to the assessment of the severity of the injury, with older adults being at greater risk for latent degenerative disease processes, and children under age 2 for immature renal and immune systems and problems with forced immobility during treatment. The date of the patient's last tetanus immunization should be determined, and initial first aid measures should be noted.

In extremity injuries the patient's occupation and left- or right-handedness are important assessment parameters for nursing management. Severity of pain should also be determined as an indication of the amount of initial sensory alteration and possible tissue damage. Assessment of pain is important in planning interventions to decrease the patient's anxiety and promote comfort.

PHYSICAL ASSESSMENT

Inspection is the most important assessment parameter in burns of the hands and feet. The entire extremity should be inspected, including integrity of the skin, tendons, joints, muscles, vascular bed, and nerve response. The exact depth of injury may not be immediately known. The nurse should observe for exposure of underlying structures. When underlying structures such as tendons are not affected, indicators of depth of skin damage are similar as for all burn injuries.

The percentage of total hand or foot surface injured should be estimated, as well as the location of the injury. Palmar damage versus dorsal damage will have implications for rehabilitation, as will the amount of joint involvement.

Assessing the status of tissue perfusion is important. More superficial burns will show signs of blanching with pressure. Deeper full-thickness burns conversely show no evidence of capillary refill. This should be an ongoing assessment parameter during the early course of treatment because changes in tissue perfusion may indicate increasing tissue damage or peripheral constriction due to circumferential burns and inelastic eschar formation.

The presence or absence as well as the quality of peripheral pulses should be assessed at least hourly for the first 36 hours to determine functional blood supply to the extremity. Use of a Doppler ultrasound may be necessary if pulses are difficult to palpate.[1] It is important to monitor pulse rate over time because it serves as an indicator of both tissue perfusion status and cardiovascular status. Weak or absent radial or pedal pulses may indicate circulatory constriction. In electrical injuries, arrhythmias may be present, indicating cardiac instability and a need for monitoring.

Types of Injuries

(Refer also to Chapter 3, Types of Burns, page 28.)

The types of heat tissue injuries are classified by causative agents and are chemical, electrical, flame, and frostbite. Assessment criteria for flame injury are as described in the previous section.

Industrial chemical accidents frequently involve the hands and feet. Appearance varies, based on the causative agent, from soft and serous to leatherlike. Without aggressive management, tissue destruction may continue up to 72 hours postinjury. Treatment for most chemicals focuses on removing the damaging agent by flushing with copious amounts of fluids.

The hands and feet are frequent sites of current exit and entry wounds in electrical injury. Local tissue destruction is often less than the underlying tissue destruction that may have occurred to other body organs. The appearance of the wound is usually circumscribed, dry, charred, and depressed, involving cutaneous, subcutaneous, and possibly deeper tissue (Color Plates 29 and 30).

Frostbite is the necrosis of tissue due to extreme cold, either from overexposure or direct contact, and is seen in the colder regions of the country. Hands and feet are the most vulnerable to frostbite, as are the ears and face. The area appears pale and waxy with some swelling. It becomes necrotic with black eschar forming and possible bone damage (Color Plate 31). Circulation to the extremity distal to the injury may be compromised. The treatment of choice is rapid rewarming, with water immersion of the affected part being the most effective method. Water kept at from 38.7 to 40.6°C (100 to 105°F) for 20 to 30 minutes is acceptable.[2] The most important concern is to revitalize tissue without causing further damage. Therefore, rubbing is contraindicated, as is overexposure of the hand or foot to heat sources such as campfires or space heaters.

DIAGNOSTIC STUDIES

If a large surface area of hands and feet is involved, or if the injury accompanies burns of other body areas, laboratory work discussed previously such as complete blood count (CBC) and blood urea nitrogen (BUN) should be obtained. Discussed here are those studies of most specific importance for injury to the hands and feet.

X-rays: To determine bone and joint injury.
Intravenous fluorescein: Useful in assessing the functional circulation of the skin and in reliability discriminating between full- and partial-thickness injury.[3]
WBC: May indicate infection during course of recovery.
Albumin, hemoglobin, and myoglobin: Indicate deep tissue damage and are especially important in electrical injuries in which urine may be reddish-black.
ECG: For indicating dysrhythmias and myocardial ischemia which may occur with electrical injuries.
Photographs of burns: Provide baseline and ongoing documentation of the injury and healing.

NURSING CARE PLAN: BURNS OF THE HANDS AND FEET

Nursing Priorities

1. Support tissue perfusion
2. Maintain function through positioning and appropriate range of motion (ROM) exercises
3. Minimize/control pain
4. Prevent infection
5. Assist patient in meeting dependency needs
6. Meet psychosocial needs of the patient and significant others

Nursing Diagnosis: Tissue Perfusion, Alteration In

(Refer to Chapter 9, Tissue Perfusion, Alteration in, page 164)

May Be Related To:

- Decreased circulating blood volume from the fluid shift and the tourniquet effect of circumferential burns
- Vascular injury from deep partial- and full-thickness burns

Possibly Evidenced By: Diminished capillary refill; skin that is cool, pale, clammy; lack of sensation to affected extremity; deep pain; diminished or absent peripheral pulses; swollen extremity; tight skin; compartment pressure greater than 30 mm of H_2O.

Desired Patient Outcomes: The patient will experience normal capillary refill and skin color in uninjured areas; pulses maintained and equal; normal sensation.

Interventions	Rationale
INDEPENDENT	
• Assess color, sensation (for temperature, pressure), movement and peripheral pulses for quality and presence (Color Plates 32, 33, and 34). Utilize a Doppler device as needed.	• These parameters are indicated of circulatory status of the extremity. A diminished supply of O_2 to tissues resulting from impaired tissue perfusion causes tissue death.
• Elevate extremity. If hand, elevate above the level of the heart. If foot, maintain patient in supine position with foot elevated.[4]	• Support physiologic mechanisms to decrease or minimize edema and promote venous return.
• Remove anything circumferentially surrounding the extremities such as rings, blood pressure cuff, bracelets.	• With edema formation, pressure may reduce perfusion resulting in further tissue damage.
• Investigate complaints of deep or throbbing ache or numbness.	• These are indicators of decreased perfusion.
• Encourage and assist in active and passive range of motion exercise.	• Promotes circulation through muscle activity.
COLLABORATIVE	
• Assist with escharotomy or fasciotomy, if indicated (Color Plate 35).	• Enhances circulation by relieving constriction caused by edema formation under inelastic eschar and relieves vascular occlusion.
○ This is usually done in the first 48 hours postinjury.	
○ Incisions are continued over involved joints.	

Nursing Diagnosis: Tissue Perfusion, Alteration In (*Continued*)

Interventions

○ When digits are involved in addition to extremity excisions, excisions are made on each side of the burned digit.
○ The patient should experience no direct discomfort, as the incisions are made only down to normal tissue and full-thickness burns destroy nerve endings.

Rationale

Nursing Diagnosis: Skin Integrity, Impairment Of, Actual

(Refer to Chapter 4, Skin Integrity, Impairment Of, page 64)

May Be Related To:

• Burn wound
• Graft site
• Donor site

Possibly Evidenced By: Disruption of skin surface and destruction of skin layers.

Desired Patient Outcomes: The patient will experience restoration of skin integrity through natural healing or surgical grafting with maximum restoration of function.

Interventions

INDEPENDENT

• Promote good hygiene, comfort, and prevent physical injury through dressings.

• Observe for signs of necrosis or tissue death (increased pain, separation of graft edges, increased redness, or burning.)
• Cleanse wound and change dressing.

○ After washing and rinsing and before reapplying dressing, obtain wound culture at least weekly.
○ Loose eschar may be removed at this time either on dressing or manually.

Rationale

• Wound healing depends on adequate nutritional support and protection of the wound for new tissue growth or grafting.
• Increasing tissue damage may indicate poor perfusion, inadequate nutrition, or infection.

• Allows for wound examination. Manual cleansing debrides wound, promotes healing, and decreases wound contamination.
• Accepted goals of dressing change include:
1. Minimizing infection
2. Removing dead tissue

Interventions	**Rationale**

Interventions:

○ Apply dressing as ordered. If impregnated with a topical agent, avoid contact with uninjured skin.
• For extremities and digits, avoid wrapping circumferentially, if possible. Vertical strips should be applied.
• Prevent skin surface contact (e.g., wrap each burned finger or toe separately[5]).

• Prevent unnecessary trauma to wound area (use cradles; moisten dressings before removal only if adherent; and dress carefully).

COLLABORATIVE

• Refer to dietitian/nutritional support team to establish nutritional needs.

• Work collaboratively with occupational and physical therapy (OT/PT) team to maximize functional ability of hand or foot.
• Encourage active and passive ROM exercises to burned extremity from early postburn course.

• During dressing application:
  ○ Put hand in a position to maintain joint function and minimize contractures (wrist dorsiflexed; metacarpophalangeal joints flexed; interphalangeal joints extended or slightly flexed 20 degrees; thumb in moderate abduction[6]).
  ○ Position foot in functional (90 degrees) position with use of splint rather than footboard to maintain constant positioning.
• Exercise unburned foot and especially the unburned hand.[7]

Rationale:

3. Maintaining integrity of uninjured skin

• As edema forms or drainage saturates the gauze and dries, constriction may result, with circulation impairment.
• Prevents adherence of one wound surface to another it may be touching and promotes healing.
• Additional trauma can further increase severity of injury and prevent wound closure.

• Wound healing depends on necessary nutritional requirements being met based on patient weigh, age, body surface area, and percent of body surface injured.
• Rehabilitative care begins at the time of admission.

• Exercise maintains joint mobility and strengthens muscle tone. Input from the entire burn team is necessary to plan and safely implement exercise plan. Only an experienced therapist should perform passive ROM exercises to prevent damage to healing tissues. Exercise is generally contraindicated in the early periods following grafting. Maintaining immobilization of graft areas promotes healing.
• Goal of positioning is to promote optimal functioning and prevention of "claw hand" deformity (Color Plate 36).

• Studies indicate loss of strength and coordination in unburned extremities at discharge.

Nursing Diagnosis: Mobility, Impaired Physical

(Refer to Chapter 9, page 174, for etiology, manifestations, desired patient outcomes, and interventions.)

Nursing Diagnosis: Sensory-Perceptual Alteration: Tactile

May Be Related To:

- Decreased sensation in scar tissue due to poor innervation
- Altered tissue perfusion with burns of the extremities
- Injury to nerve endings

Possibly Evidenced By: Reported change in sensory acuity.

Desired Patient Outcomes: Patient is aware of altered stimuli response and is able to compensate for it.

Interventions

INDEPENDENT

- Assist patient in determining difference in sensory response between burned and unburned tissue.

- Advise patient against exposure to extremes of hot or cold environments and surfaces.

- Advise against restrictive clothing and jewelry.

Rationale

- Knowledge of difference can increase patient's awareness of need for protective measures in extreme hot and cold environments.
- Decreased tactile response may inhibit appropriate safety response, causing localized vasoconstriction or vasodilation and subsequent tissue damage.
- Constriction prevents adequate venous return, impairing circulation and resulting in possible tissue damage.

Nursing Diagnosis: Self-Care Deficit

May Be Related To:

- Burns to hands, which may limit functional capacity to feed, bathe, dress, toilet oneself; due to pain of burn, edema, or restrictive dressings

Desired Patient Outcomes: Patient's care needs are met by others, but with increased ability for self-care patient ultimately demonstrates ability to complete self-care tasks.

Possibly Evidenced By: Inability to provide personal self-care.

Interventions	Rationale

INDEPENDENT

• Assist with mobility, bathing, feeding, and other self-care activities in an unhurried manner. Refer to PT and/or OT for possible alternative devices that can maximize self-care abilities.

• When patients cannot meet their own needs, they must be helped by others. Patients may already be experiencing decreased self-esteem due to inability to care for self. An unhurried pace will allow for communication and assistance in self-care to best of patient's ability.

• Promote comfort and prevent complications by positioning.

• Restful position with minimal pressure on any point promotes comfort and decreases potential for complications related to pressure. Splints and braces individual to the patient are modified regularly to avoid pressure points.

Nursing Diagnosis: Anxiety

(Refer to Chapter 7, page 98 for etiology, manifestations, desired patient outcomes, and interventions.)

Nursing Diagnosis: Infection, Potential For

(Refer to Chapter 9, page 171, for etiology, manifestations, desired patient outcomes, and interventions.)

Nursing Diagnosis: Nutrition, Alteration In, Less Than Body Requirements

May Be Related To:

• Inability to feed self

(Refer to Chapter 9, page 172, for etiologies, manifestations, desired patient outcomes, and interventions.)

Nursing Diagnosis: Pain

(Refer to Chapter 9, page 169 for etiology, manifestations, desired patient outcomes, and interventions.)

Nursing Diagnosis:
Social Isolation

(Refer to Chapter 7, page 90, for etiology, manifestations, desired patient outcomes, and interventions.)

Nursing Diagnosis: Coping,
Ineffective Family/Individual

(Refer to Chapter 7, page 92, for etiology, manifestations, desired patient outcomes, and interventions.)

Nursing Diagnosis:
Post-Trauma Response

(Refer to Chapter 7, page 93, for etiology, manifestations, desired patient outcomes, and interventions.)

Nursing Diagnosis: Fear

(Refer to Chapter 7, page 94, for etiology, manifestations, desired patient outcomes, and interventions.)

Nursing Diagnosis: Grieving

(Refer to Chapter 7, page 94, for etiology, manifestations, desired patient outcomes, and interventions.)

Nursing Diagnosis:
Adjustment, Impaired

(Refer to Chapter 7, page 95, for etiology, manifestations, desired patient outcomes, and interventions.)

Nursing Diagnosis: Powerlessness

(Refer to Chapter 7, page 96, for etiology, manifestations, desired patient outcomes, and interventions.)

Nursing Diagnosis: Family Process, Alteration In

(Refer to Chapter 7, page 97, for etiology, manifestations, desired patient outcomes, and interventions.)

Nursing Diagnosis: Parenting, Alteration In

(Refer to Chapter 7, page 105, for etiology, manifestations, desired patient outcomes, and interventions.)

Nursing Diagnosis: Self-Concept, Disturbance In

(Refer to Chapter 7, page 89, for etiology, manifestations, desired patient outcomes, and interventions.)

Nursing Diagnosis: Knowledge Deficit

(Refer to Chapter 9, page 176, for etiology, manifestations, desired patient outcomes, and interventions.)

REFERENCES

1. Brunner, L and Suddarth, D: Medical/Surgical Nursing, ed 6. JB Lippincott, Philadelphia, 1988, p 627.
2. Callaham, M: Hypothermia. In Kravis, T and Warner, C (eds): Emergency Medicine. Aspen Systems, Rockville, Maryland, 1983, p 433.
3. Hummel, R: Burn Therapy. John Wright – PSG, Boston, 1982, p 255.
4. Kenner, C, Guzzetta, C, and Dossey, B: Critical Care Nursing: Body-Mind-Spirit, ed 2. Little, Brown, & Co, Boston, 1985, p 832.
5. Moorhouse, M, Geissler, A, and Doenges, M: Nursing Care Plans. FA Davis, Philadelphia, 1984, p 281.
6. Artz, C, Moncrief, J, and Pruitt, P: Burns: A Team Approach. WB Saunders, Philadelphia, 1979, p 502.
7. Covey, M, et al: Return of hand function following major burns. Journal of Burn Care and Rehabilitation 8:224, 1987.

BIBLIOGRAPHY

Campbell, C: Nursing Diagnoses and Interventions in Nursing Practice. John Wiley & Sons, New York, 1984.

Carpentino, L. Handbook of Nursing Diagnosis. JB Lippincott, New York, 1984.

Howell, E, Widra, L, and Hill, M: Comprehensive Trauma Nursing. Scott, Foresman, and Company, Glenview, IL, 1988.

McLane, A (ed): Classification of Nursing Diagnosis. CV Mosby, St Louis, 1987.

Unit FOUR

CARE OF THE SPECIAL BURN PATIENT

Chapter 13

MELVA KRAVITZ
ELIZABETH I. HELVIG

CARE OF THE PREGNANT PATIENT WITH BURNS

NURSING ASSESSMENT

Mortality

Pregnant burn clients are uncommon because of two predominant characteristics of the hospitalized burn population: (1) approximately 80 percent of all burn victims are men or children, and (2) not all adult female burn patients are of childbearing age. Women who are of childbearing age when sustaining a major burn injury are estimated to have a pregnancy rate of 4 percent.[1] There is no difference in the cause of burns between pregnant and nonpregnant women nor does pregnancy reduce the likelihood of a woman sustaining burns severe enough to require hospitalization.[2] The lifestyle of pregnant women is generally to remain active and continue prepregnancy daily routines until near-term.

The mortality rate for the mother-child unit is altered drastically when the burn is greater than 50 percent total body surface area (TBSA). An analysis of 50 patients with burns in pregnancy revealed only 2 of 14 patients survived burns of 50 percent or greater TBSA.[3] In another report of 30 pregnant burn patients, 20 patients with burns less than 50 percent TBSA survived, whereas the remaining 10 patients, with greater than 50 percent TBSA burns, died.[4] Fetal survival is also related to the extent of the mother's burn. In this group of 30 pregnant women, there were 17 fetal survivors. Sixteen of the 17 fetal survivors belonged to mothers with TBSA burn of less than 50 percent. If the injury of the gravid patient is lethal, the pregnancy will usually terminate spontaneously prior to her death. In a group of 11 pregnant women with burns ranging from 3 to 93 percent TBSA, all mothers survived and eight babies survived.[5] Five of the women burned in the first trimester of pregnancy revealed that fetal mortality was high, with one mother aborting the fetus 45 days after the injury and another producing a stillbirth at 33 weeks. Fetal mortality during the first trimester did not appear to be directly related to the extent of the injury since two of five patients with burns less than 20 percent TBSA aborted. Premature delivery or stillbirth usually occurs within the first

225

5 days but a wide range of possibilities exists. In one group, six of seven lethally burned patients terminated their pregnancies from 2 to 36 days after injury.[6] In a case report a 17-year-old primapara, 16 weeks pregnant, sustained a 65 percent mostly full-thickness burn injury that resulted in maternal survival and the pregnancy progressing to term.[7]

In a report of 30 cases, there were eight cases in which maternal injury became lethal with all fetuses born spontaneously prior to maternal death, but seven were stillborn. The largest burn survived by both mother and fetus was 58 percent TBSA. No fetus survived if the burn covered greater than 60 percent of the mother's body surface area.[8] Spontaneous vaginal delivery occurred within 5 days after the burn in 9 of the 12 cases of fetal death. The remaining three stillborn fetuses were delivered spontaneously on the 7th, 13th, and 54th postburn days, respectively. A positive relationship was also found between the extent of maternal burn and the risk of premature labor leading to delivery. A 30 percent TBSA burn was found to be strongly related to the finding of premature labor. Seven of nine preterm deliveries occurred within 5 days after burn injuries of 24 to 97 percent TBSA.

In another study, maternal mortality was found to be 37 percent (7 of 19) when the burn involved 60 percent or more body surface area, whereas there were no maternal deaths in burns of less than 60 percent. Maternal deaths were directly related to respiratory problems, sepsis, renal failure, and liver failure. Infant mortality was 47 percent (9 of 19) and related to hypoxia, hyponatremia, sepsis, and prematurity.[9]

Etiology

The cause of burn injury to pregnant women appears to be no different than that in nonpregnant women, and pregnancy does not reduce the likelihood of major burn accidents. Most pregnant women sustain burns from flames, explosion injuries (motor vehicle accidents, house fires), hot liquids, or contact with a hot surface. Electrical injuries are rare. Pregnant women suffer burns on the job or away from home in the same proportion as nonpregnant women of childbearing age.[11] Today's pregnant women, like most women, are more exposed to dangers because more are working outside the home, often in jobs that are more hazardous and/or require travel.

Accidental injury is estimated to occur in 6 to 7 percent of all pregnancies. A prospective study of over 3000 pregnant patients indicated that motor vehicle accidents were a frequent cause of injury to pregnant patients. Motor vehicle injuries cause death nearly 10 times more frequently than other accidents for women in the reproductive years, with falls, burns, and firearm injuries being the next most frequent causes.[12] Fatigue, fainting spells, and hyperventilation commonly occur owing to the unpredictable physiologic changes of pregnancy. These factors, combined with the possible alterations in mobility associated with pregnancy, can lead to harmful situations.[13]

Burn injuries in pregnancy are caused by fires in buildings (house, trailer, and so on); motor vehicle accidents; aircraft accidents; ignition of flammable liquids or gases; hot water and grease; ignition of clothing by household appliances; ignition of clothing from flame; and lightning.[14] In a report of three cases, two pregnant women were burned in house fires and the third in a gas explosion at home.[15] In a report of 30 cases, most burns occurred at home and involved house fires (10), hot water (9), flammable liquids or gases (7), grease (2), or household appliances igniting clothing (2).[16] Burn injury in a different group of 30 pregnant women was due to flame burns in each case.[17]

The trimester status of 113 women was reported from the literature as 36 women (32 percent) in the first trimester, 45 (40 percent) in the second, and 32 (28 percent) in the third trimester.[18]

ANATOMIC/PHYSIOLOGIC CONSIDERATIONS

When dealing with the pregnant burned patient, there are really two separate patients being treated: the mother and the fetus. For the purpose of clarity of presentation, their care will be discussed separately but their conditions remain interchangeable until delivery or death of the fetus.

The pregnant patient undergoes physiologic and psychologic changes of enormous magnitude. A system review will reveal major changes, which will be discussed both as a normal response to pregnancy and as a pathophysiologic response to the burn injury.

Cardiovascular System

In the first trimester, the cardiac output begins to rise 20 to 30 percent during the first 10 weeks and reaches a peak at 24 weeks. The rise is gradual, at a rate to reach about 6 liters per minute at 10 weeks followed by an increase to about 7 liters per minute by 24 weeks, where it is maintained to term. This 40 to 50 percent increase in cardiac output may become an 80 to 100 percent increase if there are twins. The heart rate rises by 15 to 20 beats per minute during pregnancy to an average peak of about 80 to 95 beats per minute at term. While cardiac rate and output rise, the blood pressure remains normal in the first trimester.[19] However, blood pressure often falls during the second trimester, primarily the diastolic pressure, dropping an average of 5 to 15 mmHg. By the start of the third trimester, a rise toward normal occurs and persists to term.

Positional hypotension and diminished right ventricular return occur in the second and third trimesters when a pregnant patient lies on her back in the supine position because the uterus exerts pressure on the inferior vena cava, impeding venous return. For the burn patient, it may be critical to tip the right hip and buttock upward approximately 15 degrees into a slight left lateral decubitus position in order to restore or promote venous return. This maneuver may increase cardiac output by as much as 30 percent at term. If the patient has other injuries than the burn that preclude turning her, manually pushing the uterus to the left and holding it there may produce the same effect. Venous pressure rises progressively in the lower extremities secondary to the pressure on the inferior vena cava by the uterus and may lead to increased bleeding in accompanying leg injuries.

Peripheral vascular resistance is diminished, especially during the second and third trimesters and at term, and may lead to vasodilation instead of vasoconstriction in burned pregnant patients. This may be related to the placental production of vasodilating prostaglandins. This means that cold, clammy skin as a clinical sign of shock will be absent and that a larger volume of resuscitation fluid will be required for organ perfusion. Urine output of 30 to 50 ml per hour remains the hallmark of adequate fluid resuscitation in pregnant patients. All peripheral vasopressors, although they may restore maternal mean arterial pressure, further decrease uterine blood flow. The centrally acting vasopressors ephedrine and mephentermine may simultaneously restore maternal blood pressure and uterine blood flow.[20]

Blood plasma volume increases significantly by the middle of the second trimester and reaches a 50 percent or 40 to 70 ml/kg increase in total circulating maternal plasma volume by 34 weeks. Plasma volume increases out of proportion to the red blood cell (RBC) mass increase of 25 to 30 ml/kg, with a resultant physiologic dilutional anemia. In addition, total body water volume is increased by 6 to 8 liters, mostly in the placenta, amnionic fluid, and myometrium. The retained fluid will be even greater if peripheral edema is present. About 900 mEq of sodium is retained in pregnancy.[21] Central venous pressure measurements tend to be slightly higher in healthy pregnant women in comparison to healthy nonpregnant women but infusion of equal amounts of fluid leads to approximately equal incremental changes in central venous pressure. However, when shock is present, a significantly greater volume of fluid is required to restore the intravascular volume of the pregnant patient.

Immediately after delivery, the cardiac output is increased to 60 percent of normal until the excess volume can be excreted by the kidneys. The increased blood volume may permit a patient pregnant beyond the first trimester to lose 30 to 35 percent of her circulating blood volume before demonstrating clinical signs of hypovolemic shock. Prior to delivery, the fetus may be the first to respond to the loss of maternal blood volume since a decline in fetal heart rate may be due to either fetal hypoxemia or maternal hypovolemia.[22] The electrocardiogram is usually normal in the first and second trimester, but then exhibits marked changes as the heart is pushed up and rotated forward by the enlarging uterus in the third trimester. Persistent neck vein distention will be noted.

CARDIOVASCULAR PATHOPHYSIOLOGY

Pregnant women with major burn injury develop burn shock of a severity common to other burn patients. Since the fetus, uterus, and placenta are not considered vital organs, blood is preferentially shunted away from these organs and conserved for maternal vital organ flow. Maternal hypovolemia can cause fetal hypoxia and ischemic changes in the placenta. Maternal hypotension may lead to decreased uterine blood flow, fetal distress or death, and the onset of labor.

Early and adequate fluid resuscitation of the mother should ensure adequate placental, uterine, and fetal blood flow.[23] It should be anticipated that maternal resuscitation fluid requirements will be in excess of 4 ml/kg per percent TBSA burn in the first 24 hours, and adequate urine output must be maintained at all times to ensure adequate perfusion to the fetus. Hypovolemic shock may lead to acute ischemic changes in the placenta with subsequent fetal hypoxia and acidosis. After initial fluid resuscitation, the daily maintenance fluid volume will remain in excess of predicted volumes because of the greater plasma volume and persistent decreased peripheral resistance associated with normal pregnancy. Careful attention must be paid to hematocrit and hemoglobin in addition to circulating volume. The status of the fetus is assessed using electronic fetal monitors continuously.

Pulmonary System

As pregnancy progresses the diaphragm is elevated and the chest wall flares, resulting in a fixed, elevated rib cage and decreased chest wall compliance. The tracheobronchial tree is dilated and conductance is greatly increased. Pulmonary compliance remains unchanged while pulmonary resistance is reduced by half. Minute ventilation increases substantially with up to a 70 percent increase in tidal volume accompanied by a decrease of 15 to 20 percent in residual volume.[24] Total lung capacity is unchanged during pregnancy but is reduced in the first 2 weeks after delivery.

Increased levels of progesterone in pregnancy lower the threshold of the respiratory center to carbon dioxide thereby increasing minute ventilation by as much as 50 percent at term. Alveolar ventilation is increased by as much as 65 percent and oxygen consumption by 15 percent. A persistent compensated respiratory alkalosis and reduced buffering capacity results in a maternal decrease in pCO_2 to about 30 mmHg, an increase in pO_2 to about 105 mmHg, a compensatory decrease of approximately 4 mEq/liter in serum bicarbonate, and a pH within normal limits.[25] Hypoventilation may produce respiratory acidosis with a pCO_2 of 40 mmHg, which is a normal value in the nonpregnant woman. The effects of a decrease in maternal oxygenation are magnified in the fetus because the fetus exists at a pO_2 much lower than that of the mother; thus, a decrease in maternal oxygenation results in an additional decrease in the already marginally oxygenated fetus. Fetal hypoxic deaths occur at maternal levels of pO_2 that are compatible with maternal survival.[26]

PULMONARY PATHOPHYSIOLOGY

Smoke inhalation injury and hypoxia occur in pregnant patients and are managed similarly to a comparable injury in a nonpregnant patient with the exception of the use of more aggressive oxygen therapy to prevent fetal hypoxia. The intubated patient receives minute ventilation to maintain a pCO_2 in the 30 mmHg range and oxygen concentrations to maintain a pO_2 level of about 105 mmHg. Increased serum carbon monoxide levels may be present immediately postburn, as carbon monoxide freely crosses the placenta to bind with fetal hemoglobin molecules.[27] The diagnosis of carbon monoxide poisoning is made from the nursing history, physical signs and symptoms, and arterial blood gas (ABG) analysis. The most common incidence of carbon monoxide poisoning in burn patients is associated with house fires. The physical signs and symptoms are those of hypoxia. Laboratory ABG analysis will frequently reveal a normal partial pressure of oxygen in carbon monoxide poisoning but further analysis will reveal low oxygen saturation. Pulse oximetry is not useful in carbon monoxide poisoning because it measures the percentage of saturation of available binding sites (not including sites bound by carbon monoxide) and is thus falsely elevated.[28] Pulmonary edema is a common finding subsequent to carbon monoxide poisoning.

Patients with large surface burns without inhalation injury should also receive supplemental oxygen therapy to reduce the chance of hypoxia for the mother and fetus.[29] One technique to improve maternal oxygenation in the conscious patient is to place her in a semisitting position or on her left side. If the patient's condition requires the supine position, elevation of the right hip followed by manual displacement of the uterus to the left will promote vena caval blood flow and improved oxygenation.[30]

Pneumonia may be a more frequent complication in third trimester pregnancy as the efforts to limit atelectasis are less effective due to a fixed chest wall. Five of 19 patients in one series were reported to have developed pulmonary complications prior to pregnancy termination. One patient had a bilateral pleural effusion which responded to thoracentesis. Four women developed bilateral bronchopneumonia shortly before the loss of their fetuses.[31] In a series of 30 patients, three sustained an inhalation injury, five developed pneumonia, one developed pleural effusion, and one developed acute respiratory distress syndrome. In the inhalation injury group, maternal survival was one of three and fetal survival was zero of three.[32]

Abdominal Alterations

As pregnancy progresses, compartmentalization of the small intestine into the upper abdomen occurs and a general hypomotility of all smooth muscle results in delayed gastric emptying.[33] Sonography examination of the abdomen can demonstrate fetal cardiac movement, detect fetal heart tones, identify the location of the placenta, provide information to estimate fetal size, and often identify soft tissue masses that may represent retroplacental or pelvic hematomas. In the presence of intercurrent abdominal trauma with suspected intraperitoneal bleeding, a diagnostic Lazarus-Nelson peritoneal lavage kit may be used to tap the abdomen laterally rather than through the midline.[3]

Even if an exploratory laparotomy is indicated, a cesarean section is not necessary if the maternal hemorrhage can be controlled. A cesarean section is required if the risk of hypoxia or fetal distress outweighs the risk of prematurity, the uterus is ruptured, the gravid uterus interferes with adequate surgical therapy, or there is immediate or impending maternal death.

The amniotic fluid may be tested for signs of potential or possible fetal distress and fetal maturity. The presence of meconium suggests prior fetal anoxia although the condition may have resolved, erythrocytes suggest intrauterine bleeding, and white blood cells or bacteria suggest the presence of infection. The amniotic fluid may be tested for the lecithin/sphingomyelin (L/S) ratio to predict the maturity of the fetal lung.[35] Amniocentesis on an Rh-negative unsensitized patient must be followed by a full dose (300 mg) of RhoGAM, especially if the tap is bloody.[36] Patients who receive RhoGAM during pregnancy must repeat the full dose at or immediately after delivery. Electronic fetal monitoring permits the early detection of fetal hypoxia.

Gastric changes occur during pregnancy, producing lower tone of the esophageal sphincter, increased frequency of nonpropulsive contractions, and some stomach atony. Gastric acid and pepsin secretion are decreased and vitamin B_{12} is not readily absorbed in the stomach. Esophagitis or hiatal hernia, or both, is common.

ABDOMINAL PATHOPHYSIOLOGY

Abdominal trauma is managed as conservatively as possible and cesarean section is performed only in true emergencies. The gastrointestinal changes accompanying pregnancy result in decreased motility and esophageal reflux, thus making the delivery of enteral nutrition in the amount required by burn patients more difficult. These patients need continuous drip jejunal feedings to best meet metabolic demands. Because gastric motility is decreased and gastric emptying time is prolonged during pregnancy, these women are at greater risk for aspiration if unconscious or receiving general anesthesia. The prophylactic use of cimetadine against Curling's ulcer in pregnant patients has not been explored. Since gastric acid secretion is reduced in pregnancy, a conservative approach using antacids to control gastric pH is indicated as the first method of choice.

Electrolyte, Glucose, and Hematologic Alterations

Hypernatremia occurs in pregnancy due to the increased secretion of adrenocortical steroids, which enhances sodium reabsorption at the renal tubules. The administration of fluid to maintain serum sodium between 140 and 150 mEq/liter is used to regulate sodium balance. Hyponatremia in pregnant burn patients can result from dilution, losses through the burn wound, gastrointestinal drainage, diarrhea, diuresis, silver nitrate dressings, and prolonged hydrotherapy with tap water.

Hyperkalemia may not be seen in patients with burn injury unless extensive red blood cell hemolysis has occurred. A finding common to all patients with major burn injury is hypokalemia due to increased losses of potassium and increased cellular demands. The serum levels for the fetus are identical to those of the mother, so appropriate potassium replacement is necessary. Monitoring and corrective therapy for all electrolytes are performed as necessary to achieve physiologic balance.

Mild glucose intolerance during pregnancy is fairly common, as is the spilling of sugar into the urine. Diabetes in pregnancy effects about 2 percent of pregnant women; however, the incidence of the diabetes of stress associated with burn injury may increase with both burn and pregnancy. Serum glucose levels are monitored and appropriate dietary and/or insulin regimens initiated. The non–insulin-dependent diabetic is not at increased risk of perinatal death from her disease unless her glucose tolerance decreases and she becomes insulin dependent, but the risk of fetal macrosomia increases. The glucose intolerance associated with burn injury may require insulin treatment. Oral hypoglycemic drugs are teratogenic, so intravenous insulin is required. The need for a high-calorie high-protein diet with a large burn injury may increase the insulin requirement. The parameter is to maintain the patient's plasma glucose at around 100 mg% in order to allow development of a normal-sized fetus.[37] Management of stress-induced glucose intolerance in pregnant patients has not been reported in the literature.

Hematologic changes in burned pregnant women follow the course of nonpregnant burn patients. Although disseminated intravascular coagulation (DIC) is a possibility in pregnant patients and in burn patients, the effects do not appear to be cumulative since only one review lists DIC as a factor in one maternal death.[38]

RISK VARIABLES

Current experience indicates that maternal survival is usually accompanied by fetal survival in the presence of adequate oxygenation and volume support of both maternal and fetal cardiopulmonary systems. Taylor and colleagues[39] reviewed 19 cases and concluded the following:

1. Pregnancy does not alter maternal outcome after thermal injury.
2. Maternal survival is usually accompanied by fetal survival.
3. If the gravida's injury is lethal, the pregnancy will usually terminate spontaneously prior to her death.
4. Obstetric intervention is indicated only in the gravely ill woman whose complications (hypotension, hypoxia, or sepsis) jeopardize the life of the fetus.
5. A better understanding of the complications of major burns and the care available in modern burn units should improve the prognosis for burned pregnant patients.

Early attention to volume replacement and oxygen support in prehospital therapy will decrease the stress of the maternal-fetal unit upon arrival. Immediate transfer to a burn center is indicated for pregnant burned women.

If conditions are not favorable to meet fetal oxygen or circulatory demands, especially if the mother's percentage of total body burn is massive, emergency delivery plans must be made because spontaneous labor may occur. Spontaneous labor that will produce a 32-week-old or older infant is allowed to proceed under close observation by both a burn team and an obstetric/pediatric team. Whenever possible, delivery should occur in a burn center with a level III (tertiary care) newborn intensive care unit. Spontaneous labor that will deliver a 24- to 32-week fetus should be considered for pharmacologic inhibition of labor (tocolysis) while the underlying cause of fetal distress such as hypoxia or hypovolemia can be treated.[40] However, the administration of beta-mimetic tocolytic agents such as ritodrine or terbutaline may lead to myocardial ischemia, pulmonary edema, hyperglycemia, and hypokalemia. Tocolytic therapy using parenteral magnesium sulfate might be better tolerated because magnesium has less cardiovascular and metabolic effects than the other agents. Although fetuses delivered before 24 weeks' gestation usually do not survive labor is allowed to proceed. Vaginal delivery is the method of choice even in the presence of perineal burns. Cesarean section is used only in true medical emergencies when the life of the mother or child, or both, is at risk.

SPECIAL NURSING CONSIDERATIONS

Psychologic Aspects

In cases of major burn trauma, the patient often withdraws emotionally while all efforts are focused on survival. This phenomenon also occurs in massively burned pregnant women who may have little energy to devote to following the course of their pregnancy in the early postburn period. However, the nurse should offer information periodically even though the patient may not respond at the time. As the patient survives the emergent period, more awareness becomes apparent and answers must be ready. Experience has shown us that, in most cases, patients can deal with reality and should be given hopeful information only when such hope exists. The care plan must address issues such as fetal demise or the death of a delivered infant. Patients with less-extensive injuries may focus on the pregnancy and its burn implications, but depending on how the patient feels about the pregnancy, emotional reactions may differ. Some patients may be relieved while others may be horrified at the thought of fetal demise. Careful evaluation of the emotional status of the patient and her feelings and those of her significant others regarding the pregnancy must be carefully assessed early.

After delivery of the infant, maternal-child bonding is prolonged if the delivery occurs early in the hospital course and visitation is not possible. Every effort must be made to encourage bonding, such as the nurse's taking daily Polaroid pictures of the infant and making daily visits to the nursery to report on the infant's status. The addition of the needs of an infant to the rehabilitative phase of burn care requires early and detailed discharge planning. The infant delivered near term may be ready for discharge weeks to months prior to maternal discharge, thus complicating the facilitation of maternal-child bonding.

Wound Care

Standard wound care is delivered despite maternal-fetus management. There is no contraindication to general anesthesia for skin grafting and early wound closure remains the primary goal of burn therapy.[41] Standard topical agents are applied even though their effect on the fetus is unknown due to the low incidence of use in pregnancy. Antibiotics are chosen that do not have teratogenic effects. Tetanus toxoid is administered per unit protocol.

Old Burns and Pregnancy

It is unusual for old burns to cause problems in subsequent pregnancies. On occasion, a band of abdominal scarring may be severe enough to require surgical release with coverage of the defect using split-thickness skin grafts. In the only reported case in which this type of procedure was performed, the patient was already at 24 weeks' gestation and went into spontaneous labor and fetal delivery on postoperative day 3. Another physician performed decompression surgery in two women because of maternal pain in the third trimester, followed by split-thickness autograft to the defect, with no precipitation of early labor.[42]

Nutritional Support

Nutritional requirements increase during pregnancy, with an increase in oxygen consumption of about 15 percent at term. The use of indirect calorimetry[43] to assess needs accurately is indicated in all pregnant patients. Standard nutritional support therapy is used to meet predicted and actual energy expenditures (see Chapter 6).

NURSING CARE PLAN: CARE OF THE PREGNANT PATIENT WITH BURNS

Nursing Priorities

1. Maintain maternal-fetal oxygenation
2. Position mother to prevent vena caval compression and optimize cardiac output
3. Monitor hemodynamic status of patient—maintain adequate blood-plasma volumes
4. Monitor mother and fetus for early signs of distress
5. Prepare for emergency delivery of fetus
6. Provide emotional support for mother and significant others
7. Evaluate and nutritionally support the hypermetabolic rate
8. Prevent complications
9. Promote wound healing
10. Prepare for discharge

Nursing Diagnosis: Breathing Pattern, Ineffective

May Be Related To:

- Elevation of the diaphragm and the rib cage with decreased chest wall compliance
- Decrease in respiratory rate or depth

Possibly Evidenced By: Shortness of breath, dyspnea, nasal flaring, cyanosis, tachypnea, abnormal arterial blood gases, altered chest excursion, use of accessory muscles.

Desired Patient Outcomes: Patient will ventilate effectively and maintain normal blood gases.

Interventions	Rationale
INDEPENDENT	
• Encourage good posture and full expansion of thoracic cavity. Place arms on a bedside table in front of the patient when positioned in a chair to maintain elevation and promote thoracic expansion.	• Increased progesterone lowers pCO_2 and raises pO_2, causing a sensation of hyperventilation. Pressure of the uterus on the diaphragm elevates diaphragm by as much as 4 cm and decreases chest wall compliance.
• Elevate head of bed 45 degrees if comfortable for the mother.	• Decreased functional residual capacity (FRC), caused by the elevated diaphragm, is attenuated when positioned in semi-Fowler's rather than sitting.[44]
• Encourage patient to cough, turn, and deep-breathe to minimize potential to pneumonia.	• Pneumonia is a frequent complication of the burn patient in late pregnancy due to limited chest wall excursion.
• Closely monitor respiratory rate and depth.	• The decreased FRC plus high oxygen consumption leads to a dramatic fall in oxygenation during periods of hypoventilation.[45]

Nursing Diagnosis: Breathing Pattern, Ineffective (*Continued*)

Interventions	Rationale
• Minimize hyperventilation secondary to pain and anxiety.	• Maternal hyperventilation can lead to an increased respiratory alkalosis, which shifts the oxygen dissociation curve to the left, thereby reducing the oxygen available to the fetus.[46]

Nursing Diagnosis: Gas Exchange, Impaired: Maternal and Fetal

May Be Related To:

• A decrease in maternal oxygenation magnified in the fetus (fetal hypoxic deaths may occur at pO_2 levels compatible with maternal survival)

Possibly Evidenced By: Dyspnea, confusion, restlessness, hypoxia, cyanosis, fetal bradycardia, fetal distress.

Desired Patient Outcome: Mother and fetus will maintain adequate oxygenation.

Interventions	Rationale
INDEPENDENT	
• Monitor signs of hypoxia (increased respiratory rate, restlessness, tachycardia, diaphoresis, hypertension, arrhythmias). Investigate complaints of pain and signs of anxiety. Assess for fetal distress.	• Provides for recognition of signs of hypoxia.
• Hyperoxygenate ventilated patients prior to suctioning.	• Maintains pO_2 levels at all times.
COLLABORATIVE	
• Administer supplemental oxygen.	• Elevated diaphragm decreases the mother's FRC; fetal distress occurs rapidly in the presence of hypoxia.
• Treat the acute flame-injured pregnant patient with 100 percent oxygen and obtain carboxyhemoglobin levels.	• Assesses for hypoxia secondary to carbon monoxide poisoning (confusion or lethargy, decreased coordination, headache, nausea and vomiting, depressed ST segments on ECG, coma); prophylactically treats while awaiting carboxyhemoglobin results.
• Monitor chest x-rays, ABGs, clinical signs of pulmonary congestion (tachypnea, wheezes, consolidation), fever, and	• "Pneumonia of all etiologies is the second most common cause of nonobstetric maternal mortality."[47]

Interventions	**Rationale**
sputum cultures to detect early signs of pneumonia and adult respiratory distress syndrome (ARDS).	
• Monitor respiratory therapy when mechanical ventilation is indicated for the presence of progressive retention of carbon dioxide, uncompensated respiratory acidosis, PaO_2 of less than 60 mmHg on greater than 50 percent FIO_2, impaired mental status, or difficulty clearing secretions.	• Mechanical ventilation may be required to maintain oxygenation and thus viability of fetus.
• Monitor effectiveness of positive end-expiratory pressure (PEEP) in the ventilated patient to improve maternal/fetal oxygenation.	• PEEP can be used to correct hypoxemia refractory to high concentrations of oxygen by increasing FRC and preventing alveoli closure.
• Prepare for insertion of pulmonary artery catheter; in the unstable patient, use of a Swan-Ganz catheter to draw mixed venous oxygen gases may be advised.	• Evaluates tissue oxygen delivery and utilization.
• Monitor oxygen saturation levels; monitor hemoglobin level.	• Oxygen delivery is dependent upon arterial oxygen saturation and cardiac output plus hemoglobin.
• Monitor plasma colloid osmotic pressure (COP) and prevent IV fluid overload.	• Low plasma COP and hypervolemia will contribute to the development of pulmonary edema.

Nursing Diagnosis: Cardiac Output, Alterations In: Decreased (Potential)

May Be Related To:

• Supine positioning leading to inferior vena caval occlusion

Possibly Evidenced By: Fatigue, dyspnea, changes in hemodynamic status, cyanosis, hypotension, bradycardia, weakness, syncope.

Desired Patient Outcomes: Patient will maintain a cardiac output necessary to preserve function of the fetus and maternal organs.

Interventions	**Rationale**
INDEPENDENT	
• Position pregnant patient in left lateral position. If supine positioning is necessary, elevate right hip 15 degrees and manually move fetus to the left.	• Supine recumbency in late pregnancy causes inferior vena caval occlusion and decreased venous blood return to the heart, resulting in maternal hypotension and bradycardia. The fetus should be positioned to avoid this "supine hypotensive syndrome."

Nursing Diagnosis: Cardiac Output, Alterations In: Decreased (Potential) (Continued)

Interventions	Rationale
• Monitor vital signs, intake and output, electrolytes, hematocrit, and blood urea nitrogen levels.	• These measurements are important in evaluating status of hydration and changes in patient condition.
• Ace-wrap legs and dangle patient when moving from the supine to standing position.	• Light-headedness and syncope may occur with changes in position due to obstruction of venous return. Ace wraps promote venous return.
• Monitor fetal heart activity. A daily nonstress test may be ordered in pregnancies of more than 30 weeks.	• Fetal tachycardia may be caused by maternal fever or dehydration, hypoxia, stimulation of the fetus, maternal anxiety, fetal tachydysrhythmias, or pharmacologic interventions (such as administration of parasympathetic blockers to the mother).[48]
• Minimize stresses that increase heart rate (exercise, fever, and shivering) during late pregnancy.	• Increased heart rate in late pregnancy will decrease end-diastolic ventricular filling volume, thereby decreasing stroke volume (pregnant patients may be at maximum Starling curve and unable to increase cardiac output to meet increased energy demands).

COLLABORATIVE

• Measure pulmonary artery pressure, pulmonary capillary wedge pressure, and cardiac outputs as needed to evaluate cardiovascular status.	• Use of Swan-Ganz catheter may be helpful to evaluate cardiac, pulmonary, and vascular status of the pregnant burn patient. In early pregnancy, the increased cardiac output is due to an increased stroke volume; in late pregnancy it is primarily due to increased heart rate.

Nursing Diagnosis: Fluid Volume, Deficit

May Be Related To:

• Burn shock or septic shock.

Possibly Evidenced By: Decreased blood pressure, increased pulse, decreased urine output, elevated hematocrit, weight loss, decreasing mental status, weakness, decreased skin turgor, dry mucous membranes, fetal distress.

Desired Patient Outcomes: Patient and fetus will not develop circulatory compromise secondary to the development of shock. Patient will maintain fluid and electrolyte balance within normal limits.

Interventions	**Rationale**

INDEPENDENT

- Evaluate for peripheral and circumoral cyanosis or pallor, confusion, dyspnea, capillary refill, peripheral pulses, skin turgor, mucous membranes, and thirst.
- Monitor ECG, vital signs including central venous pressure (CVP) (pulmonary capillary wedge pressure and cardiac output using Swan-Ganz catheter if needed), serum and urine electrolytes, and intake and output (maintain urine output of 0.5 to 1 ml/kg hourly by indwelling Foley catheter).

- Monitor fetal heart rate.

- Turn mother on left side if any change in fetal heart rate.

COLLABORATIVE

- Assess arterial blood gases.

- Signs of peripheral vasoconstriction and impaired circulation may be apparent prior to changes in vital signs.

- These values serve as guidelines for adequacy of fluid resuscitation. Confusion, decreasing CVP, changes in vital signs (increased heart rate and changes in blood pressure), and decreasing urine output are indicative of shock. Pregnant burn patients require a greater volume of resuscitation fluid than do nonpregnant burn patients.
- Hypovolemic shock will lead to decreased circulation to the placenta and fetus, leading to hypoxia and distress. Following rupture of membranes, an internal fetal monitor may be placed. Fetal heart rate decelerations without beat-to-beat variability is indicative of fetal hypoxia and acidosis.[49]
- Intrauterine resuscitation measures are maximized by promoting well-oxygenated circulation to the fetus.

- Dropping pO_2 and high pCO_2 levels are indicative of respiratory failure; increasing metabolic acidosis reflects poor tissue perfusion.

Nursing Diagnosis: Tissue Perfusion, Alteration In (Edema Formation)

May Be Related To:

- Massive edema formation secondary to burn injury, hypoproteinemia, and/or dependent positioning.
- Venous congestion secondary to pressure on vessels, pre-eclampsia, or sodium and water retention due to hormonal changes.

Possibly Evidenced By: Increased heart rate; thready pulse; cool, pale, and clammy skin; diminished or absent peripheral pulses; poor capillary refill; decreased urine output; anxiety; restlessness; lethargy; decreased pulmonary artery and central venous pressures.

Desired Patient Outcome: Patient will demonstrate adequate tissue profusion.

Nursing Diagnosis: Tissue Perfusion, Alteration In (Edema Formation) (*Continued*)

Interventions	Rationale
INDEPENDENT	
• Elevate burned extremities; ambulate as permitted by clinical condition.	• Minimizes edema; promotes venous return.
• Monitor pulses in extremities to assess adequate blood flow.	• Massive edema formation, particularly in areas of circumferential full-thickness burn, may compromise arterial flow to the extremity.
• Avoid binding clothing and dressings; always wrap dressings distally to proximally.	• Maximizes venous return and prevents stasis.
• Increase protein and fluid intake during pregnancy.	• Provides amino acids for building of tissues and fluids for expansion of blood volume and elimination of waste products.
• Weigh patient daily.	• An increase of 0.5 to 0.7 kg per day indicates fluid retention.
• Monitor for edema formation, increased blood pressure (systolic increase of 30 mmHg over baseline or diastolic increase of 15 mmHg over baseline persisting over 6 hours), and proteinurea.[50]	• This triad of symptoms is indicative of pre-eclampsia, which may be life-threatening to the pregnant patient. Hypovolemia, oliguria, and seizures may occur.
• Place oral airway, oxygen, and suction supplies at the bedside. Attach patient to fetal monitor.	• Pre-eclamptic patients may develop convulsions with fetal bradycardia and maternal pulmonary edema.
• Monitor and protect patient if seizures occur.	• Convulsions represent the more advanced eclampsia phase.
• Differentiate between water intoxication and seizures due to eclampsia.	• Water intoxication seizures occur in the presence of decreased sodium levels, muscle weakness and cramping, and decreased respiratory rate. Seizures due to eclampsia occur in the presence of vasoconstriction, elevated blood pressure, and oliguria, possibly leaving the mother comatose or leading to cerebral hemorrhage.
• In patients with pregnancy-induced hypertension, observe for severe sustained abdominal pain with rigid abdomen, change in fetal heart tones, and vaginal bleeding.	• Placenta abruptio may occur as a result of vasospasm and decreased perfusion of intervillous space.
COLLABORATIVE	
• In the presence of pre-eclampsia, place patient on bedrest, monitor hourly vital	• Bedrest improves urine output and decreases edema. Renal function may be-

Interventions	Rationale
signs and intake and output (with specific gravity, sugar and acetone, and protein levels evaluated), in addition to creatinine levels. Monitor deep tendon reflex and patient's general condition (alertness, presence of edema) every 2 to 4 hours.	come compromised and must be evaluated every 1 to 2 hours.
• The following drugs may be used to treat pre-eclampsia:	
○ Apresoline, 20 to 40 mg rapid intravenous (IV) injection (monitor fetal heart rate since a fall in maternal blood pressure may result in fetal hypoxia).	○ Causes vasodilatation and decreased blood pressure; increases cardiac output and renal blood flow. Maintain a systolic pressure of at least 80 mmHg to ensure adequate perfusion to fetus.
○ Magnesium sulfate ($MgSO_4$) is withheld if deep tendon reflexes are absent, respiratory rate is less than 10 to 14, or urine output is less than 30 ml/hr.	○ Use to control seizures: Causes vasodilatation, relaxation of smooth muscles, increased cerebral and uterine blood flow, and increased urine output. Should not be given to digitalized patients. Calcium gluconate will reverse effects of $MgSO_4$.
• Request obstetric and pediatric consult.	• Emergency delivery may be necessary.

Nursing Diagnosis:
Grieving, Anticipatory

May Be Related To:

- Loss of idealized, trouble-free pregnancy
- Loss of independence, separation from family, disfigurement, and the potential loss or damage to the fetus and her own life
- Changed relationship with her family, friends, and work relations

Possibly Evidenced By: Distress, sorrow, denial of potential loss, guilt, alterations in activity level, changes in eating habits, altered sleep and communication patterns.

Desired Patient Outcome: Patient will identify problems of grieving process. Patient will identify and express feelings appropriately.

Interventions	Rationale
INDEPENDENT	
• Establish a relationship with the patient based on compassion and honesty.	• Mother will have individualized feelings about her pregnancy which may include anger, ambivalence, guilt, or joy in varying degrees. She needs support at this time of potential loss.
• Actively listen to the patient when she voices concerns; support those concerns.	• Verbalization helps patients to work through anxieties. Enables health care personnel to identify fears and to give patient the appropriate information and resources to deal with those fears.

Nursing Diagnosis:
Grieving, Anticipatory
(*Continued*)

Interventions	Rationale
• Encourage patient to work through the stages of the grieving process.	• Expect patient to demonstrate shock, denial, despair, and anger prior to being able to absorb information and to begin to deal with her grief.
• Provide factual information at a level the patient can understand, as requested or needed by the patient.	• Differentiating between fact and fears will help patient establish reality and better enable her to make decisions.
• Encourage touch by family and nursing care personnel.	• Therapeutic touch can provide great comfort to those suffering grief and isolation.

COLLABORATIVE

• Consult psychologic counseling services.	• Professional counseling may be helpful in this time of many anxieties.

Nursing Diagnosis: Coping, Ineffective Family, Compromised (Potential)

May Be Related To:

• Disruption of family unit secondary to hospitalization
• High stress in the home secondary to financial concerns, grief, ambivalence toward the fetus, potential loss of the fetus, and/or anxiety about the safety of the mother

Possibly Evidenced By: Verbalizations; withdrawal; disproportionate protective behavior by significant other(s).

Desired Patient Outcome: Family members will deal effectively with the crisis of injury and hospitalization.

Interventions	Rationale
INDEPENDENT	
• Provide support and compassion regarding the possibility of maternal and/or fetal death.	• Reactions are individualized. Promote expression of feelings.
• Encourage family members to verbalize concerns.	• Family members and health care workers can deal with issues that are important to the family member.
• Provide family with information regarding burn injuries and burn rehabilitation as it relates to pregnancy.	• Knowledge deficit will increase anxiety.

Interventions	Rationale

- Encourage children in the home to voice feelings about the accident and the pregnancy.

- Help family explore alternate child care arrangements for other children in the home as needed.

- Children often feel responsible for bad happenings in the home due to a fear that thinking negative thoughts can cause negative actions.
- Family may have difficulty scheduling work, child care, and visits to the hospital.

COLLABORATIVE

- Refer family to social services to explore financial and personal ramifications of parent's hospitalization.
- Consider psychologic intervention for children in the home.

- Identification of resources can decrease anxieties and improve ability to cope with crisis.
- Separation anxiety, fears, and guilt may lead to isolation, depression, and anger.

Nursing Diagnosis: Pain

May Be Related To:

- Burn wounds and donor sites
- Mouth lesions
- Abdominal pain secondary to complications of pregnancy

Possibly Evidenced By: Verbalizations, whimpering, crying, resistance to movement, guarding.

Desired Patient Outcome: Patient will be comfortable during clinical course.

Interventions

INDEPENDENT

- Assess patient's response to pain.
- Mouth lesions may be relieved by rinsing with warm saline several times daily; use of a soft toothbrush.
- Teach patient the use of diversion, self-hypnosis, and relaxation therapy to cope with pain without pharmacologic interventions.

COLLABORATIVE

- Administer narcotics carefully, in small doses, to minimize respiratory depression. Monitor maternal respirations.

Rationale

- Intervention should be individualized.
- Sore, bleeding gums and hyperplasia are a symptom of hyperemia from increased blood volume.
- Use of nonpharmacologic pain reduction methods are effective in burn care and have no deleterious effects on the fetus.

- Depression of maternal respirations may lead to fetal hypoxia. Narcan reverses condition when due to narcotic intoxication.

Nursing Diagnosis: Nutrition, Alterations In: Potential For Less Than Body Requirements

May Be Related To:

- Increased metabolic demands

Possibly Evidenced By: Weight loss, decreased plasma proteins, decreased albumin, decreased caloric intake, decreased muscle mass, negative nitrogen balance, decreased iron.

Desired Patient Outcome: Patient will maintain her preburn weight with appropriate weight gain during the hospitalization to support fetal growth. The patient will remain in positive nitrogen balance.

Interventions	Rationale
INDEPENDENT	
• Provide frequent small meals.	• Enlarged uterus may cause gastric pressure and reflux.
• Encourage increased calorie and protein intake to meet increased energy expenditure needs. Due to the markedly increased metabolic demands of burn injuries, supplemental formulas are usually necessary.	• Pregnancy demands an increase of about 300 kcal/day over basal needs during the second two trimesters. Protein needs increase by about 30 g per day to maintain fetal development.
• Weigh patient daily.	• Monitors weight gain and loss.
COLLABORATIVE	
• Assess nutritional status, including:	
◦ Daily nutritional assessment	◦ Provides information regarding mother's nutritional status.
◦ Evaluation for glycosuria	◦ Identifies stress and hyperglycemia.
◦ Ultrasound and fundal height measurements	◦ Evaluates fetal growth.
◦ Fetal heart rate monitoring and/or mother's evaluation of fetal activity	◦ Evaluates fetal well-being.
• Supplement diet with vitamins, iron, and trace elements.	• Needed in greater amounts during pregnancy.
• Administer supplemental high-protein, high-calorie diet tube feeding. Evaluate tolerance in terms of residuals, diarrhea, elevated glucose levels, spilling of urine glucose, and nausea and vomiting.	• Enlarged uterus and gastrointestinal pressure may decrease tolerance for enteral intake.

Nursing Diagnosis: Bowel Elimination, Alteration In: Constipation

May Be Related To:

- Use of supplemental iron products
- Decreased smooth muscle motility secondary to increased progesterone levels
- Pressure on or displacement of intestines secondary to uterine enlargement
- Antacid use

Possibly Evidenced By: Hard-formed stool, straining at stool, decreased bowel sounds, back pain, frequency less than pattern, nausea, discomfort.

Desired Patient Outcome: Patient will maintain preburn elimination patterns.

Interventions

INDEPENDENT

- Encourage warm fluids in the morning.

- Encourage daily bowel elimination routine by ambulating patient to the bathroom at the same time each day, as patient's condition permits.

COLLABORATIVE

- Work with dietitian to develop high-protein, high-calorie diet that is low in fat and high in fiber.
- Stool softeners or bulk laxatives that are not irritating to the bowel may be ordered; do not give mineral oil.

Rationale

- Contributes to regularity in bowel elimination.
- Encourages daily pattern of elimination.

- Bulk aids passage of fecal contents; fats depress peristalsis.

- Mineral oil interferes with absorption of fat-soluble vitamins.

Nursing Diagnosis: Potential For Infection

May Be Related To:

- Changes in genital and urinary tract
- Loss of skin integrity
- Impaired pulmonary function

Possibly Evidenced By: Elevated temperature; positive cultures.

Desired Patient Outcome: Patient will achieve timely wound healing, with infections either prevented or controlled.

Interventions

INDEPENDENT

- Assess burn wounds daily for cellulitis, purulent drainage, odor, eschar lysing,

Rationale

- Early detection of infection is essential for prompt treatment.

Nursing Diagnosis: Potential
For Infection (*Continued*)

Interventions	Rationale

deepening of the wound, blackening or petechia in the eschar, or other wound changes.
- Monitor patient for early signs of sepsis: changes in vital signs (increase heart rate, tachypnea, change in blood pressure), decreasing urine output, confusion, hyperglycemia or hypoglycemia, decreasing platelet count, acidosis.

- Septic shock must be detected early and treated aggressively to minimize maternal and fetal compromise.

COLLABORATIVE

- Perform all invasive procedures using sterile technique.
- Perform wound cultures (preferably biopsies of the eschar) three times each week on open wounds for microorganism identification and quantification with determination of sensitivity and resistance patterns.
- Administer antibiotics based on sensitivity and resistance, using the following guidelines:
  ○ Sulfonamides are contraindicated late in pregnancy

  ○ Aminoglycosides use should be limited to life-threatening situations
  ○ Tetracycline use should be avoided if possible in the second and third trimester.
  ○ Penicillin and its derivatives appear safe for mother and fetus.
  ○ Cephalosporins have not been extensively studied in pregnancy. May require higher doses to maintain therapeutic levels.
  ○ Chloramphenicol, clindamycin, and metronidazole are contraindicated in pregnancy.[51]

- Prevention of nosocomial infections.

- Antibiotic choice should be based on microorganism's sensitivity patterns.

- Minimizes the development of resistant organisms.

○ Sulfonamides cross the placenta; in case of delivery, will compete with bilirubin for albumin binding sites (increased risk of kernicterus).
○ May have ototoxic and nephrotoxic effects on fetus.
○ Tetracyclines form a complex that is incorporated into structures being calcified; will stain infant's teeth.

○ Estolate form of erythromycin may cause hepatotoxicity.

○ Chloramphenicol causes "gray baby syndrome"; clindamycin has not been widely used in pregnancy; metronidazole may have teratogenicity and may have carcinogenic effects.

Nursing Diagnosis: Skin Integrity, Impairment Of, Actual

(Refer to Chapter 4, page 64, for etiology, manifestations, desired patient outcomes, and interventions.)

Nursing Diagnosis: Social Isolation

(Refer to Chapter 7, page 90, for etiology, manifestations, desired patient outcomes, and interventions.)

Nursing Diagnosis: Coping, Ineffective Family/Individual

(Refer to Chapter 7, page 92, for etiology, manifestations, desired patient outcomes, and interventions.)

Nursing Diagnosis: Post-Trauma Response

(Refer to Chapter 7, page 93, for etiology, manifestations, desired patient outcomes, and interventions.)

Nursing Diagnosis: Fear

(Refer to Chapter 7, page 94, for etiology, manifestations, desired patient outcomes, and interventions.)

Nursing Diagnosis: Anxiety

May Be Related To:

- Uncertainty of outcome of pregnancy
- Health of fetus

Possibly Evidenced By: Constant questions about the condition of the fetus; reluctance to discuss or ask questions about the fetus

Desired Patient Outcome: The patient will be able to discuss and ask questions about the fetus, and yet maintain an interest and involvement in other areas.

(Refer to Chapter 7 for other etiologies, manifestations, desired patient outcomes, and interventions.)

Nursing Diagnosis: Grieving

(Refer to Chapter 7, page 94, for etiology, manifestations, desired patient outcomes, and interventions.)

Nursing Diagnosis: Adjustment, Impaired

(Refer to Chapter 7, page 95, for etiology, manifestations, desired patient outcomes, and interventions.)

Nursing Diagnosis: Powerlessness

(Refer to Chapter 7, page 96, for etiology, manifestations, desired patient outcomes, and interventions.)

Nursing Diagnosis: Family Process, Alteration In

(Refer to Chapter 7, page 97, for etiology, manifestations, desired patient outcomes, and interventions.)

Nursing Diagnosis: Parenting, Alterations In

(Refer to Chapter 7, page 105, for etiology, manifestations, desired patient outcomes, and interventions.)

Nursing Diagnosis: Self-Concept, Disturbance In

(Refer to Chapter 7, page 89, for etiology, manifestations, desired patient outcomes, and interventions.)

Nursing Diagnosis: Knowledge Deficit

(Refer to Chapter 9, page 176, for etiology, manifestations, desired patient outcomes, and interventions.)

REFERENCES

1. Smith, B, Rayburn, W, and Feller, I: Burns and pregnancy. Clin Perinatol 10:383, 1983.
2. Matthews, RN: Obstetric implications of burns in pregnancy. Br J Obstet Gynaecol 89:603, 1982.
3. Matthews, RN: Obstetric implications of burns in pregnancy. Br J Obstet Gynaecol 89:603, 1982.
4. Amy, BW, et al: Thermal injury in the pregnant patient. Surg Gynecol Obstet 161:209, 1985.
5. Deitch, EA, et al: Management of burns in pregnant women. Surg Gynecol Obstet 161:1, 1985.
6. Taylor, JW, et al: Thermal injury during pregnancy. Obstet Gynecol 47:434, 1976.
7. Stilwell, JH: A major burn in early pregnancy with maternal survival and pregnancy progressing to term. Br J Plast Surg 35:33, 1982.
8. Rayburn, W, et al: Major burns during pregnancy: Effects on fetal well-being. Obstet Gynecol 63:392, 1984.
9. Taylor, JW, et al: Thermal injury during pregnancy. Obstet Gynecol 47:434, 1976.
10. Matthews, RN: Obstetric implications of burns in pregnancy. Br J Obstet Gynaecol 89:603, 1982.
11. Smith, BK, Rayburn, WF, and Feller, I: Burns and pregnancy. Clin Perinatol 10:383, 1983.
12. Crosby, WM: Traumatic injuries during pregnancy. Clin Obstet Gynecol 26:902, 1983.
13. Baker, DP: Trauma in the pregnant patient. Surg Clin North Am 62:275, 1982.
14. Bernardo, LM: Burns in pregnancy. Emergency Medical Services 15:21, 1986.
15. Stage, AH: Severe burns in the pregnant patient. Obstet Gynecol 42:259, 1973.
16. Rayburn, W, et al: Major burns during pregnancy: Effects on fetal well-being. Obstet Gynecol 63:392, 1984.
17. Amy, BW, et al: Thermal injury in the pregnant patient. Surg Gynecol 161:209, 1985.
18. Bernardo, LM: Burns in pregnancy. Emergency Medical Services 15:21, 1986.
19. Haycock, CE: Emergency care of the pregnant traumatized patient. Emerg Med Clin North Am 2:843, 1984.
20. Patterson, RM: Trauma in pregnancy. Clin Obstet Gynecol 27:32, 1984.
21. Harris, BA: Pregnancy with complications. Emergency Medicine 1:22, 1984.
22. Crosby, WM: Traumatic injuries during pregnancy. Clin Obstet Gynecol 26:902, 1983.
23. Bernardo, LM: Burns in pregnancy. Emergency Medical Services 15:21, 1986.
24. Sorensen, VJ, et al: Trauma in pregnancy. Henry Ford Hosp Med J 34:101, 1986.
25. Barron, WM: The pregnant surgical patient: Medical evaluation and management. Ann Intern Med 101:683, 1984.
26. Crosby, WM: Traumatic injuries during pregnancy. Clin Obstet Gynecol 26:902, 1983.
27. Longo, LD: The biological effects of carbon monoxide on the pregnant woman, fetus, and newborn infant. Am J Obstet Gynecol 129:69, 1977.
28. Spear, RM and Munster, AW: Burns, inhalation, injury and electrical injury. In Rogers, M (ed): Textbook of Pediatric Intensive Care. Williams & Wilkins, Baltimore, 1987, p 1323.
29. Deitch, EA, et al: Management of burns in pregnant women. Surg Gynecol Obstet 161:1, 1985.
30. Bernardo, LM: Burns in pregnancy. Emergency Medical Services 15:21, 1986.
31. Taylor, JW, et al: Thermal injury during pregnancy. Obstet Gynecol 47:434, 1976.
32. Amy, BW, et al: Thermal injury in the pregnant patient. Surg Gynecol Obstet 161:209, 1985.
33. Davison, JS, Davison, MC, and Hay, DM: Gastric emptying time in late pregnancy and labour. Br J Obstet Gynaecol 77:37, 1970.
34. Lazarus, HM and Nelson, EA: Refining the technique of diagnostic peritoneal lavage. ER Reports 1:111, 1980.
35. Baker, DP: Trauma in the pregnant patient. Surg Clin North Am 62:275, 1982.
36. Harris, BA: Pregnancy with complications. Emergency Medicine 1:22, 1984.
37. Harris, BA: Pregnancy with complications. Emergency Medicine 1:22, 1984.
38. Amy, BW, et al: Thermal injury in the pregnant patient. Surg Gynecol Obstet 161:209, 1985.
39. Taylor, JW, et al: Thermal injury during pregnancy. Obstet Gynecol 47:434, 1976.
40. Deitch, EA, et al: Management of burns in pregnant women. Surg Gynecol Obstet 161:1, 1985.
41. Brown, SL: The pregnant patient: Postanesthetic considerations. J Post Anesthesia Nsg 1:17, 1986.
42. Matthews, RN: Old burns and pregnancy. Br J Obstet Gynaecol 89:610, 1982.

43. Saffle, JR, et al: Use of indirect calorimetry in the nutritional management of burned patients. J Trauma 25:32, 1985.
44. Berkowitz, RL (ed): Critical Care of the Obstetric Patient. Churchill Livingstone, New York, 1983, p 78.
45. Berkowitz, RL (ed): Critical Care of the Obstetric Patient. Churchill Livingstone, New York, 1983, p 80.
46. Berkowitz, RL (ed): Critical Care of the Obstetric Patient. Churchill Livingstone, New York, 1983, p 344.
47. Berkowitz, RL (ed): Critical Care of the Obstetric Patient. Churchill Livingstone, New York, 1983, p 356.
48. Knuppel, RA and Drukker, JE: High Risk Pregnancy. WB Saunders, Philadelphia, 1986, p 239.
49. Friedman, EA, Acker, DB, and Sachs, BP: Obstetrical Decision-Making, ed 2. BC Dekker, Philadelphia, 1987, p 200.
50. Queenan, JT (ed): Management of High Risk Pregnancy, ed 2. Medical Economics Books, Oradell, New Jersey, 1985, p 407.
51. Knuppel, RA and Drukker, JE: High Risk Pregnancy. WB Saunders, Philadelphia, 1986, p 121.

Chapter 14

LISA MARIE BERNARDO
KATHLEEN SULLIVAN

CARE OF THE PEDIATRIC PATIENT WITH BURNS

MORTALITY

A burn injury is a traumatic experience for a person at any age. Relative to the extent of the burn injury, the child may also face the loss of an intact and healthy body, the loss of normal activities such as play or school, and, most devastating of all, the loss of a parent or sibling. The thoughtful, knowledgeable, sensitive nursing care that the burn-injured child receives has a profound impact on the child's survival and quality of life (Fig. 14–1).

Burns are the leading cause of pediatric injury-related deaths in the home; they rank just behind motor vehicle collisions and drowning as an injury-related cause of death outside the home.[1] In children 1 to 4 years of age, burns are the leading cause of death in the home and the second leading cause, after motor vehicle fatalities, overall.[2] From 1970 to 1984 (excluding 1981 and 1982), an average of 3212 children under age 15 died each year from injuries sustained in the home.[3] Fires and burns were the main cause of fatality in children aged 1 to 14, suffocation being the leading cause of home injury-related fatality in children under age 1.[4] Older children (ages 13 to 18 years) have better survival rates; survival is progressively worse the younger the child.[5]

Three fourths of all fire-related deaths are due to home fires;[6] children under age 5 are at greatest risk.[7,8] The largest percentage of these fires are due to adults who smoke carelessly; only 2 percent are caused by children playing with matches or lighters.[9]

Electrocution is another cause of burn-related death in children. As reported in McIntire, the Consumer Product Safety Commission (CPSC) estimates that 30 children under age 5 and 40 children between the ages of 5 and 14 die each year from electrocution.[10]

Etiology

The etiology of unintentional burn injury in children is the same as in all age groups; that is, flame, scald, contact, electrical, chemical, and ultraviolet radiation.

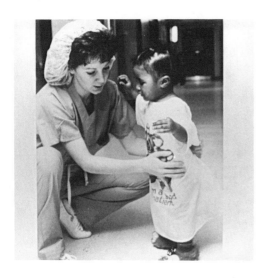

FIGURE 14–1. A nurse assists a preschool child in balance and coordination following a burn injury. (Courtesy of Burn Center, The Mercy Hospital of Pittsburgh, Pittsburgh, Pennsylvania.)

Scalds from hot liquids (Fig. 14–1) are the most common cause of nonfatal burns in children under age 3;[11,12] they are usually limited to small body areas.[13] A review of 247 emergency department (ED) records and 80 inpatient records of pediatric burn patients from July 1981 through June 1984 was done at the Kapiolani Women's and Children's Medical Center in Honolulu.[14] The results showed that most burns occurred in children aged 8 months to 3 years. More than half of these injuries (53 percent) were from scalds (coffee or tea 35 percent; other 24 percent; soup or other food 17 percent; saimin (Hawaiian noodle soup), 9 percent; and tap water 3 percent). The remaining burns were from heating appliances (16%), fire (8%), and other causes (23%). Of the fire-related injuries (8 percent) none was the result of a house fire. This is probably attributed to the warm climate of Hawaii.

Another study reviewed the medical records of 464 children under age 16 admitted to the Harborview Medical Center Burn Unit between 1979 and 1984.[15] Scalds were the most common cause of burn injury in children (54 percent), with flame burns the second most common cause (33 percent). Eighty-two percent of the scald injuries were seen in children under age 4; 86 percent of the flame injuries were seen in children over age 4 (p <0.01 with regard to etiology of burn injury).[16]

Flame injuries are more common in older children;[17–19] however, the most severe injuries occur in infants unable to escape fires.[20] McIntire cites the CPSC statistics in which 66 percent of all ED visits for fireworks-related injuries involved children under age 15; 60 percent of these injuries were burns.[21]

Nonfatal electrical burns usually involve infants and toddlers aged 6 months to 39 months; 66 percent of these injuries involve the oral cavity.[22] Chemical burns include ingestion of lye or disc batteries.

Contact burns occur when children come into contact with oven doors, furnace gratings, irons, radiators, and so on. Ultraviolet radiation burns are seen primarily in infants and young children who are left exposed to the sun, tanning lamps, and the like, for prolonged periods of time.

Intentional burn injuries are found in children of all ages. Approximately 10 percent of child abuse cases involve burn injuries.[23,24] Because younger children cannot protect themselves from the perpetrator, they are at the greatest risk for any form of abuse or neglect. Intentional burns can be inflicted by the parent or other caregiver (e.g., babysitter, sibling, other relative). The caregiver may burn the child to "punish" or "discipline" him or her. The etiologies are the same for unintentional and intentional burns.

TABLE 14–1. Differences Between Unintentional and Intentional Burn Injuries in Children

Etiology	Unintentional	Intentional
Flame		
Cigarette burns	Small, reddened areas; first-degree burns found usually on arms, legs; usually from dropping ashes	Punched in, round; full-thickness burns found on hands, feet
House fire		Neglect from leaving children alone in the home
Scald		
Hot foods or liquids	Splash pattern over body	Well-defined pattern concentrated in one area; oral burns from being fed with very hot food or formula
Bath water	Nonimmersion splash pattern; first- or second-degree	Forced immersion; well-defined pattern, usually seen on buttocks and perineum with deep partial thickness burns; symmetrical full-thickness burns to hands, feet; resembling "gloves" or "socks"
Contact	Very small area with second- or third-degree burn	Large, well-demarcated area of burning object (iron, electric range burner, radiator)
Chemical		Feeding the child chemicals (lye, household cleaners)

Therefore, the nurse must be aware of the possibility of abuse in any child who incurs a burn injury. Table 14–1 highlights the differences in burn patterns between intentional and unintentional burn injuries. One highly unusual form of abuse reported in the literature involved placement of a 5-week-old infant and a 14-month-old toddler in microwave ovens.[25] Although these burns occurred on separate occasions to unrelated children, their burn patterns were the same. Microwave oven burns are found on skin surfaces closest to the microwave-emitting devices; they are well demarcated, may have tissue layer sparing, and do not resemble electrical burns because the surface is not charred.[26]

ANATOMIC/PHYSIOLOGIC CONSIDERATIONS

When caring for the burn-injured child, the nurse must remember the child's developmental needs as well as the physiologic needs. An extension of the child is the family, who needs emotional support and care throughout the child's hospitalization. A systematic physiologic and developmental review will clarify the unique differences in caring for the burn-injured child.

Cardiovascular System

The cardiovascular system is a sensitive indicator of adequate systemic perfusion. Changes in a child's heart rate are early indicators of distress. In the older child, tachycardia is the first response to hypoxemia; in the neonate, bradycardia occurs as a response to hypoxemia.[27] Tachycardia may also occur from fear, pain, anxiety, fever, and shock. Tachycardia is the most effective way for the child to increase cardiac output. A decreased cardiac output occurs in the burned child because of inadequate preload (hypovolemia) due to third spacing.[28] Bradycardia in a previously tachycardic child is a warning that cardiac arrest is imminent. Therefore, the child must be closely observed and evaluated for any changes in heart rate so the underlying cause can be effectively treated—medicate for pain, readjust intravenous (IV) fluids, and so forth.

Blood pressure measures the ability of the heart to perfuse the body adequately. The child can maintain a normal blood pressure as long as vasoconstriction, tachycardia, and increased contractility occur. Hypotension results when the body can no longer compensate. In children, hypotension is a late sign of cardiovascular decompensation.[29] Therefore, it is important to know normal blood pressure values for each group as well as the burn injured child's own normal range (Table 14–2). A decrease of 10 mmHg in the systolic blood pressure should be a warning to evaluate the child further.[30]

Probably the best method for evaluating perfusion in the child is by assessing the peripheral pulses. All pulses should be equal and symmetrical; discrepancies may be due to hypothermia or may possibly be an early sign of decreased stroke volume.[31] Circumferential burns can also result in unequal pulses due to compression on the arteries. While acrocyanosis is normal in neonates, cyanosis to the feet and hands in children is an indicator of decreased cardiac output. Severe vasoconstriction creates a pallid color. Frequent assessment of the peripheral vascular system helps prevent complications from developing (e.g., shock, loss of limb function).

Respiratory System

Anatomic and physiologic differences exist in the pediatric and adult respiratory systems. It is crucial that these differences be recognized, because ventilatory compromise can occur if the young child is treated with airway support methods appropriate for adults.

Four major differences in the pediatric airway are:

1. The larynx is positioned relatively cephalad.
2. The epiglottis protrudes into the pharynx and is U-shaped.
3. The vocal cords are short and concave.
4. The cricoid cartilage is the narrowest part of the airway in children under age 8. (In older children and adults, the vocal cords are the narrowest part of the airway.[32])

The lower airway passages, which are narrower and more flexible in infants and young children, may easily obstruct with mucous plugs, foreign bodies, or edema. The ribs and sternum are more cartilaginous and more pliable. Breath sounds are easily transmitted; these may appear equal and bilateral when they are not. Therefore, when auscultating for breath sounds, the nurse must also observe for equal and symmetrical chest expansion. This chest wall movement will confirm if the lung fields are being ventilated bilaterally. The younger child relies on the diaphragm for breathing as the intercostal muscles and rib cage become more developed. If the diaphragm cannot move freely because of increased intra-abdominal pressure or increased intrathoracic pressure, respiratory efforts become ineffective.[33] Also, constricting eschar to the abdomen or thorax can compromise ventilation; escharotomies are performed as needed to allow for adequate chest and abdominal expansion.

Physiologically, the child has a reservoir of oxygen that is too small to provide protection during stress;[34] this is likely to result in respiratory distress. The child also has

ASSESSMENT OF EXTENT OF BURNS

1 YEAR
18
9 — 9
36
14 — 14
9 — 9

5 YEARS
9
36
14 — 14
16 — 16

15 YEARS
9
10
36
18 — 18
9 — 9

NOTE: Numbers indicate both sides of trunk and/or extremities

TABLE 14-2. Pediatric Trauma Reference.

Airway, Breathing, Vital Signs

AGE	WEIGHT (KG)	HEART RATE	BLOOD PRESSURE	RESPIRA-TIONS	ENDOTRACHEAL TUBE (UNCUFFED)	LARYNGOSCOPE BLADE	SUCTION CATHETER	CHEST TUBE	URINARY OUTPUT (ML/KG/HR)
Birth	3.5	140	65/40	40	3.5	1 Miller	6F	12F	1.0–2.0
6 mo	6	120	85/60	30	4.0	1½ Wis-Hipple	8F	12F	1.0–1.5
1 yr	10	120	90/60	30	4.5	1½ Wis-Hipple	8F	16F	1.0–1.5
3 yr	14	100	95/60	25	5.0	2 Miller	8F	20F	1.0
6 yr	20	90	100/60	22	6.0	2 Miller	10F	24F	1.0
12 yr	40	80	110/60	16	7.0 (Cuffed)	3 Miller	12F	28F	1.0
						3 Macintosh			

(Capillary Refill <2 seconds)

Volume Replacement

AGE	AVERAGE WEIGHT (KG)	IV BOLUS/SHOCK			MAINTENANCE
		WHOLE BLOOD (20 ML/KG)	PACKED CELLS (10 ML/KG)	LACTATED RINGER'S (20 ML/KG)	$D_5\frac{1}{4}$ NSS (ML/HR)
Birth	3.5	70	35	70	14
6 mo	6	120	60	120	24
1 yr	10	200	100	200	40
3 yr	14	280	140	280	48
6 yr	20	400	200	400	60
12 yr	40	800	400	800	80

Partial listing from Pediatric Trauma Reference, Benedum Pediatric Trauma Program, Children's Hospital of Pittsburgh, Pittsburgh, PA, with permission.

a greater metabolic rate and demand, where oxygen consumption is 6 to 8 ml/kg per minute;[35] this demand can become greater with a burn injury.

Respiratory injury is ominous for the pediatric population and is a major cause of mortality, morbidity, and extended hospitalization.[36] Causes of respiratory injury in children are the inhalation of hot air (steam) or toxic fumes (carbon monoxide, smoke),and the ingestion of caustic substances (lye). The respiratory tract may be injured with caustic ingestions because the child may choke and aspirate the substance; also, the substance can burn through the oropharynx and esophagus into the respiratory tract.

The inhalation of hot, smokey air during a house fire causes burns to the upper airway structures. Thermal injury is most often limited to the upper airway because it acts as a heat exchanger and humidifier of inhaled gases.[37] This heat creates edema; because of the already anatomically narrow airway, a small amount of edema can quickly cause obstruction. This edema occurs quickly and peaks at approximately 6 to 8 hours postinjury.[38] Therefore, early endotracheal intubation and administration of 100 percent humidified oxygen are indicated. Mechanical ventilation is considered because the work of breathing required by the intubated child will cause fatigue, resulting in inadequate respiratory effort and hypoxemia.

Signs and symptoms of respiratory injury are the same in children as in adults: burns to the face and neck; carbonaceous sputum; singed eyebrows and eyelashes; dry and cracked lips, tongue, and mucous membranes; cough; stridor; hoarseness; and a history of being in an enclosed, burning space. Auscultating for wheezing and rales, as well as observing for retractions, nasal flaring, and stridor, are nursing responsibilities. Performing scrupulous pulmonary toilet is an absolute priority to ensure proper oxygenation. Following an inhalation injury, pulmonary capillaries can heal in 7 to 10 days; in children with 70 percent or greater total body surface area (TBSA) burns, several more days may be needed for healing to be appreciated.[39]

Severe pulmonary injury can increase fluid requirements in the resuscitative phase up to 37 percent beyond the calculated requirements.[40] One consideration is to maintain the diastolic blood pressure at 60 mmHg or above, and to keep the urine output at 0.5 to 1.0 ml/kg per hour in the child who weighs less than 30 kg.[41] Common respiratory complications include pulmonary edema, tracheobronchitis, bronchopneumonia, and alveolar-capillary block syndrome.[42] The nurse is constantly vigilant for signs of pulmonary edema in case of fluid overload. This pulmonary edema associated with inhalation injury is the result of increased pulmonary blood flow and increased capillary permeability and is noncardiac.[43] Monitoring central venous pressure (CVP), pulmonary capillary wedge pressure (PCWP), and carbon monoxide as well (CO), as auscultating breath sounds astutely, observing for chest expansion, and assessing oxygenation status (arterial blood gases [ABGs], level of consciousness) are paramount in the prevention of pulmonary complications.

Metabolism and Thermoregulation

In the young child under age 2, problems related to metabolism and thermoregulation include hypothermia, metabolic acidosis, and hypoglycemia.[44] Hypothermia is a problem in children because of their larger surface area to body weight. They lose more heat from evaporation and convection than do adults. Cold-stressed neonates and infants under 6 months old cannot shiver to generate body heat. They must break down brown fat to maintain their body temperature.[45] This is not efficient for the infant, as there is an increase in energy expenditure and an increase in oxygen consumption during this process, known as "nonshivering thermogenesis."[46,47]

In the infant or young child who is burned, this loss of body heat through the open wounds becomes even more crucial. To minimize energy expenditure for heat production, the environmental temperature is kept warm enough for the child. A temperature of 28° to 33°C has been found to minimize the metabolic expenditure for the body to maintain its core temperature as well as to maximize comfort.[48] The nurse intervenes to decrease metabolic demands by keeping the child warm during dressing changes and at rest, planning daily activities that include undisturbed rest and sleep periods, administering pain medications as needed, and providing emotional support and comfort.

Hypoglycemia can be seen in younger children who are stressed. This is due to the small amount of glycogen stores in the liver. During stressful experiences, such as illness or injury, these stores are quickly depleted. It is important to note that hypoglycemia or hyperglycemia are early signs of sepsis in infants, while glycosuria is an early sign of infection in children.[49] Closely monitoring the burned child's blood glucose levels and other metabolic components allows for detection of abnormalities before complications arise. Metabolic acidosis can be detected on admission. It occurs because the buffering capacity is less in children under age 2.[50] Sodium bicarbonate given intravenously will help to raise the arterial pH.[51]

Surface area is one of the major determinants of water turnover, caloric expenditure, and other metabolic indicators. Insensible water loss from evaporation is greater in the burned child because of the larger surface-to-weight ratio.[52] Fluid administration and laboratory studies are closely monitored, as is the child's weight, to determine if this insensible water loss is under control.

Gastrointestinal and Renal Systems

The stomach of a child 2 years of age has a 500-ml capacity; emptying time is 3 to 6 hours.[53] These facts become important during resuscitative methods. The child may have eaten dinner and later been injured. Because of the stress of the burn, coupled with the delayed emptying time, gastric distention develops. Gastric decompression is indicated in children under age 2 or in children with a burn larger than 20 percent TBSA.[54,55] Further, gastric dilatation is compounded during air transport when atmospheric pressure is lower and altitude is higher.[56] Monitoring and recording gastric fluid aspirates, as well as administering antacids to prevent stress ulcers, is a vital nursing responsibility.

The kidneys are not fully developed until approximately 1 year of age; therefore, filtration and absorption in infants are relatively poor.[57] The ability of the kidneys to concentrate urine increases with age. It is very important during fluid resuscitation that an accurate output record is maintained. Inserting a Foley catheter to measure urine output is essential in a child with a greater than 20 percent TBSA burn.[58]

Neurologic System

Cerebral edema can occur in burn-injured young children.[59,60] It appears that the child's brain is prone to edema and irritability.[61] This may be related to the fluid shifts from the intravascular compartment during fluid resuscitation, as well as the large volume of IV fluids administered during this time. Keeping the child's head and neck midline, as well as elevated approximately 30 degrees, helps reduce intracranial pressure (ICP). Increased ICP, with its potential for brainstem herniation, is always a concern with cerebral edema. Frequent neurologic checks, including level of consciousness, symmetry of movement, ability to follow commands, pupil size and reactivity, and speech (if not intubated) are some important indicators for determining cerebral function.

NUTRITIONAL REQUIREMENTS

Caloric requirements are best estimated from the body surface area. Ultimately, they are obtained based upon growth pattern, sense of well-being, and satiety.[62] Daily caloric requirements in the first year are approximately 80 to 120 kcal/kg, decreasing approximately 10 kcal/kg for each succeeding 3-year period.[63] During periods of increased growth, such as puberty, the amount of calories consumed should increase.[64]

The burned child has smaller nutritional reserves and greater caloric and protein requirements per kilogam than does the burned adult.[65] When calculating nutritional requirements, the child's daily requirements based on growth, plus added requirements for the burn wound, must be considered. One method to calculate nutritional requirements is as follows:[66]

> <2 years 80 kcal/kg + 30 kcal/% burn
> 3–6 g protein/kg per day
> >2 years: 60 kcal/kg + kcal/% burn
> 2–8 g protein/kg per day

Similar methods are found in the literature.[67,68] It must be remembered that calculations are an estimate; how well the child is doing in terms of weight gain and wound healing are more accurate indicators of nutritional status. Methods to ensure adequate nutrition include oral, enteral, and parenteral feedings, including lipids and hyperalimentation (see Care Plan, p. 265). Daily weights, limb circumference measurements, and calorie counts are ways to measure the effectiveness of nutritional intake.

FLUID REQUIREMENTS

External abnormal losses from the burn wound are as follows:[69]

> 140 mEq/liter Na
> 5 mEq/liter K
> 110 mEq/liter Cl
> 3–5 g% protein

It is important to replace losses volume for volume for physiologic readjustment. Laboratory studies for minerals, electrolytes, and total protein must be constantly monitored, with fluids adjusted as needed.It is not uncommon for the child with an electrical burn or inhalation injury (as well as any other trauma) to require additional fluid replacement.[70]

Any burns greater than 10 to 15 percent TBSA in children require fluid resuscitation, as well as any-size burns accompanied by smoke inhalation.[71] There are different methods of fluid calculation for resuscitation in children, which include the Modified Brooke formula and the Parkland formula (see later). These formulas are only a guide to administering fluids during resuscitation. Adequate fluid resuscitation is guided by the child's physiologic parameters of level of consciousness (alert), adequate capillary perfusion, vital signs within a normal range (slightly elevated BP and heart rate), absence of metabolic acidosis, hourly urine output at 1 ml/kg in children under age 1 and at 0.5 ml/kg in children over age 1 with normal urine osmolality and specific gravity.[72–76] Colloid administration during resuscitation is controversial. Its usage is directed by the burn physicians at the receiving burn center. The child's maintenance fluids (preferably $D_5\frac{1}{2}NS$) must also be calculated and added to the resuscitation fluids.

MODIFIED BROOKE FORMULA

3 ml/kg per % burn in the first 24 hours (glucose may be added, but beware of stress hyperglycemia)[76]
5% dextrose in 0.5 normal saline plus colloid as needed in the second 24 hours

PARKLAND FORMULA

Ringer's lactate 4 ml/kg per % burn in the first 24 hours
5% dextrose in 0.5 normal saline plus colloid as needed in the second 24 hours

While intravenous cannulation may be difficult in the unburned child, inserting an IV in the burned child is a true challenge. It is best to obtain IV access in an unburned area.[77,78] If that is not possible, IV insertion into a burned area can be obtained as long as the area is not circumferentially burned. Peripheral sites that are acceptable are the arm, hand, leg, and foot. In the infant, scalp veins may not be preferable especially with an inhalation injury or facial burns due to the edema formation during fluid resuscitation. Also, these IV sites tend to be rather precarious and may dislodge during transport. Central cannulation is an option for experienced professionals. Central access can be obtained through the femoral, internal, and external jugular veins and through the subclavian vein in older children.[79] Central line monitoring may be necessary in the extensively burned child where PCWP or CVP must be closely monitored to avoid fluid overload. The IV cannulas are sutured into place and covered with an antimicrobial cream and a sterile dressing. The IV sites are then monitored for signs and symptoms of infiltration and infection.

The intraosseous method for fluid and medication administration is gaining popularity. This temporary route can be helpful in initial fluid resuscitation until adequate venous access is obtained. Regardless of the route of fluid administration, the nurse is responsible for accurately administering and monitoring fluid intake. Infusion pumps, mini-drip set-ups, and Buretrols are adjuncts that assist the nurse in accurately measuring fluid administration.

RISK VARIABLES

Children are at an exaggerated risk for burn injury because they have a less acute perception of danger, less control of elements within their environment, and a limited ability to react promptly and properly to a fire or other type of burn situation.[80] For example, the frightened toddler may hide from a fire instead of escaping. Because of their limited cognitive problem solving abilities, children believe that if hidden, the fire will not "find" them and they will be safe.

The family's life events also are associated with burn injuries in children. These events include financial strains, tense marital relations, and family illness.[81] Presumably, the family becomes involved in these events, leaving little time or energy to share with their children.

The vulnerability of infants, toddlers, and preschoolers to burn injury is related to the ability of the caregiver (parent, guardian) to provide a safe environment for the growing child. Caregivers who are not knowledgeable about their child's safety needs (leaving matches within reach, leaving pothandles turned outward on the stove) or who permit their child to remain unsupervised (leaving young children alone in the house for hours or days) place their offspring at great risk for injury.

Infants are particularly vulnerable to scald burns if they are held by the caregiver who is drinking or eating hot foods (Color Plate 37). Tub water that is not checked for a safe temperature can result in burns to the infant. As infants grow and begin to crawl, stand, and cruise, they become at risk for scald injuries due to spilling hot liquids onto themselves. Because of the federal regulations for flame-retardant sleepwear, flame burns from ignited clothing are not often seen, except when the family makes their own sleepwear.

Toddlers are beginning to explore their environment by searching and reaching. They can walk and run, but their coordination is poor. Curiosity abounds; therefore, it is common to see splatter burns from pulling down cups of hot liquids from the table. Biting on electrical cords and mouthing electrical sockets can occur as molars and baby teeth appear. Placing objects or fingers into electrical outlets can also occur. Contact burns to the hands may occur as toddlers try to support themselves using the open hot oven door. Ingestions of household chemicals can cause burns to the mouth, respiratory tract, and upper gastrointestinal tract.

Preschoolers imitate family members' activities. Motor skills are more refined. Cognitive functioning and understanding the concepts of right and wrong are beginning. Safety education can be learned at this age. Anxiety, guilt, nightmares, and fear of bodily injury are prominent. Scald burns may occur by children turning on the bath water by themselves. Pulling pots down from the stove (trying to cook like Mommy/Daddy) or playing with matches (trying to smoke like Mommy/Daddy; imitating older siblings) are other ways burns may occur. Chemical burns to the respiratory tract can result if the child mixes and then inhales household chemicals (trying to clean like Mommy/Daddy).

School-aged children have more social contacts outside of the home. They are beginning to make friends and play more independently. Motor functioning is more coordinated.Cognitive abilities include reasoning, understanding time, and knowing the consequences of actions. Peer pressure and dares can be a cause of burn injury. Burns occur because of inappropriate play with chemistry sets, mixing flammable fluids (gasoline, kerosene), trying to light ovens or barbecues, or setting off fireworks. Electrical burns resulting from contact with high-tension wires, changing fuses, repairing outlets, and using hair dryers or electric radios in the bathroom are also possible.

Adolescents are moving into adulthood and are taking on added responsibilities in the home. Working at a job brings new potential for burn injury from lawnmowers, gasoline pumps, or cooking in fast food restaurants (grease burns). Burns may result from working on electrical wiring, working on car engines in enclosed spaces, or climbing structures with high-tension wires "on a dare." Contact burns may occur on the leg from contact with a motorcycle muffler. Although adolescents can escape house fires, they may go back inside a burning house to save someone else. Playing sports in open fields during electrical storms can result in lightning injuries. Gunpowder burns may also result from firing weapons or making pipe bombs. Sneaking cigarettes in enclosed spaces that have chemical fumes may result in an explosion and flame burn. Gasoline sniffing, leading to subsequent explosion, is documented in the literature.[82] Adolescents' sense of omnipotence may foolishly lead them into potentially dangerous situations in which burns can occur.

NURSING CARE PLAN: CARE OF THE PEDIATRIC PATIENT WITH BURNS

Nursing Priorities

1. Maintain patent airway
2. Maintain strict fluid management to replace fluid losses but not over-hydrate
3. Minimize and control bacterial contamination to promote healing and prevent complications
4. Minimize pain and suffering

5. Maintain adequate nutritional support to meet caloric and nitrogen demands for proper healing
6. Maintain joint mobility
7. Assist the child and caregiver to deal with grief and loss associated with alterations in body image and disfigurement
8. Maintain a holistic approach to nursing care by meeting the needs of the patient physically and psychosocially
9. Initiate discharge planning on admission, modifying as necessary
10. Educate child and caregiver in the prevention of burns

Nursing Diagnosis: Airway Clearance, Ineffective

(Also refer to Chapter 9, page 162, Airway Clearance, Ineffective)

May Be Related To:

- Exposure to intense heat, causing upper airway burn, edema, and resultant airway obstruction
- Eschar formation on neck or chest, which may restrict optimum respiratory effort
- Smoke inhalation injury (refer to Chapter 18)

Possibly Evidenced By: Hoarseness, croup, carbonaceous sputum, facial burns, singed nasal hairs, dyspnea, wheezing, cyanosis, circumoral and circumnasal edema.

Desired Patient Outcomes: Child will maintain adequate levels of oxygenation (paO_2 80 to 100 mmHg) and will have unlabored respirations; lung sounds will be clear and present in all lobes.

Interventions	Rationale
INDEPENDENT	
• Observe for respiratory distress and airway compromise: breath sounds, stridor, nasal flaring, retractions, wheeze, cough, cyanosis, and thick secretion; auscultate lungs at least every 4 hours.	• Airway edema and bronchospasm can cause airway obstruction.
• Suction as needed.	• Maintains a clean, patent airway.
• Position child as comfortably as possible; arms at sides, not crossed on chest.	• Added pressure can decrease lung expansion.
• Encourage cough and deep breathing, incentive spirometry, blowing feathers and bubbles every 2 to 4 hours.	• Promotes lung expansion. Assists in ventilation. Assists in mobilizing secretions.
• Monitor arterial blood gases (ABGs)	• Assists in modification of treatment.
• Monitor intake and output (I&O).	• Assists in modification of fluid therapy.
COLLABORATIVE	
• Humidified air may decrease respiratory distress.	• Cool, moist air can assist thin secretions and soothe edematous mucosa.
• Chest physiotherapy should be done before meals.	• Mobilizes secretions. Promotes drainage of secretions.
• Administer mucolytic agents as prescribed.	• Assists in liquifying secretions.

Nursing Diagnosis: Fluid Volume Deficit, Potential

May Be Related To:

- Large fluid losses related to denuded skin
- Shifting of plasma and plasma proteins into interstitial spaces due to vasodilatation and increased capillary permeability
- Hypovolemic shock, metabolic acidosis, and electrolyte imbalances resulting from third spacing
- Inadequate estimation of percentage of burn injury
- Decreased fluid intake

Possibly Evidenced By: Decreased blood pressure, increased pulse, decreased urinary output, weight loss, lethargy, decreased central venous pressure, decreased urine specific gravity, elevated hematocrit.

Desired Patient Outcomes: Child will not become hypovolemic and develop burn shock (first 48 hours). The patient will maintain electrolyte balance. Fluid excess is controlled.

Interventions

INDEPENDENT

- Monitor I&O hourly.

- Weigh daily. If child in diaper obtain diaper dry weight, and subtract wet weight from dry weight to obtain urine output.
- Record hourly urine specific gravity.

- Monitor vital signs and hemodynamic parameters hourly. Compare normal values for age group (Table 14–2).
- Monitor sensorium.

- Monitor electrolytes.

- Maintain IV patency.

COLLABORATIVE

- Administer IV fluids as prescribed.

- Assist in placement of monitoring lines.

Rationale

- Fluid overload can cause edema. Serves as a guide for fluid loss and replacement. Minimum volume of urine per hour:
  <age 2 years: 10–20 ml
  2–5 years: 20–30 ml
  >5 years: 30–50 ml
  Urine output should be at least 0.5 ml/kg per hour.

- Increase in weight may indicate fluid overload and/or increasing edema formation.

- Serves as a guide for fluid loss and replacement.
- Serves as a guide for fluid replacement. CVP is an important indicator of fluid needs.
- Changes in sensorium can indicate a hydration problem.
- Changes occur with fluid and electrolyte deficits and excesses.[83]
- Necessary for replacement therapy and vascular access.

- Fluid resuscitation in burn therapy begins immediately and is based upon the depth and percentage of burn and the child's weight (Table 14–2).
- Serves as a guide for fluid replacement.

Nursing Diagnosis: Fluid Volume, Alteration In: Excess, Potential

May Be Related To:

- Pulmonary edema due to overzealous fluid therapy, or primary lung and airway damage; may also be due to increased pulmonary blood flow and increased capillary permeability[84]
- Return of normal capillary function with protein remaining in vascular space

Possibly Evidenced By: Edema, weight gain, fluid intake greater than output, shortness of breath, dyspnea, anxiety, restlessness, elevated pulmonary artery and central venous pressures, decreased hematocrit and hemoglobin, low urine specific gravity.

Desired Patient Outcomes: Child will maintain adequate fluid and electrolyte balance.

Interventions

(Refer to Chapter 9, page 167, Fluid Volume Deficit.)

Nursing Diagnosis: Infection, and Sepsis, Potential For

(Also refer to Chapter 9, p. 171, Infection, Potential For.

May Be Related To:

- Loss of skin integrity
- Accumulation of eschar and drainage
- Decreased resistance to infection
- Multiple dressing changes and tubbings

Possibly Evidenced By: Elevated temperature, positive wound cultures, changes in wound status (odor, redness, tenderness, swelling, and amount and type of drainage).

Desired Patient Outcomes: Child will not develop sepsis: optimum healing will result.

Interventions	Rationale
INDEPENDENT	
• Shave hair around burn area to 1-inch margin.	• Hair is a medium for bacterial growth.
• Use clean technique during tubbing and aseptic technique during dressing changes.	• Decreases bacterial contamination.
• Tub younger children. Older adolescents may prefer shower.	• Younger children are less frightened in a tub than in a shower. Cleansing of wound is more easily controlled in tub with a younger child. If child was scalded in a tub, will need to use play therapy, allowing child to "test" tub water before submerged, so he or she is reassured burning will not happen again during tubbing.

Nursing Diagnosis: Infection, and Sepsis, Potential For (Continued)

Interventions	Rationale
• In child, clean minor burn first, most extensive burn area last.	• More painful part done last when end of procedure will quickly follow.
• Heat lamp should be on in room during tubbing and dressing change.	• Children, especially infants, are more prone to radiant and evaporative heat losses. Increased fluid loss and heat loss will be minimized or decreased in a heated environment.
• Using sterile technique, use tweezers to remove loose, flaked eschar and any gauze threads from old dressing.	• All eschar needs to be removed as it loosens, to promote granulation, healing, and preparation of vascular bed for grafting.[85,86]
• Evaluate wound. Assess for presence of: ∘ Edema ∘ Purulent drainage ∘ Indications of healing ∘ Granulation tissue	• Allows for early detection of complications, as well as identification of progress in wound healing.
• Inspect extremities to ensure adequate neurovascular status maintained.	• If dressings were applied too tightly, neurovascular compromise can result; inelastic eschar can also result in neurovascular compromise.
• Evaluate wound for clean, vascular bed, granulation tissue.	• Presence will indicate wound's readiness for grafting—final stage of burn therapy.[87]
• Reapply dressings using aseptic technique—tubbing, debridement—then apply antimicrobial agent to dressing and lay over wound. Cover with gauze, and wrap.	• Aseptic technique must be maintained throughout procedure.
• Avoid "buttering" technique (using gloved hand to apply agent directly to wound) as this is quite painful to child.	• This technique is quite painful to the child.

Nursing Diagnosis: Pain

(Also refer to Chapter 9, page 169, Pain)

May Be Related To:

• Exposed nerve endings in partial-thickness burns
• Donor site

Possibly Evidenced By: Verbalizations, wimpering, crying, screaming, withdrawal, facial grimaces; patient may resist moving the affected area; vital signs may be increased

Desired Patient Outcomes: The child will experience maximum pain relief and be as comfortable as possible.

Interventions	Rationale

INDEPENDENT

- Assess child's pain before, during, and after procedure.

- It may be difficult to distinguish real versus remembered pain. The pain, regardless of origin, should be treated as real.[88] Can use a series of faces— smiling, smiling broadly, neutral, frowning, crying—and have young child point to face that best describes his or her pain. Child can also use color— pink, red, dark red—to indicate pain intensity.

- Evaluate possible pattern of pain and requests for pain medications.

- Pain relief will be more effective if medications are given prior to development of excruciating pain.

- Assess physiologic responses to pain: increased BP, pulse, and respiratory rate. Know age-appropriate values and behaviors and child's baseline values.

- Physiologic responses change according to pain intensity.

- Reassure the child:
  ○ That pain medication will help relieve pain
  ○ That pain will begin to decrease

- The patient needs to believe in the prescribed pain relief.

- Evaluate effectiveness of analgesics.

- Need to monitor for proper relief. Very difficult to do in young infant; observe nonverbal signs and vital signs.

- Offer age-appropriate diversional activities (e.g., play therapy, games, music, TV)

- Assists the patient to focus on other things other than pain.

- Teach pain relief techniques:
  ○ "He-hoo" train breathing
  ○ Pant like dog

- Can make somewhat of a game of this so child can participate and experience some relief.

- Explain all potentially painful procedures and their importance (e.g., tubbing, ROM, dressing changes).

- Decreases fear of unknown. Allows patient to prepare and allows for more control.

COLLABORATIVE

- Medicate prior to dressing change with appropriate medication.

- Medicate prior to treatment so medication is in effect before treatment started.

- If possible, tailor medication to child's needs.

- Often small, frequent doses of medication are most effective. Medications ineffective for a child's pain need to be identified, so a medication that will result in pain relief may be ordered.

- Discuss child's response to pain medication with physician and identify most effective method of medication administration to provide relief for the individual child.

Nursing Diagnosis: Pain
(*Continued*)

Interventions	Rationale
• Cover wounds as soon as possible.	• Decreases nerve exposure and therefore pain. Child will become less anxious when dressings are on and when child knows painful dressing change is over.

Nursing Diagnosis: Fear, Potential For

May Be Related To:

• Loss of control during dressing change
• Anticipated pain (e.g., ROM, tubbing, dressing change)

Possibly Evidenced By: Apprehension, crying, screaming, withdrawal, nightmares; sympathetic stimulation: cardiovascular excitation, vomiting.

Desired Patient Outcomes: The child's fear is minimized; child demonstrates few or no manifestations of pain; child is able to maintain some control.

Interventions	Rationale
INDEPENDENT	
• Explain all treatments and procedures.	• Lessens fear of the unknown.
• Explain rationale for all treatments and procedures (e.g., dressing changes are needed to remove old skin so child will get better).	• Child needs to know this is the reason, and that dressing changes are not punishment for misdeeds; child needs to develop trust.
• Give the child a choice (within limits) if appropriate, such as "Do you want to do your dressing now, or in 15 minutes?"	• This will provide some small measure of control for the child.
• Have all needed supplies and equipment assembled before bringing child to treatment room.	• Decreases the time for the dressing change.
• Provide dressing changes, tubbings, and debridements that are gentle yet thorough, efficient but unhurried.	• Will convey nursing skill at performing the dressing.
• Use a soft washcloth, made very soapy with cleansing agent.	• The soft, soapy cloth will cause less pain.
• Let child know it is all right to cry or yell, *when it hurts.*	• The nurse's gentle firmness can help control the child's emotional excess.
• Provide reassurance. Nurse should point out progress daily; e.g., it is easier to remove dressing; there is less eschar; burn is healing.	• Child will not be able to identify small areas of improvement.

Interventions	Rationale

COLLABORATIVE

- Consult with child development therapist as appropriate.

- A child's response to fear varies with developmental level. Therapist can assist child to cope as well as provide health care workers with appropriate guidelines.

Nursing Diagnosis: Nutrition, Alteration In: Less Than Body Requirements

(Also refer to Chapter 9, page 172, Nutrition, Alteration In: Less Than Body Requirements and Chapter 6)

May Be Related To:

- Protein wasting from burn wound
- Hypermetabolic state
- Inability to ingest and digest food
- Refusal to ingest food

Possibly Evidenced By: Weight loss, decreased plasma proteins, decreased caloric intake to meet high nutritional needs, negative nitrogen balance, decreased muscle mass.

Desired Patient Outcome: Child will ingest adequate amount of calories and protein needed for healing.

Interventions	Rationale

INDEPENDENT

- Carefully monitor caloric and protein intake. Monitor I & O.

- Interview child and parents to identify child's specific food likes and favorites. Work to include these in child's diet with many varieties.
- Provide child's special food requests; child should get snack when desired.

- Schedule treatments as much as possible at times other than meal time. Encourage Gatorade, and high-protein, high-calorie snacks.
- Encourage child to eat meals with other children or with family member.
- Provide adaptive devices to utensils as needed so the child can feed self.

- Caloric and protein requirements need to be met to maintain a positive nitrogen balance and provide calories needed for healing.[89]
- Child needs to ingest 70 to 100 kcal/kg and 3 to 5 gm protein/kg. Breast-fed infant can continue to be breast fed, but may need supplemental bottle feedings.
- Overall the child will feel anorexic; providing favorite foods may improve appetite.
- Upsetting child at meal time adds to anorexia.

- Provides a more normal social atmosphere.
- This independence and control may entice the child to eat.

Nursing Diagnosis: Nutrition, Alteration In: Less Than Body Requirements (*Continued*)

Interventions

- Monitor daily weights carefully. Do not weigh child in diaper or dressings.
- Assess bowel sounds; observe for signs and symptoms of gastrointestinal disorders.

- Provide positive reinforcement for good eating habits.

COLLABORATIVE

- Consult with dietitian to plan patient's diet.
- Medicate with analgesics prior to meal time as necessary.

Rationale

- Assesses fluid volume changes and caloric intake adequacy.
- Gastrointestinal problems occur due to severe injuries and high-level stress. Child is prone to develop paralytic ileus, which may cause gastric dilatation and vomiting.
- Encourages good eating habits. Allows patients to feel good about their efforts.

- Allows for appropriate interventions.

- A patient in severe pain will be too consumed with pain or too weak to eat.

Nursing Diagnosis: Mobility, Impaired Physical

(Also refer to Chapter 9, page 174, Mobility, Impaired Physical)

May Be Related To:

- Inhibited movement due to intense pain
- Development of hypertrophic tissue and contractures

Desired Patient Outcomes: Child will return to optimal physical function; contractures and hypertrophic tissue will be prevented.

Possibly Evidenced By: Limited ROM and contractures

Interventions

- Apply burn dressings with extremities in a functional position; be certain no two skin surfaces touch.
- Provide active and passive ROM every 4 hours while awake. For a child, make into a game:
  - Tape on wall for child to reach with finger or toe
  - Bouncing a large ball
  - Throwing a ball through a hoop
  - Small child can ride a tricycle

Rationale

- Prevents or limits development of contractures and scar tissue.

- Prevents or limits loss of motion and development of contractures.[90] Exercise in form of a game will increase child's compliance.

Interventions	Rationale
• Change position of patient every 2 hours; ambulate as early as possible; young child can ride tricycle if legs burned.	• Prevents or limits skin breakdown caused by pressure.
• Initiate the rehabilitative process on admission.	• Prevents loss of function. Enlists patient participation from onset.

COLLABORATIVE

• Medicate with analgesics as necessary prior to exercise and ambulation.	• Decreased pain facilitates mobility.
• Consult with physical therapist and occupational therapist.	• Coordinates activities of daily living.
• Apply splints per order. Identify on splint the appropriate placement of device on patient. Indicate times, if any, when splints may be removed.	• Prevents or limits contracture formation. Instructions written on splint allow appropriate application.
• Have child measured for pressure garments as appropriate. Instruct child and family on use (Color Plates 38 and 39).	• Prevents hypertrophic scarring.

Nursing Diagnosis: Self-Concept, Disturbance In: Body Image

(Also refer to Chapter 7, page 89, Psychosocial Considerations.)

May Be Related To:

• Burn wound and healing process
• Hypertrophic scarring

Desired Patient Outcomes: The child will verbalize understanding of body changes.

Possibly Evidenced By: Verbalizations, withdrawal, refusal to look at wounds.

Interventions	Rationale
INDEPENDENT	
• Help prepare child and family for what child will look like: ○ Mirror available in child's room ○ Mirror available in treatment room ○ Have child and family look at small area of burn wound, gradually larger areas (Fig. 14–2).	• Enables child and family to set own pace, to look at burns when ready.

Nursing Diagnosis: Self-Concept, Disturbance In: Body Image (*Continued*)

Interventions	Rationale

- Provide a realistic appraisal for the child:
  - Nurse's acceptance of child essential; facial expressions and use of touch can be therapeutic (Fig. 14–3).
  - Older child needs opportunities to express concern, and needs to know others outside protective hospital environment can react negatively to the child's appearance.
- Deal openly with the child's concerns.

- Provide opportunities for the child to express concerns; e.g., discussions with older children and adolescents, use of doll or puppet play for younger children.
- Encourage child to get out of bed and into play area and halls so he or she can see and be seen by others.

COLLABORATIVE

- Consult with psychiatrist, psychologist, and/or child development therapist, school teacher as appropriate.

- Nurse's acceptance will help child deal with appearance;[91] child needs to know that most people will accept but that some can be frightened by the child's appearance.

- Nurses need to be sure they are dealing with the child's concerns—not their own.
- Child needs opportunities to express his or her feelings and concerns. Should be encouraged to do this.

- Prevent child from isolating self in room.

- Coordinates interventions with child and family.

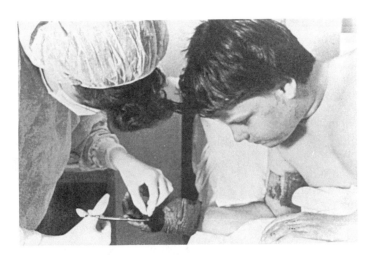

FIGURE 14–2. The adolescent's concern for body image is apparent as this patient intently observes the nurse removing his hand dressing. Note the upper arm donor sites and the healing burns to the face. (Courtesy of Burn Center, The Mercy Hospital of Pittsburgh, Pittsburgh, Pennsylvania.)

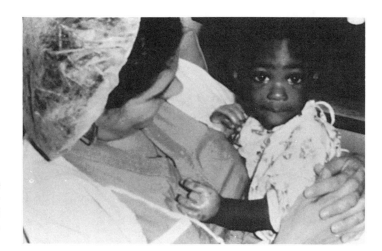

FIGURE 14-3. A nurse's use of touch with a toddler. (Courtesy of Burn Center, The Mercy Hospital of Pittsburgh, Pittsburgh, Pennsylvania.)

Nursing Diagnosis: Coping, Ineffective Individual

(Also refer to Chapter 7, page 92, Psychosocial Considerations.)

May Be Related To:

- Situational crisis of injury
- Changes in role; changes in body image

Possibly Evidenced By: Verbalizations, lack of appetite, insomnia, chronic depression or anxiety, destructive behavior toward self.

Desired Patient Outcomes: Child's coping abilities are identified; psychologic needs are adequately met.

Interventions	Rationale
INDEPENDENT	
• Encourage child to play out or talk about the accident.	• Assists child to verbalize guilt that may exist, especially if the child caused the burn.
• Encourage the child to do this by asking about the event.	• This will let the child know he or she can talk about what happened and will help eliminate pent-up anxiety.
• Provide clear, simple explanation about all aspects of care.	• The child needs to develop trust in the caregivers. Information should be provided in small, meaningful segments that do not overwhelm.

• Assess child for indications of depression; then:
  ○ Encourage verbalizations and play
  ○ Contact by mail, phone, and visits with siblings and peers
  ○ Provide appropriate activities for child's developmental level
	• Denial and withdrawal may be responses; caregiver will need to try to get child involved in normal activities.[92]

Nursing Diagnosis: Coping, Ineffective Individual (*Continued*)

Interventions

- Encourage child to do as much of own care as possible. Child can direct nurse's activities, tell the nurse what aspects of care to do and when to do them (within limits).
- Talk to children about their life after discharge; will need to know others may stare, point, laugh at, or be afraid of appearance.
- Encourage child to get back to school; socialization with peers.

Rationale

- These will enhance child's self-esteem.

- People who do not understand appearance alterations may be afraid and may respond by avoidance or laughter.

- Optimum rehabilitation will occur when child resumes previous level of activity.

Nursing Diagnosis: Family Process, Alteration In

(Also refer to Chapter 7, page 97, Psychosocial Considerations)

May Be Related To:

- Situation crisis of injury
- Hospitalization

Possibly Evidenced By: Verbalization, inability to deal with traumatic experience, ineffective decision-making process.

Desired Patient Outcomes: Family copes effectively with fears and concerns.

Interventions

INDEPENDENT

- Talk with family about their feelings so they can verbalize possible feelings of anger, guilt, fear, rejection of patient, frustration.
- Involve family in doing nonpainful aspects of care: play and activities, combing hair, bringing favorite toys and objects from home.
- Encourage involvement in family support groups for families of burn victims.
- Assess family relationships.
- Assess parenting skill level.

Rationale

- Child's appearance is greatly altered; cause of accident will impact family's emotional response.

- Family frustration can be decreased as they become involved in care.

- Provides outlet for emotion. Allows family to develop strength and meet needs.
- Identifies needs of individual members.
- Considers intellectual, emotional, and physical strengths and weaknesses.

Nursing Diagnosis:
Knowledge Deficit

(Also refer to Chapter 9, page 176, Knowledge Deficit.)

May Be Related To:

- Inability to understand instructions on care of burned child at home
- Lack of information on burn prevention

Possibly Evidenced By: Inability to answer questions related to burn wound care and outpatient regimen; inability to provide return demonstration of wound care.

Desired Patient Outcomes: Child and family will know how to care for burns at home; child and family will identify ways to prevent burn injuries.

Interventions	Rationale
INDEPENDENT	
• Assess child and family learning styles and gear teaching to their level; use charts, pictures, and equipment.	• Enhances learning and understanding of information.
• Areas to be taught include:	• Care at home must be done to prevent complications.
○ Burn care dressing changes	
○ Need for exercise and activity	
○ Dietary requirements	
○ Need for compliance with wearing pressure garment, braces, and/or splints	○ Pressure suit essential to prevent growth of uneven scar tissue.
• Family and child need to understand emotional responses of child; fear, anger, depression, and withdrawal seen in hospital may exacerbate after child is discharged.	• These are psychologic sequelae of burns in children.[93]
• Information is discussed at intervals with family to reinforce teaching. Family needs to understand potential changes in child's socialization.	• Family level of understanding must be assessed.
• Child should be aware that people who do not understand may be afraid of their appearance and avoid them or laugh at them. Children can be encouraged to talk about their burns with close peers.	• Family must also be aware of potential long-term emotional sequelae of burns so they can assist child in coping.
• Older child may be reluctant to return to school; will need encouragement and limit-setting to do this.	• Child's altered body image may cause this reluctance; will need family support, and possibly professional support to cope.[94]
• Adolescent's concerns may focus on appearance, loss of function, concerns about future, and changes in socialization.[95,96]	• Nurses need to prepare the adolescent and family that these may result, and through discussion and education prepare them to deal with these concerns.

Nursing Diagnosis: Knowledge Deficit (Continued)

Interventions	Rationale
• Child and family will be taught ways of preventing future burn accidents (developmental level–specific burn accidents discussed previously in this chapter).	• Anticipatory guidance and accident prevention information must be included in family teaching.

Nursing Diagnosis: Skin Integrity, Impairment Of, Actual

(Refer to Chapter 4, page 64, for etiology, manifestations, desired patient outcomes, and interventions.)

Nursing Diagnosis: Tissue Perfusion, Alteration In: Peripheral

(Refer to Chapter 9, page 164, for etiology, manifestations, desired patient outcomes, and interventions.)

Nursing Diagnosis: Social Isolation

(Refer to Chapter 7, page 90, for etiology, manifestations, desired patient outcomes, and interventions.)

Nursing Diagnosis: Post-Trauma Response

(Refer to Chapter 7, page 93, for etiology, manifestations, desired patient outcomes, and interventions.)

Nursing Diagnosis: Anxiety

(Refer to Chapter 7, page 98, for etiology, manifestations, desired patient outcomes, and interventions.)

Nursing Diagnosis: Grieving

(Refer to Chapter 7, page 94, for etiology, manifestations, desired patient outcomes, and interventions.)

Nursing Diagnosis: Adjustment, Impaired

(Refer to Chapter 7, page 95, for etiology, manifestations, desired patient outcomes, and interventions.)

Nursing Diagnosis: Powerlessness

(Refer to Chapter 7, page 96, for etiology, manifestations, desired patient outcomes, and interventions.)

Nursing Diagnosis: Parenting, Alteration In

(Refer to Chapter 7, page 105, for etiology, manifestations, desired patient outcomes, and interventions.)

REFERENCES

1. McIntire, M (ed): Injury Control for Children and Youth. American Academy of Pediatrics, Elk Grove, IL, 1987, p 121.
2. Carvajal, HF: Burns. In Behrman, RE and Vaughan, VC (eds): Nelson Textbook of Pediatrics, ed 13. WB Saunders, Philadelphia, 1987, p 223.
3. Pollock, D, McGee, D, and Rodriguez, J: Deaths due to injury in the home among persons under 15 years of age, 1970–1984. Centers for Disease Control, CDC Surveillance Summaries. MMWR 37:14(SS-1), 1988.
4. Ibid, p 16.
5. East, MK, et al: Epidemiology of burns in children. In Carvajal, HF and Parks, DH (eds): Burns in Children: Pediatric Burn Management. Yearbook Medical Publishers, Chicago, 1988, p 7.
6. McIntire, p 121.
7. Ibid, p 121.
8. McLoughlin, E and Crawford, J: Burns. Pediatr Clin North Am 32:61, 1985.
9. McIntire, pp 122, 123.
10. Ibid, p 150.
11. Carvajal, p 223.
12. East, et al, p 5.
13. Carvajal, p 223.
14. Yamamoto, L and Wiebe, R: Survey of childhood burns in Hawaii. Pediatr Emerg Care 1:120, 1985.
15. Parish, RA, et al: Pediatric patients in a regional burn center. Pediatr Emerg Care 2:165, 1986.

16. Ibid, p 166.
17. East, et al, p 5.
18. Coren, CV: Burn injuries in children. Pediatr Ann 16:331, 1987.
19. Jacoby, F: Nursing Care of the Patient with Burns, ed 2. Mosby, St Louis, 1976, p 118.
20. Coren, p 331.
21. McIntire, p 207.
22. Ibid, p 152.
23. Schmitt, BD and Kempe, CH: Abuse and neglect of children. In Behrman, RE and Vaughan, VC (eds): Nelson Textbook of Pediatrics, ed 13. WB Saunders, Philadelphia, 1987, p 80.
24. Kelley, S: Child abuse and neglect. In Kelley, S (ed): Pediatric Emergency Nursing. Appleton-Lange, Norwalk, 1988, p 8.
25. Alexander, RC, Surrell, JA, and Cohle, SD: Microwave oven burns to children: An unusual manifestation of child abuse. Pediatrics 79:255, 1987.
26. Ibid, p 259.
27. Chameides, L (ed): Textbook of Pediatric Advanced Life Support. American Heart Association, American Academy of Pediatrics, Elk Grove, IL, 1988, p 5.
28. Hazinski, MF: Nursing Care of the Critically-Ill Child. CV Mosby, St Louis, 1984, p 91.
29. Chameides, p 5.
30. Ibid, p 5.
31. Ibid, p 6.
32. Ibid, p 21.
33. Ibid, p 21.
34. Thompson, A: Respiratory distress. In Fleisher, G and Ludwig, S (eds): Pediatric Emergency Nursing, ed 2. Williams and Wilkins, Baltimore, 1988, p 274.
35. Chameides, p 21.
36. Kneut, C: Burns. In Kelley, S (ed): Pediatric Emergency Nursing, ed 2. Appleton Lange, Norwalk, Connecticut, 1988, p 160.
37. Lybarger, PM: Inhalation injury in children: Nursing care. Issues Compr Pediatr Nurs 10:35, 1987.
38. Ibid, p 35.
39. Ibid, p 37.
40. Ibid, p 37.
41. Charnock, EL and Meehan, JJ: Postburn respiratory injuries in children. Pediatr Clin North Am 27:661, 1980.
42. Carvajal, p 226.
43. Herndon, DN, et al: Treatment of burns in children. Pediatr Clin North Am 32:1327, 1985.
44. Gordon, MD: Nursing care of the burned child. In Artz, CP, Moncrief, JA, and Pruitt, BA (eds): Burns: A Team Approach. WB Saunders, Philadelphia, 1979, p 393.
45. Hazinski, p 3.
46. Ibid, p 3.
47. O'Neill, JP: Burns in children. In Artz, CP, Moncrief, JA, and Pruitt, BA (eds): Burns: A Team Approach. WB Saunders, Philadelphia, 1979, p 342.
48. Herndon et al, p 1316.
49. Hazinski, p 5.
50. Gordon, p 393.
51. Ibid, p 393.
52. O'Neill, p 341.
53. Whaley, LF and Wong, DL: Nursing Care of Infants and Children, ed 3. CV Mosby, St Louis, 1987, p 1407.
54. Vasileff, WG and Whitaker, LA: Plastic surgical emergencies: Facial injuries and burns. In Ludwig, S and Fleisher, G (eds): Textbook of Pediatric Emergency Medicine, ed 2. Williams and Wilkins, Baltimore, 1988, p 1058.
55. Coren, p 335.
56. Bailey, WC: Burns. In Ehrlich, FE, Heldrich, FJ, and Tepas, JJ: Pediatric Emergency Medicine. Aspen Publications, Rockville, MD, 1987, p 435.
57. Whaley and Wong, p 1159.
58. Bailey, p 435.
59. Solomon, p 166.
60. Jacoby, p 121.
61. Ibid, p 121.
62. Barness, LA: Nutrition and nutritional disorders. In Behrman, RE and Vaughan, VC: Nelson Textbook of Pediatrics, ed 13. WB Saunders, Philadelphia, 1987, pp 114, 115.

63. Ibid, p 115.
64. Ibid, p 115.
65. Solomon, p 167.
66. Rowe, PC (ed): The Harriet Lane Handbook, ed 11. Year Book Medical Publishers, Chicago, 1987, p 265.
67. Solomon, p 168.
68. Gordon, p 399.
69. Robson, AM: Parenteral fluid therapy. In Behrman, RE and Vaughan, VC: Nelson Textbook of Pediatrics, ed 13. WB Saunders, Philadelphia, 1987, p 193.
70. Gordon, p 392.
71. Herndon et al, p 1311.
72. Kneut, p 154.
73. Coren, p 338.
74. Jacoby, p 120.
75. Gordon, p 392.
76. Rowe, p 264.
77. Solomon, p 162.
78. Kneut, p 154.
79. Chameides, p 37.
80. McLoughlin and Crawford, p 62.
81. Surveyer, JA and Halpern, J: Age-related burn injuries and their prevention. Pediatr Nurs 7:29, 1981.
82. Cole, M, et al: Gasoline explosions, gasoline sniffing: An epidemic in young adolescents. Journal of Burn Care and Rehabilitation 7:6, 1986.
83. Coren, C: Burn injuries in children. Pediatr Ann 16(4):335, 338, 1987.
84. Herndon, D: Treatment of burn in children. Pediatr Clin North Am 32(5):1326, 1985.
85. Steele, S: Child Health and the Family. Masson Publishers, New York, 1981, p 263.
86. Whaley, L and Wong, D: Nursing Care of Infants and Children, ed 2. CV Mosby, St Louis, 1982, pp 1088, 1091.
87. Solomon, J: Pediatric burns. Critical Care Clinics 1(1):170, 1985.
88. Schnurrer, J: Evaluation of pediatric pain medications. Journal of Burn Care and Rehabilitation 6(2):105, 1985.
89. Solomon, J: Ibid, p 167.
90. Scipien, G: Comprehensive Pediatric Nursing. McGraw-Hill, New York, 1986, p 1342.
91. O'Brien, K: A return-to-school program for the burned child. Journal of Burn Care and Rehabilitation 6(2):108, 1985.
92. Sutherland, S: Burned adolescents' descriptions of their coping strategies. Heart Lung 17(2):153, 1988.
93. Scipien, G: Comprehensive Pediatric Nursing, ed 3. McGraw-Hill, New York, 1986, p 1343.
94. O'Brien, K: Ibid, pp 109–110.
95. Sutherland, S: Ibid, p 153.
96. Sullivan, K: Cognitive responses of adolescents to a major burn injury and its treatment. Unpublished PhD. Dissertation, University of Pittsburgh, 1985, p 94.

BIBLIOGRAPHY

Abston, S: Burns in children. Clin Symp 28:2, 1976.
Alexander, R, Surrell, J, and Cohle, S: Microwave oven burns to children: An unusual manifestation of child abuse. Pediatrics 79:255, 1987.
Archambeault-Jones, C: The child with burns. In Tackett, J and Hinsburg, M (eds): Family Centered Care of Children and Adolescents. WB Saunders, Philadelphia, 1981.
Arneson, S: How children cope with disfiguring changes to their appearance. Am Matern Child Nurs 3, 1978.
Bailey, W (ed): Pediatric Burns. Year Book Medical Publishers, Chicago, 1979.
Bernstein, N: Emotional Care of the Facially Burned and Disfigured. Little, Brown & Co, Boston, 1976.
Coren, C: Burn injuries in children. Pediatr Ann 16:328, 1987.
Durtschi, J: Burn injury in infants and young children. Surg Gynecol Obstet 150, 1980.

Gonzales, E: Psychosocial adjustment of children following hospitalization for acute burns. Journal of Burn Care and Rehabilitation 5:138, 1984.

Gordon, M: Nursing care of the burned child. In Artz, C, Moncrief, J, and Pruitt, B (eds): Burns: A Team Approach. WB Saunders, Philadelphia, 1979, p 390.

Gordon, M, et al: Burn care protocols—nutritional support. Cook County Hospital Burn Unit, Chicago, University of Kansas–Burn Center. Journal of Burn Care and Rehabilitation 7:351, 1986.

Hildreth, M and Carvajal, HF: A simple formula to estimate daily caloric requirements in burned children. Journal of Burn Care and Rehabilitation 3:78, 1982.

Jacoby, R: Nursing care of the patient with burns, ed 2. CV Mosby, St Louis, 1976.

Kavanaugh, C: A new approach to dressing change in the severely burned child and its effect on burn-related psychopathology. Heart Lung 12:612, 1983.

Lybarger, P: Inhalation injury in children: Nursing care. Issues Comprehens Pediatr Nurs 10:33, 1987.

Manley, L, Haley, K, and Dick, M: Intraosseous infusion: Rapid vascular access for critically ill or injured infants and children. J Emerg Nurs 14:63, 1988.

McLaughlin, E and Crawford, J: Burns. Pediatr Clin North Am 32:61, 1985.

Merrell, SW, et al: Fluid resuscitation in thermally injured children. Am J Surg 152:664, 1986.

O'Brien, K and Wit, S: A return-to-school program for the burned child. Journal of Burn Care and Rehabilitation 6:108, 1985.

O'Neill, J: Burns. Top Emerg Med 4:28, 1982.

Petrillo, M and Sanger, S: Emotional Care of Hospitalized Children, ed 2. JB Lippincott, Philadelphia, 1980.

Roberts, J: Emergency tips from the literature. Emerg Med 2:15, 1988.

Robinson, M and Seward, P: Electrical and lightening injuries in children. Pediatr Emerg Care 2:186, 1986.

Schnurrer, J, Marvin, J, and Heimbach, D: Evaluation of pediatric pain medications. Journal of Burn Care and Rehabilitation 6:105, 1985.

Smith, M and Goodman, J. Child and family concepts of nursing practice. McGraw-Hill, New York, 1982.

Solomon, J: Pediatrics burns. Critical Care Clinics 1:159, 1985.

Surveyer, J and Halpern, JS: Age-related burn injuries and their prevention. Pediatr Nurs Sept/Oct 29, 1981.

Sutherland, S: Burned adolescents' descriptions of their coping strategies. Heart Lung 17:150, 1988.

Chapter 15

LORNA L. SCHUMANN

CARE OF THE GERIATRIC PATIENT WITH BURNS

NURSING ASSESSMENT

Mortality

The geriatric burn patient is a high-risk patient who offers multiple patient care challenges for the burn team. The elderly are at risk because of their decreased ability to cope with the prolonged physiologic and psychologic stresses associated with major burns. The percentage of elderly burn victims is higher than other age groups by comparison. The figures in the literature vary, with 12 to 20 percent of admissions being patients over age 60.[1]

Kravitz and colleagues[2] reported that 58 percent of their elderly burn patients during the period from January 1978 to January 1984 were men. They found that the peak season for burn injuries in the elderly was during the fall and winter months. Thirty-two percent of the injuries occurred between 4:00 P.M. and 10:00 P.M. The most common causes of burns, in order of ranking, were flame burns, scalds, chemicals, contact with hot objects, and contact with electricity. The mortality rate for this population was 35 percent, with a mean burn size of 44 percent TBSA for those who died. The primary cause of death was cardiac insufficiency (71 percent). The study also found that 68 percent of the population had previously documented cardiopulmonary disease, which decreased their survival chances and made clinical management difficult.

The April-June, 1984 issue of the Statistical Bulletin[3] reported that the population of elderly adults over the age of 65 in the United States makes up 12 percent of the total population. During that same year, elderly catastrophic deaths (accidents taking five or more lives) from fire were 152, with 73 percent of those fires occurring in family dwellings. The national elderly burn-related mortality[4] figure for 1980 was 1662. Residential fires were the most common sites of fires for the elderly. Baptiste and Feck[5] found that scald burns occurred in 27 percent of their elderly burn population.

Factors that increase the morbidity and mortality rates are pre-existing illnesses, side effects of medication, malnutrition, associated injuries, and physiologic degeneration seen in the normal aging process such as decreased reaction time, impaired sensory system (vision, hearing, smell, touch), impaired immune response, and delayed wound healing.[6-9] In Chapter 9, Figures 9–1 and 9–2 present data from the National Burn Information Exchange (NBIE)[10] related to burn patient survival by age groups for individuals according to total percent burn and percent of full-thickness area burned. Those individuals who fall in the age categories of 60 to 74 and 75 and up consistently have lower survival rates. For instance, a patient with a 40 percent burn has less than a 10 percent chance of survival if he or she is 75 years old compared with a 95 percent chance of survival for a 25-year-old with the same percent burn. In addition, the difference by age groups according to the percent of full-thickness burns reveals that a 75-year-old burn victim with a 30 percent full-thickness burn has a survival rate of 5 percent. In comparison, a 25-year-old burn victim with the same size full-thickness burn has an 88 percent survival rate.[11]

National Burn Information Exchange[12] figures show that 81 percent of burn victims over age 70 are burned because of their own actions. Approximately 70 percent of these injuries occur in the home.[13]

Etiology

Nationally the leading cause of burns in the elderly is scalding.[14,15] A review of the literature shows regional variations in the leading cause of burns in the elderly. Long[16] states that the leading cause of burns at Brooke Army Medical Center in Texas is mishandling of volatile fuels (36 percent of the patients). Gas explosions (18 percent) and smoking in bed (13 percent) rank second and third, respectively, in causes of geriatric burns. Edlich and associates[17] from the University of Virginia Burn Center found that flame burns were the major cause of serious burns (36.7 percent). Scald burns were the second major cause of burns (total of 34.1 percent) in their elderly population. Scald burns were divided into three categories: steam (2.4 percent), liquid (23.5 percent), and grease (8.2 percent). They also determined that scalds were the major cause of injury in minor burns (steam 3.7 percent, liquid 18.9 percent, grease 10.4 percent).[18] Feck and Baptiste[19] found that hot tap water caused 27 percent of the burns in elderly in a New York burn study. Jay and coworkers[20] also found scalds to be the major cause of burns in the elderly in a California study.

The elderly are at risk related to their decreased reaction time, loss of mobility, and loss of sensation from aging. The decreased mobility may have the greatest impact on the severity of burns in the elderly. The decreased reaction time also leads to increased severity of the burn that may have been much less if the individual had been able to extricate himself or herself from the burning agent sooner.

Other factors that are influential in burns in the elderly are injuries involving ignition of clothing. In 1967, Congress passed the Flammable Fabrics Act Amendment to require children's sleepwear to contain flame-resistant materials. Flame-retardant clothing and sleepwear for children is available through size 14. Of course, this does not protect adults or children who have home-sewn clothes. Flame-retardant clothing is more expensive and less durable than homemade clothes.

Matches, cigarette smoking, and kitchen ranges are common causes of fabric ignition. It is not uncommon to see the elderly burned from falling asleep while smoking in bed. In 1981, 65,000 fires were caused by cigarettes. Cigarettes are the leading cause of fire fatalities.[21] Other common scenarios are ignition of clothing while cooking over a gas range, lighting a furnace (Color Plate 40) and using gasoline or other flammable solvents to clean with (Color Plate 41).

ANATOMIC/PHYSIOLOGIC CONSIDERATIONS

The complications that increase morbidity and mortality figures in the elderly burn victim reflect a magnification of physiologic changes seen in the normal aging process. Aging may be defined as:

> . . . a decline in physiologic competence that inevitably increases the incidence and intensifies the effects of accidents, disease, and other forms of environment stress.[22]

The external physiologic factors seen in the normal aging process that affect life expectancy are variable and can be classified into two major categories — those that are permanent and those that are reversible. Permanent factors include sex, longevity of grandparents, longevity of parents, and childhood diseases that produce a lasting effect (e.g., streptococcal infection producing cardiac murmur).

Reversible factors that tend to decrease longevity are: city dwelling, unmarried status (divorced, single, or widowed), smoking, high lipoprotein concentration, and uncontrolled diabetes.[23]

Many of these factors also have a major effect on the morbidity and mortality of the elderly burn victim. Many other age-related changes seen in the elderly do not appear to influence mortality in the elderly. Among these are factors such as graying or loss of hair, decreased height, slowing of electrical activity in the brain unless it affects psychomotor reactions, loss of teeth, and wrinkling of the skin. Other aging and disease factors have a major effect on survival in the elderly burn victim. For example, pre-existing cardiopulmonary disease reduces the elderly person's ability to withstand the rapid changes in fluid volume associated with burns.

Age-Related Cardiovascular Changes

The cardiovascular system is affected both by aging and the significant advancing of atherosclerosis and arteriosclerosis seen in European and North American populations. As a result of these factors hypertension is prevalent among the elderly population.[24,25] The increase in systolic blood pressure reflects reduced vascular elasticity. The increase in diastolic blood pressure is not as great as that seen in systolic blood pressure.

Other cardiovascular changes that affect burn mortality and morbidity include decreased cardiac output, decreased beta-adrenergic responsiveness, decreased intrinsic heart rate, decreased blood flow, decreased vascular permeability, and increased prevalence of postural hypotension. The decreased cardiac output is a result of several factors, including the inability of the heart to respond to the stress of a burn. Stimulation of beta-adrenergic receptors normally produces an increase in heart rate. With aging this response diminishes. Autopsies on elderly persons have shown increased density and sclerosis of cardiac collagen. Fibrous tissue and accumulated fatty deposits are noted in the myocardium and rings of the aortic and mitral valves. The elderly heart weighs less than that of a younger adult with the same body size. Also, it is brown as a result of the accumulation of lipofusion deposits.[26] Amyloid, a protein substance, is found deposited in the myocardium and between myocardial fibers. It was found on autopsies in 42 percent of 300 elderly persons.[27] Amyloid may cause heart failure due to restrictive cardiomyopathy.

Changes within the electrical conducting system of the heart lead to a decreased intrinsic heart rate. Fibrosis of the sinoatrial (SA) node and loss of pacemaker (P) cells account for this change. There is also an increase in elastin, collagen, and fat in the atrial myocardium between the SA node and the atrioventricular (AV) node. These changes may account for the irritable myocardium and increased presence of dysrhythmias in the elderly. The end result is reduction in cardiac output which is a product of heart rate and stroke volume.[28]

The multiple physiologic changes seen in the aging cardiovascular system are a major challenge in the treatment of the elderly burn victim. Fluid resuscitation to prevent hypovolemia without overtaxing the cardiovascular and renal systems is a major concern. Restoration of fluid volume postburn is essential to organ perfusion and cellular oxygenation. It is necessary to replace blood and plasma losses in order to accomplish adequate circulating volume and prevent hypoxemia. The routine fluid resuscitation with 3 to 4 ml/kg of body weight times the percent burn is commonly given. Half of the fluid is given in the first 8 hours postburn and the remainder over the next 16 hours. Adequate perfusion is assumed if the hourly urine output is maintained between 30 to 70 ml.[29] A further, more accurate measure of adequate perfusion is cardiac output, which requires the insertion of a thermodilution catheter in an already immunodeficient patient susceptible to sepsis.

Cardiac monitoring should be instituted upon admission. Sinus tachycardia is common in all burn patients and may be a problem that requires rapid digitalization and careful monitoring. Tachycardia greater than 140 beats per minute may indicate fluid volume overload or a compensatory mechanism to overcome hypovolemia. Blood pressure support with vasopressors may also be necessary to maintain adequate renal and cerebral perfusion. Nursing care is directed at maintaining adequate fluid volumes to ensure proper perfusion and oxygenation while preventing complications.

Age-Related Pulmonary Changes

Respiratory system changes due to the normal aging process include loss of lung parenchymal elasticity and the ability to recoil, loss of muscular elasticity of the chest wall, degeneration of intervertebral discs and vertebrae, decreased arterial oxygen saturation, and decreased pulmonary capillary circulation. The loss of parenchymal elasticity is found in all areas except the pleural and septal tissues. It leads to a decrease in tidal volume and vital capacity and an increase in functional residual capacity, which is a combination of residual volume and expiratory reserve volume. In addition, the loss of chest wall expansion leads to a total reduction in lung volume of about 30 percent by the eighth decade.[30]

The decrease in arterial oxygen saturation may be due to ventilation-perfusion (V/Q) mismatch and decreasing pulmonary capillary circulation with aging. Decreased oxygen saturation tends to disappear with deep breathing.[31]

For the burn patient these changes put the person at risk for hypoxemia and potential lung infection (pneumonia). The pulmonary system can be further taxed by an inhalation injury, fluid overload, open wounds, a suppressed immune response, and frequent surgical procedures.

Management of the pulmonary system requires frequent assessment of lung sounds (at least every 4 hours), monitoring of vital signs, chest x-rays, blood gases, complete blood count (CBC), and sputum cultures. Oxygen administration is usually required in order to provide adequate oxygen levels. Oxygen may be administered via nasal prongs or face mask, and in severe cases ventilator support may be necessary. The patient is monitored for pulmonary edema and pulmonary emboli.

Age-Related Nervous System Changes

Nervous system changes seen in the elderly probably have a greater impact on susceptibility to burn rather than morbidity and mortality factors. Changes within the brain itself include weight loss, patchy loss of nerve cells within the cortical layers of the brain,[32] 25 percent loss of cerebellar cortical cells,[33] decreased nerve conduction velocity, decreased memory recall, decreased speed of response to questions, and slowing of electroencephalogram (EEG) electrical activity in the brain.[34]

Age-Related Sensory Organ Changes

Sensory organ changes with aging are common impairments. It appears that these losses are due in part to the need for an increase in threshold stimulation required for stimulation. Taste, smell, vision, hearing, and pain require higher levels of stimulation to elicit a response similar to that of a younger individual. The loss of taste and smell influence the elderly's desire to eat. They tend to prefer highly seasoned foods or tart tastes.[35] These are important factors in meeting the critical nutritional needs of the burned patient.

Visual losses in the elderly include decreased visual acuity, decreased adaptation to darkness, loss of accommodation, and decreased visual fields.[36] These changes are accounted for by loss of adaptation of the lens related to loss of elasticity and increasing lens density. Loss of vision may impair the ability of the burn victim to provide self-care activities such as self-administration of medications, preparation of food, and wound care.

Hearing loss in the elderly is common. It is due to degeneration of hair cells and supporting cells in the cochlea, loss of auditory neurons, and atrophy of various structures. Impairments range from loss of high frequencies to the more severe loss of the ability to understand speech. The nurse needs to speak clearly and slowly, validating for understanding.

With aging there is a decrease in pain sensation and sensitivity to touch. An increased pain threshold may negatively affect the patient's response time to the pain of burn injury, thus increasing the depth of burn.

Age-Related Changes in the Immune System

The altered immune response seen in the elderly puts them at high risk for infection. A pre-existing malnourished state may further impair the immune response to burn trauma and infection. With advancing age there are decreasing numbers of leukocytes and decreasing effectiveness of their response to infection.[37] In addition, there is a decline in the cell-mediated T-cell responses to proliferate and respond appropriately to an infectious process.[38]

As with any burn patient, nursing care will focus on preventing and controlling infection. Frequent routine antiseptic care of intravenous lines, Foley catheters, and other invasive devices must be provided. Administration of antibiotics and antimicrobial agents should be undertaken when the infecting organism has been identified and sensitivity testing is complete. Prophylactic administration of antibiotics is discouraged due to the potential for a superinfection.

RISK VARIABLES

As we approach the 21st century the average life expectancy continues to increase and the percentage of elderly within the American population is increasing. The 1984 population statistics show that the elderly (those over the age of 65) comprise approximately 12 percent of the total population. The projected figures for the years 2000 and

2050 are 13 percent and 22 percent, respectively.[39] In 1959, the life expectancy at birth of a boy was 67.6 years and of a girl 74.2 years. In comparison, the life expectancy at birth of a boy born in 1984 was 71.8 and of a girl was 78.2.[40]

Moral and ethical issues arise as to initiating extensive therapy in severe burns where chances of survival are deemed very poor. A prediction of the mortality rate can be made by adding the percent burn to the patient's age. Percentages greater than 120 percent have a grave prognosis.[41] Allowing the patient to make the choice of foregoing extensive therapy, while providing measures to control pain and discomfort is one method of dealing with this situation.

Certain factors exist in the elderly population that increase or exaggerate their risk above that of other age groups after a major burn injury. Pre-existing cardiac or pulmonary disease and decreasing hepatic and renal function related to the aging process and/or disease processes are conditions that influence the elderly patient's ability to respond to the stress of a major burn.[42-44] In Chapter 9, figure 9–3 shows NBIE probit curves of survival by frequency of past medical problems. Although medical problems appear in all age groups, experience demonstrates that the greatest number of medical problems exist in the elderly group. The curves demonstrate that better survival rates are observed in groups with fewer past medical problems. For example, in the category for 50 percent TBSA burns, the survival rate for groups with three or more disease processes was 39 percent, compared with groups that had no previous history of disease who had a survival rate of 81 percent.[45] Patients with one past medical history (PMH) problem and a 50 percent burn had a survival rate of 65 percent, and those with two PMH had a survival rate of 50 percent.[46]

Of the 21,440 patient's records reviewed, 5600 had a total of 9538 identifiable medical disease processes. The most common medical problem was cardiovascular disease (20 percent), followed in order by pulmonary disease (11 percent), central nervous system problems (11 percent), emotional disorders (10 percent), alcoholism (10 percent), and metabolic problems such as diabetes (8 percent).[47] Feller and Jones[48] have determined that each PMH problem is equivalent to an 11 percent TBSA burn. This is a critical risk factor for the elderly patient, who often has several medical problems.

These risk factors come into play during the initial burn period when proper fluid resuscitation is crucial to survival. The already compromised cardiopulmonary system may not respond well to administration of large volumes of fluid necessary to correct hypovolemia. In addition, the renal system may be overtaxed by the extreme changes in fluid volume and debris being circulated to it. Maintaining a balance in the interrelationship of these major organ systems is one of the most difficult challenges in burn medicine. This crucial balance can be illustrated, for example, by reflecting on kidney perfusion and fluid balance. Acute oliguric renal failure is five times more common in the elderly than in patients under age 40. In burn patients, achieving rapid fluid resuscitation is crucial to organ perfusion and patient survival. The margin for error in the elderly is quite narrow and requires careful monitoring of vital functions (e.g., pulmonary artery pressure monitoring).

Other conditions that increase morbidity and mortality in the elderly are pre-existing malnutrition; skin changes related to aging; impaired sensory system; decreased coordination, reaction time, and judgment; alcoholism; side effects of medications; and peripheral neuropathy.

Malnutrition in the elderly is a common problem. Dietary habits change over the years and on the whole many elderly do not eat a balanced diet. This change is due to decreases in income, decreases in taste and smell, and a decreased desire to cook for oneself and eat alone. This problem is further complicated by the growing problem of alcoholism among the elderly. Malnutrition also contributes to decreases in the immune defense response, which may permit overgrowth of life-threatening bacteria.

Skin changes in the elderly also increase the risk of significant morbidity and mortality. Skin changes with aging include loss of elasticity, increased paleness, thinning, dryness, and appearance of age spots. Elderly persons also lose subcutaneous fat and muscle bulk. Complicating these skin changes, there is also perceptual losses of sense of pain, impaired vision, delayed reaction time, decreased ability to smell, and impaired hearing. These perceptual losses are crucial in burn injury. Failure to perceive and respond quickly to direct heat or to the smoke of a fire may contribute to a greater percentage and depth of burn.

The final exaggerated risk factor in the elderly is the inability of the geriatric patient to respond adequately to the stress of the burn. Their reduced metabolic reserves make it difficult to respond appropriately to maintain homeostasis. The stress of the burn injury, fluid volume shifts, exposure to cold, surgical intervention, infection, exacerbation of pre-existing illnesses, and the psychosocial disruptions of injury and hospitalization evoke maximum metabolic responses.

Prevention of burn injury is the ultimate goal of the burn team. Outreach programs directed specifically at the elderly have been successful in decreasing burns in this population.[49] The success of such programs depends on nurses who are willing to become involved in burn health teaching in community organizations.

NURSING CARE PLAN: CARE OF THE GERIATRIC PATIENT WITH BURNS

Nursing Priorities

1. Maintain a patent airway (intubation and ventilatory support may be necessary)
2. Manage associated life-threatening injuries
3. Maintain strict fluid management to replace fluid losses but not overload a compromised cardiopulmonary system
4. Obtain baseline diagnostic studies, history, and physical data
5. Minimize pain and suffering and protect the patient from further injury
6. Minimize and control bacterial contamination to promote healing and prevent complications
7. Maintain adequate nutritional support to meet calorie and nitrogen demands for proper healing
8. Provide adequate sleep and rest cycles to prevent sensory overload and deprivation
9. Maintain a holistic approach to nursing care by meeting the needs of the patient physically, emotionally, culturally, spiritually, and psychologically
10. Maintain joint mobility by providing range-of-motion (ROM) exercises, early ambulation, and proper splinting
11. Assist the elderly patient to deal with grief and loss associated with disfigurement and loss of self-esteem.
12. Maximize potential for self-care and promote independence in activities of daily living (ADLs)
13. Initiate discharge planning on admission; modify as necessary dependent on the functioning level of the elderly patient
14. Educate the elderly in burn prevention

Nursing Diagnosis: Airway Clearance, Ineffective

May Be Related To:

- Smoke inhalation injury secondary to inhalation of heat and of toxic and/or noxious gases
- Edema secondary to burns of the face or neck
- Pre-existing pulmonary disease (e.g., chronic lung disease), as well as, related conditions such as depressed immune response, fluid overload, and immobility.

(Refer to Chapter 9, page 162, Airway Clearance, Ineffective for other etiologies manifestations, desired patient outcomes, and interventions.)

Nursing Diagnosis: Gas Exchange, Impaired

(Refer to Chapter 9, page 163, Gas Exchange, Impaired for etiologies, manifestations, desired patient outcomes, and interventions.)

Nursing Diagnosis: Fluid Volume Deficit, Potential

May Be Related To:

- A rapid shift of plasma and plasma proteins, sodium, and chloride into the interstitial spaces secondary to increased capillary permeability and vasodilation
- Evaporative losses from the wound surface
- Untreated fluid shifts
- Decreased fluid intake
- Pre-existing dehydration

(Refer to Chapter 9, page 165, Fluid Volume Deficit, Potential for manifestations, desired patient outcomes, and interventions.)

Nursing Diagnosis: Fluid Volume, Alteration In, Excess, Potential

May Be Related To:

- Decreased urinary output secondary to the physiologic aging process
- Return of normal capillary function with protein remaining in the vascular spaces
- Decreased cardiac output secondary to congestive heart failure (CHF) in the elderly

Possibly Evidenced By: Increased blood pressure, tachycardia, weight gain, increased urine output, edema, restlessness, shortness of breath, hyperpnea, hyponatremia, hypokalemia, and metabolic acidosis.

Desired Patient Outcomes: The patient will maintain adequate fluid and electrolyte balance. The patient's serum albumin level and weight will remain within the normal range. Tissue perfusion will be maintained and hypervolemia prevented.

Interventions	Rationale
INDEPENDENT	
• Monitor blood pressure, pulse, and hemodynamic pressures.	• Increased levels reflect fluid excess. Tachycardia over 140 beats per minute may indicate overload and heart failure.
• Monitor for signs and symptoms of pulmonary edema and hypoxemia.	• Increased fluid in the pulmonary tree may prevent adequate oxygenation.
• Weigh patient daily.	• A gain in daily weight is an indication of fluid retention.
• Monitor serum sodium, osmolarity, potassium levels, and blood count.	• Hemodilution of electrolytes may occur with fluid volume excess. Serious complications can occur with low levels of sodium and potassium. Hemoconcentration in the elderly may not be well tolerated due to decreased cardiopulmonary reserves.
COLLABORATIVE	
• Administer intravenous (IV) fluids and electrolytes as prescribed.	• Proper fluid and electrolyte replacement is based on the severity of the burn and the individual needs of the elderly patient.
• Administer diuretics (such as mannitol) and albumin as necessary.	• Assists in mobilizing excess fluid volume. Effects of fluid volume mobilization in the elderly is carefully monitored.

Nursing Diagnosis: Tissue Perfusion, Alteration In

(Refer to Chapter 9, page 164, Tissue Perfusion, Alteration In for etiology, manifestations, desired patient outcomes, and interventions.)

Nursing Diagnosis: Pain

(Also refer to chapter 9, page 169, Pain.)

May Be Related To:

- Exposure of nerve endings in partial-thickness burns
- Donor site harvesting

Possibly Evidenced By: Verbalization of pain, rubbing, guarding, whimpering, crying, moaning, screaming, facial grimacing, clenched teeth, clenched fists, decreased movement, tight lips, and knotted brow.

Desired Patient Outcomes: The patient's pain is minimized or controlled as evidenced by stated relief, nonverbal cues, and vital signs.

Interventions	Rationale
INDEPENDENT	
• Assess and record the nature, location, quality, intensity, and duration of pain.	• Monitors individual responses to pain. Monitors response to therapy and changes in pain response. Pain sensation may be decreased in the elderly.
• Evaluate effectiveness of analgesics.	• Need to monitor for oversedation versus not giving enough medication to control the pain. Medication tolerance is altered in the elderly, so care should be taken to not overmedicate the elderly patient.

Nursing Diagnosis: Infection, Potential For

(Refer to Chapter 9, page 171, Infection, Potential For for etiologies, manifestations, desired patient outcomes, and interventions.)

Nursing Diagnosis: Nutrition, Alteration In: Less Than Body Requirements

(Refer to Chapter 9, page 172, Nutrition, Alteration In: Less Than Body Requirements for etiologies, manifestations, desired patient outcomes, and interventions.)

Nursing Diagnosis: Mobility, Impaired Physical

May Be Related To:

- Inhibited movement secondary to intense pain
- Development of hypertrophic tissue and contractures
- Decreased energy level in the elderly
- Decrease of total bone mass and muscle mass secondary to aging

- Loss of balance and change of center of gravity secondary to aging
- Postural hypotension

    (Refer to Chapter 9, page 174, Mobility, Impaired Physical for manifestations, desired patient outcomes, and interventions.)

Nursing Diagnosis: Fear

(Also refer to Chapter 9, page 175, Fear.)

May Be Related To:

- Hospitalization
- Disability or death
- Separation from friends and family
- Failure in the elderly
- Loss of respect (perceived or actual)

Possibly Evidenced By: Verbalization of fear, insomnia, noncommunication, clenching of teeth, wringing of the hands, and increased sweating.

Desired Patient Outcomes: The patient is able to:

- Verbalize fears and concerns, identify sources of fear
- Communicate positive feelings about self and body image
- Express hope and confidence in recovery
- Identify and use support systems
- Integrate at least one fear-reducing coping mechanism in daily behavior

Interventions

INDEPENDENT

- Speak clearly and validate understanding.

- Provide a sleep environment similar to the patient's home environment.

Rationale

- Hearing may be impaired in the elderly. Sensory overload may impair understanding of what is being communicated.
- Sleep deprivation in the elderly is common. Loss of rapid eye movement (REM) and non-REM sleep leads to confusion, decreased healing, and impaired restoration of normal physiologic mechanisms.

Nursing Diagnosis: Knowledge Deficit, Wound Healing, Burn Treatments, And The Rehabilitation Process

(Refer to Chapter 9, page 176, Knowledge Deficit for etiology, manifestations, desired patient outcomes, and interventions.)

Nursing Diagnosis: Skin Integrity, Impairment Of

(Refer to Chapter 4, page 64, for etiology, manifestations, desired outcomes, and interventions.)

Nursing Diagnosis: Social Isolation

(Refer to Chapter 7, page 90, for etiology, manifestations, desired patient outcomes, and interventions.)

Nursing Diagnosis: Coping, Ineffective Family/Individual

(Refer to Chapter 7, page 92, for etiology, manifestations, desired patient outcomes, and interventions.)

Nursing Diagnosis: Post-Trauma Response

(Refer to Chapter 7, page 93, for etiology, manifestations, desired patient outcomes, and interventions.)

Nursing Diagnosis: Anxiety

May Be Related To:

• Uncertainty about future ability to live independently

    (Refer to Chapter 7, page 98, for other etiologies, manifestations, desired patient outcomes, and interventions.)

Nursing Diagnosis: Grieving

    (Refer to Chapter 7, page 94, for etiology, manifestations, desired patient outcomes, and interventions.)

Nursing Diagnosis: Adjustment, Impaired

    (Refer to Chapter 7, page 95, for etiology, manifestations, desired patient outcomes, and interventions.)

Nursing Diagnosis: Powerlessness

    (Refer to Chapter 7, page 96, for etiology, manifestations, desired patient outcomes, and interventions.)

Nursing Diagnosis: Family Process, Alteration In

    (Refer to Chapter 7, page 97, for etiology, manifestations, desired patient outcomes, and interventions.)

Nursing Diagnosis: Self-Concept, Disturbance In

    (Refer to Chapter 7, page 89, for etiology, manifestations, desired patient outcomes, and interventions.)

REFERENCES

1. Kravitz, M, et al: Thermal injury in the elderly: Incidence and cause. Journal of Burn Care and Rehabilitation 6:16, 1985.
2. Ibid, p 17.
3. ————: Recent international changes in longevity. Stat Bull Metropol Life Insur Co 1:16, 1986.
4. ————: Accident death toll: 1984. Stat Bull Metropol Life Insur Co 2:24, 1985.
5. Baptiste, MS and Feck, G: Preventing tap water burns. Am J Public Health 70:727, 1980.
6. Lewis, JM: Prevent burn injury to older adults: Develop and implement a plan that works. J Gerontol Nurs 11:8, 1985.
7. Feck, G and Baptiste, MS: The epidemiology of burn injury in New York: Public Health Rep 94:312, 1979.
8. Long, JM: Burns in geriatric patients. In Artz, CP, Pruitt, BA, and Montcrief, JA (eds): Burns: A Team Approach. WB Saunders, Philadelphia, 1979, p 334.
9. Foyt, M: Does aging magnify the danger of burn injury? (Part 1). J Gerontol Nurs 11:22, 1985.
10. Feller, I and Jones CA: The National Burn Information Exchange: The use of a National Burn Registry to evaluate and address the burn problem. Surg Clin North Am 67:167, 1987.
11. Ibid, p 177.
12. Ibid, p 177.
13. Silverstein, P and Lack, B: Fire prevention in the United States: Are the home fires still burning? Surg Clin North Am 67:1, 1987.
14. Ibid, p 3.
15. Jay, KM, et al: Burn epidemiology: A basis for burn prevention. J Trauma 17:943, 1977.
16. Long, JM, p 335.
17. Edlich, RF, et al: Epidemiology and treatment of burn injury in Virginia. Journal of Burn Care and Rehabilitation 5:275, 1984.
18. Ibid, p 276.
19. Feck and Baptiste, p 312.
20. Jay et al, p 943.
21. McGuire, A: Cigarettes and fire deaths. NY State J Med 83:1296, 1983.
22. Timiras, PS: Developmental Physiology and Aging. Macmillan, New York, 1972, p 465.
23. Jones, HB: The relation of human health to age place and time. In Birren, JE, (ed): Handbook of Aging and the Individual. University of Chicago Press, Chicago, 1959.
24. Foyt, MM: Does aging magnify the danger of burn injury? (Part 2). J Gerontol Nurs 11:17, 1985.
25. Robertson, D: Physiologic changes and clinical manifestations of aging. In Pagliaro, AM and Pagliaro, LA (eds): Pharmacologic Aspects of Aging. CV Mosby, St Louis, 1983, p 111.
26. Ibid, p 111.
27. Pomerance, A, Slavin, G, and McWatt, J: Experiences with the sodium sulphate alcian blue stain for amyloid in cardiac pathology. J Clin Pathol 29:22, 1976.
28. Robertson, D, p 112.
29. Wachtel, TL and Fortune, JB: Fluid resuscitation for burn shock. In Wachtel, TL, Kahn, V, and Frank, HA (eds): Current Topics in Burn Care. Aspen Systems, Rockville, MD, 1983, p 41.
30. Rizzato, G and Marazzini, L: Thoraco-abdominal mechanics in elderly men. J Appl Physiol 28:457, 1970.
31. Harris, EA, et al: The normal alveolar-arterial oxygen-tension gradient in man. Clin Sci Mol Med 48:89, 1974.
32. Brody, H: Organization of cerebral cortex. III. A study of aging in the human cerebral cortex. J Comp Neurol 102:511, 1955.
33. Hall, TC, Miller, AKH, and Corsellis, JAN: Variations in the human purkinje cell population according to age and sex. Neuropathol Appl Neurobiol 1:267, 1975.
34. Kimmel, DC: Adulthood and aging: An interdisciplinary, developmental view. John Wiley & Sons, New York, 1974, p 342.
35. Ibid, p 372.
36. Ibid, p 372.
37. Caird, FI, Andrews, GR, and Gallie, TB: The leucocyte count in old age. Age Ageing 1:239, 1972.
38. Mathies, M, et al: Age-related decline in response to phytohemagglutinin and pokeweed

mitogen by spleen cells from hamsters and a long-lived mouse strain. J Gerontol 28:425, 1973.

39. ————————: Recent international changes in longevity, p 20.
40. Ibid, p 21.
41. Jacoby, FG: Nursing care of the patient with burns, ed 2. CV Mosby, St Louis, 1976.
42. Long, JM, p 335.
43. Foyt, M, p 17.
44. Feller and Jones, p 176.
45. Ibid, p 176.
46. Ibid, p 176.
47. Ibid, p 176.
48. Ibid, p 176.
49. Lewis, JM, p 8.

Chapter 16

CARE OF THE ALCOHOLIC AND SUBSTANCE ABUSE PATIENT WITH BURNS

NURSING ASSESSMENT

When managing the burn victim in the emergency department and in the acute care setting, many factors must be taken into consideration in terms of physiologic as well as psychologic support. A problem that health care providers are often faced with is the patient who exhibits unusually uncontrollable or bizarre behaviors. There are many explanations for a patient's "acting out" and it is essential in considering physiologic as well as psychologic factors precipitating such behavior so that appropriate treatment can be provided.

The health care provider may begin by ruling out physiologic factors manifested as unusual or bizarre behavior. Hypovolemia in the early postburn period results from inadequate replacement of the functional extracellular fluid in the first 12 to 18 hours postburn. Mental alertness and a clear sensorium are key indicators of adequate fluid resuscitation. The patient's confusion may be due to shock or hypovolemia. Conversely, fluid overload syndrome including water intoxication may also result in mental confusion, progressing to convulsions.

Hypoxia may also be present and manifested as confusion and disorientation. The inhalation of toxic chemicals found in smoke or fumes can cause lung irritation resulting in diminished ability of the body to gain oxygen through the lungs. Patients burned in enclosed spaces often sustain carbon monoxide (CO) poisoning, thereby reducing the amount of hemoglobin available to carry oxygen through the body. This hypoxia affects normal brain function and causes the patient to become suddenly combative and uncooperative. Prolonged, untreated periods of hypoxia due to CO poisoning will result in severe restlessness, lethargy, stupor, and eventually death.

Hypoglycemia may be another factor to consider when observing unusual behaviors, particularly in diabetic adults, alcoholics, and in children where glycogen stores last 24 hours or less. Symptoms of hypoglycemia may mimic intoxication. The dominant metabolic effect of burn injury is increased mobilization of glucose from the liver to peripheral tissues. Glycogen in the liver and muscle cells is converted to glucose. Protein is broken down providing amino acids for gluconeogenesis, and glycogen stores may be decreased.

Another factor to consider in the assessment of a combative, confused, or uncontrollable patient is the presence of pain. Burn injury is extremely painful, particularly when partial-thickness injury is involved and peripheral nerve fibers and pain receptors remain intact. Extreme pain may be manifested in combative and uncooperative behavior. Therefore, administration of analgesics is an important aspect of care and is given prompt attention. Prior to the administration of any analgesia, however, it may be necessary to rule out the possibility of drug overdose, and to determine if any drugs have been taken before giving additional sedation.

Besides the physical trauma involved in burn injury, the burn victim is also suffering from intense psychologic trauma. It is important for the nurse to consider the psychologic effect of the injury while assessing the patient. Feelings of fear, anxiety, and stress due to trauma may explain some uncooperative or "acting out" behaviors. Additionally, the burn patient may be faced with a long hospitalization, change in occupational status, financial difficulties, and permanent alteration in function and physical appearance. Expressed or anticipated needs must be responded to — not ignored, belittled, or judged. The response to psychologic or emotional care may include information giving, providing warmth and comfort, providing a sense of security, setting limits for patients who are prone to act out, or correcting a distortion of reality.

Once these physiologic and psychologic factors are ruled out as the primary causes of uncooperative or unusual behavior, the presence of alcohol or substance abuse may then become a consideration. Many individuals seen in the emergency department suffer from burns related to alcohol or drug abuse. Some 20 percent of acute medical and surgical admissions are alcohol related.[1] Not all of these patients drink to the point that they become addicted to alcohol, but many of them do, and present management problems to the staff. Some of these patients may develop alcohol withdrawal symptoms manifested by delirium tremens (DTs) and may experience extremes of terror and anxiety in addition to terrifying hallucinations.

Nielsen and coworkers[2] found a high correlation between the use of drugs and alcohol and self-inflicted burns. The methods of attempted suicide were self-immolation with flammable liquids, self-immolation without flammable liquids, soaking of an automobile seat or bed with flammable liquids, house gas explosion, and scald injuries. The extent of burn ranged from 1 to 98 percent total body surface area (TBSA), and mortality was 34 percent. Suicide has frequently been attempted by dousing oneself with gasoline and striking a match, resulting in total body ignition. These occurrences are often drug and alcohol related.

Burn injury is often sustained when the drug- or alcohol-intoxicated individual falls asleep in a bed or chair with a lighted cigarette, resulting in upholstery and clothing ignition. In this impaired state, the victim is unable to recognize that the fire has started and is unable to escape.

Barillo and associates[3] reported that ethanol was detected in 80 percent of fire fatalities and that 70 percent of the victims were legally drunk. Additionally, the blood alcohol levels of those found in bed were significantly higher than those found near an escape. Ethanol intoxication significantly impairs the ability to escape from fire and smoke and is a contributory factor in smoke-related mortality.[4]

Birky and Clarke[5] reported, from a study of fire victims, that alcohol was found in the blood of 40 percent of the fatalities, and it is the only drug that appears to be involved in fatal fires to any significant degree. Alcohol is a major problem in fatal fires from the standpoint of both the fatal outcome and the initiation of the fire.

Adolescents have been inhaling various volatile substances for decades to achieve a sense of euphoria. The most commonly abused substances in the 1960s and 1970s were glue, plastic, model cement, and aerosol products. During the past 10 years, gasoline has grown in popularity; in fact, the most common cause of burn injury in the 10- to 15-year-old age group is the accident related to gasoline.[6] Additionally, it involves young men more frequently than young women. Most patients are usually from divorced families, have low socioeconomic backgrounds, and have limited intellectual capabilities. These patients will usually not admit to sniffing gasoline when interviewed.

The acutely toxic gasoline sniffer presents with euphoria, nystagmus, nausea, vomiting, dizziness, visual hallucinations, and changes in consciousness.[7] Gasoline-related burns usually occur when the liquid spills on a flame source or when a victim lights a cigarette and the gasoline vapors ignite. The face, anterior torso, and arms are burned most often; the posterior torso and legs are burned less frequently. As a result of their altered sensorium, patients who had been sniffing gasoline had larger burns, larger percentage of full-thickness burns, and subsequently longer hospital stays that required more surgery than did those injured by gasoline in other accidents.[8]

Parenteral abuse of heroin and cocaine is also widespread in our society, crossing economic, ethnic, and social boundaries. Burn injury has been associated with the use of cocaine when the drug is smoked in a procedure called "free-basing." Free-base is made from cocaine hydrochloride by processes involving a strong alkali, such as ammonia or sodium hydroxide and ether. This free-base is extremely volatile. Many burn injuries have occurred while preparing and smoking the free-base material. Smoking the cocaine alkaloid (free-base) delivers extremely high plasma levels of the drug and increases risk of toxicity in addition to presenting a fire hazard to the person preparing it.[9]

CLIENT HISTORY

Physical Assessment

Vital Signs. Intoxication and withdrawal states lead to changes in vital signs. The primary physical signs of acute narcotic intoxication are the changes in respiratory rate and pupil size.[10] Opiates decrease respiratory rate and constrict the pupils. Cocaine intoxication dilates the pupils, increases blood pressure and heart rate, and may cause cardiac arrest.[11] Also found during acute withdrawal from opiates are pupil dilatation, hypertension, and tachycardia. It is difficult to evaluate hypertension in patients under the influence of opiates and alcohol, since withdrawal from both raise blood pressure.

Weight. Rapid and dramatic weight loss is often associated with heavy cocaine use or chronic alcoholic malnutrition.

Skin. Cutaneous signs of parenteral drug use include needle track marks over superficial veins, usually found in the anticubital fossa and on the forearm. Lesions found on the extremities that appear as shallow, round, hypopigmented depressions are created by "skin popping," or intradermal drug administration. Superficial cellulitis, old sores, and skin abscesses, a common cutaneous complication of drug abuse, also are found related to both chemical and infective reactions.[12] It is important to differentiate between a local or a systemic process when assessing soft tissue wounds, as treatment will vary. Cellulitis may require systemic antibiotics; abscesses may require surgical drainage.

Mucous Membranes. The nasal passages of all heroin and cocaine users are examined as both drugs are often administered intranasally. Erythema of the mucosa and rhinorrhea result from irritation caused by the drugs. The vasoconstrictive effects of cocaine can cause ulcers, bleeding necrosis, and perforation of the septum.

Pulmonary System. Death due to respiratory arrest and acute pulmonary congestion and edema is the most dramatic pulmonary complication of intravenous heroin. Pneumothorax can also occur as a result of needle puncture while attempting injection of the subclavian vein. Often, illegal drugs that are injected contain medications that were made for oral use and therefore contain soluble fibers such as starch and talc. Injection of these foreign materials can cause pulmonary fibrosis and foreign body granulomas.[13]

Heart. The use of cocaine causes tachycardia and ventricular dysrythmias. For the individual who has a history of heart disease, even low, presumably nontoxic doses can precipitate myocardial infarction and death.[14] If a parenteral drug user presents with complaints of fever, chills, and fatigue, infective endocarditis, a serious and common complication of parenteral drug use, is considered. The patient may also complain of vague musculoskeletal pains, arthralgias, and respiratory symptoms. Blood cultures are obtained when infective endocarditis is suspected. Additionally, echocardiography or other noninvasive imaging of the heart may be indicated.

Liver. Infectious hepatitis is the major hepatic complication of parenteral drug abuse. The patient's liver status is assessed regularly. Assessment includes detection of spider angioma, palmar erythema, and other skin manifestations of liver disease in addition to palpation of the liver. Serologic screening is completed for hepatitis B surface antigen (HBsAg) and antibodies to both the viral core (anti-HB core) and the surface protein (anti-HBs). Hepatitis B vaccine is given if the results of these tests are negative. Human immunodeficiency virus (HIV) screen is considered with appropriate consent and counseling in drug abusers.

Kidney. Glomerulonephritis from septic embolisms or immune complex deposition can develop in parenteral drug users with endocarditis and bacteremia. Heroin users are at risk for nephrotic syndrome which often leads to end-stage renal failure. The presence of dependent edema in the extremities as a result of obliterated peripheral veins complicates the assessment. Other early signs of kidney disease may include facial edema, proteinuria, hematuria, and elevated blood pressure.

Neurologic System. Obvious neurologic problems in the emergency department (ED) may be a result of drug or alcohol intoxication or withdrawal, trauma from drug administration, or infections. Seizures can also be associated with drug overdose and withdrawal states. It is important to differentiate between drug-induced seizures and other seizure disorders. An EEG is not reliable until the patient has been drug-free for several weeks.[15] Identifying the etiology of the seizure is important because chronic diphenylhydantoin (Dilantin) or phenobarbital therapy is not indicated for seizures that are associated with drugs.[16] However, phenobarbital may be useful during sedative hypnotic withdrawal as it, too, is a barbiturate. Phenobarbital is prescribed with caution for those patients with a history of substance abuse, since it is a frequently abused drug.[17]

Psychosocial Aspects

As part of the assessment, the ED nurse obtains information regarding the social background of the patient. This information is best obtained from the patient. If this is not possible, the information may be obtained from a family member or friend if present in the emergency department. Social background information includes the patient's age, sex, occupation, education, and ethnic/religious affiliation. Patients' perceptions of their drug and/or alcohol use are assessed, including the role drugs and alcohol play in their life, precipitating factors leading to use, and feelings of self worth. The support systems available to the patient are determined such as family and significant others as well as their interaction with the community. Also assessed by the nurse are the patient's coping mechanisms such as manipulative behavior, overuse of denial, projection, rationalization, feelings of depression and anxiety, problem-solving skills and drug-seeking behaviors. Finally the patient's mental status, physical appearance, mood or affect, memory, speech patterns, cognitive perceptions, and judgment orientation are evaluated.

RISK VARIABLES: VARIOUS AGENTS

Quick intervention is crucial when the alcohol-related and substance-abusive burn victim becomes toxic or moves into withdrawal. Early detection of signs and symptoms of drug and alcohol abuse in addition to signs of withdrawal are essential to treatment.

Alcohol (CNS Depressant)

Assessment. Physical and psychologic function affected; confusion; ataxia; pacing; fidgeting; flushed face; increased abdominal girth; lack of personal hygiene; poor nutritional intake; cigarette burns on hands; numbness in hands or feet; weight loss; dental caries; elevated liver enzymes.

Withdrawal Symptoms. Can begin a few hours to several days after last drink; nausea; vomiting; increased pulse and blood pressure; coarse tremor of the hands; moderate to extreme anxiety; sleep disturbances; depressed or irritable mood.[18]

It may be necessary to restrain extremities in the extremely combative, irritable patient to prevent both harm to the staff and self-inflicted injury. The patient is assured that the restraints are used to prevent personal harm. Paranoid feelings are common at this time. If the extremities have evidence of burn injury, a thin layer of dry sterile gauze is placed between the restraint and the surface of the burned extremity. Circulation is checked frequently to ensure that restraints are not obstructing distal blood flow.

Intervention. Administer, as ordered: antiemetics, anxiety agents (e.g., diazepam), thiamine and folic acid to correct or prevent nutritional deficiencies and anticonvulsants. Assess vital signs every 2 hours while awake. Provide a calm, quiet environment. Use simple, direct approach when communicating. There is some controversy concerning the use of Compazine, as some feel it may worsen withdrawal symptoms.

Stimulants (Cocaine, Amphetamines)

Assessment. Excessive activity, overtalkativeness, euphoria followed by depression (crashing), tachycardia, hypertension, needle track marks, irritability, tremors, violence, paranoia, and necrotic nasal septum; insomnia followed by fatigue and exhaustion; anorexia; cardiopulmonary arrest (with the use of cocaine); central nervous system (CNS) and respiratory complications (with drugs that are snorted); nausea, muscle tension, blurred vision, "unpredictable behavior," coma.

Withdrawal Symptoms. Headache, insomnia, and nervousness (associated with cessation of nicotine and caffeine); amphetamine withdrawal ("crashing") occurs within 24 to 72 hours after administration of the drug; cocaine withdrawal includes flulike pains, hallucinations and tremors; may be suicidal—therefore, interventions are taken to provide a safe environment.

Interventions. Promote safety and rest and maintain the patient's orientation. Enhance coping strategies by maintaining calm, reassuring communication. Remove harmful objects from the environment, provide adequate lighting to reduce shadows, reduce sensory stimulation, promote sleep and rest, and explain all procedures to the patient to reduce stress and anxiety.

Psychoactive Agents (Cannabinoids, Hallucinogens, PCP)

Assessment. Temporary "mind expansion" and alteration from use of cannabis-type preparations (marijuana, hashish) and from hallucinogens such as phencyclidine (PCP); alteration of reality orientation, mood, perception and consciousness; CNS depression or stimulation from the use of hallucinogens.

Patient may manifest alteration in time/space perception, relaxation and euphoria from marijuana; also anxiety, depression, visual and auditory hallucinations.

Chronic marijuana use may result in short-term memory loss, apathy, poor social functioning, and diminished goal achievement. Hypertension, irregular respirations, conjunctivitis, and tachycardia may also result.

Withdrawal/Overdose. Cannabis overdose is rare and of short duration (1 to 2 hours). There is no physiologic overdose emergency with cannabis or hallucinogens. Danger exists with drug-related distortions ("bad trips" and flashbacks) resulting in life-threatening situations including fear, altered perception, and poor judgment resulting in harm to self or others.

Phencyclidine (PCP, "angel dust") is an unpredictable and dangerous hallucinogen. Low oral doses cause slurred speech, nystagmus, blank staring, ataxia, and bizarre behaviors. Higher doses that are inhaled or injected can result in schizophrenic-type thought processes. Also, visual and auditory hallucinations and feelings of depersonalization, body image change, and estrangement. Many street drugs often contain PCP as a filler.[19] Physiologic effects of high-dose PCP may include convulsions, cardiovascular arrhythmias, coma, and respiratory failure.

Interventions. Maintain airway and monitor respirations, blood pressure, levels of consciousness, and other vital functions. Administer diazepam (Valium) as ordered. Maintain a quiet, dimly lit, nonthreatening environment. When PCP is involved, monitor cardiac, respiratory, and CNS function. Urine acidification with ascorbic acid and diureses promote elimination. Continuous gastric lavage (PCP is lipophilic; gastroenteric recirculation will occur). Cathartic administration may be needed to facilitate PCP elimination; anticonvulsants may be used to treat seizures. Antihypertensives such as propranolol may be used. Provide a quiet, low-stimuli environment and provide constant reassurance and reality orientation. Encourage friends to remain with the patient. When possible, avoid use of restraints. Do not use gastric lavage (except for PCP) as the patient may perceive the orogastric or nasogastric tube as threatening. However, a nasogastric tube may be necessary if the patient has burns involving greater than 20 percent of the body surface area and if bowel sounds are absent.

SPECIAL NURSING CONSIDERATIONS

In addition to the usual physiologic needs of burn victims, special considerations are warranted in light of their drug and/or alcohol problems. For instance, fluid resuscitation needs will vary depending upon the preburn physiologic condition of the patient. Alcoholics may already be fluid depleted from "binge" drinking, thereby increasing their postburn fluid requirements. On the other hand, the already cardiopulmonary-compromised drug user may not tolerate the large volume of resuscitation fluids required by the burn injured patient. Response to fluid resuscitation is monitored closely and frequently including urine output, blood pressure, heart rate, and the patient's sensorium.

Burn injury is extremely painful; however, sedation and pain medication must be given with extreme caution to the drug- or alcohol-abusive patient, particularly if the patient has already ingested drugs or alcohol prior to arrival in the ED. Additionally, drug-abusive patients may require higher doses of narcotics to achieve the desired level of analgesia. This may be particularly true during daily routine dressing changes.

Nutritional needs of the burn patient are greatly increased due to the hypermetabolic state. Additional calories may be required for the malnourished alcoholic and drug abusive individual.

DIAGNOSTIC STUDIES

In addition to the routine diagnostic studies that are essential to the assessment of all burn victims, the following studies may also be indicated when alcohol or substance abuse is suspected:

- Blood alcohol level
- Drug screen
- HIV screen for those patients who have a history of intravenous drug use
- Hepatitis screen (HBsAG, anti-HBs, and anti-HB core)

NURSING CARE PLAN: CARE OF THE ALCOHOLIC AND SUBSTANCE ABUSE PATIENT WITH BURNS

Nursing Priorities

1. Maintain airway, particularly for those patients experiencing drug and alcohol intox- ication
2. Provide a safe, non-threatening environment
3. Minimize anxiety and panic level
4. Provide emotional support for patient and significant others
5. Provide adequate sleep and rest activity
6. Minimize pain and discomfort
7. Provide adequate nutrition

Nursing Diagnosis: Breathing Patterns, Ineffective, Potential

May Be Related To:

- Various drugs, such as heroin, can cause dramatic pulmonary complications and inhibit normal breathing patterns, leading to respiratory arrest and eventually death
- Opiates may decrease respiratory rate and depth, depress the cough and gag reflexes and decrease activity
- Aspiration can occur during periods of "nodding" or loss of consciousness

Possibly Evidenced By: Verbalizations; shortness of breath; dyspnea; cyanosis; tachypnea; abnormal arterial blood gases (ABGs); use of accessory muscles; and depressed cough and gag reflex.

Desired Patient Outcomes: Patient will maintain adequate ventilation, patent airway, clear breath sounds, normal respiratory rate, and breathing patterns.

Interventions	Rationale

INDEPENDENT

• Monitor respiratory rate and rhythm.	• Inadequate respiratory rate and breathing patterns may lead to poor gas exchange and eventual respiratory arrest.
• Elevate head of bed.	• Optimizes lung expansion and respiratory function.
• Encourage coughing and deep breathing.	• Promotes lung expansion and drainage of secretions.
• Suction p.r.n.	• Assists in airway clearance.

COLLABORATIVE

• Administer humidified oxygen as needed.	• Prevents hypoxemia and acidosis.
• Monitor ABGs.	• Baseline is used for comparison of further studies and serves as a guide for treatment. Indicates ventilatory status.
• Obtain serial chest x-rays.	• Initial assessment may indicate aspiration pneumonia and provides a baseline to compare further studies.
• Prepare for possible endotracheal intubation.	• Provides a patient airway in the event of respiratory arrest due to drug overdose.
• Insert nasogastric tube.	• Prevents nausea and vomiting and further aspiration.

Nursing Diagnosis: Injury To Self Or Others, Potential For

May Be Related To:

• Seizure activity and environmental misperceptions

Possibly Evidenced By: Previous suicidal attempts, or reports of suicidal ideation/plan, and feelings of powerlessness or hopelessness; verbalizations.

Desired Patient Outcomes: The patient will not exhibit self-destructive behavior and will not attempt to harm others.

Interventions	Rationale

INDEPENDENT

• Provide calm, isolated environment.	• Quiet atmosphere in the presence of withdrawal symptoms will reduce anxiety. Isolation will be required to minimize contamination of burn wounds.
• Provide good lighting.	• Reduces shadows, prevents falls and overstimulation. (*Note:* lights should be dim during PCP withdrawal to decrease agitation.)

Nursing Diagnosis: Injury to Self Or Others, Potential For (*Continued*)

Interventions	Rationale
• Provide constant reassurance and reality orientation.	• Reduces confusion, fear, anxiety, and/or hallucinations.
• Remove harmful objects from the patient's reach.	• As the patient may react rather quickly, sharp objects that can be used to cause harm to self or others are removed from the environment.

COLLABORATIVE

• Administer medications such as haloperidol (Haldol) as ordered and Ativan for alcoholics.	• Reduces anxiety, confusion, and depression.
• Promote urine acidification (urine pH 4.5 to 5.5) with ascorbic acid and diuresis.	• Promotes elimination of PCP.

Nursing Diagnosis: Infection, Potential For

(Also refer to Chapter 9, p 171, Infection, Potential For.)

May Be Related To:

• Repeated IV drug injections, antitussive effects of opioids, infectious hepatitis, bacterial endocarditis, and glomerulonephritis

Possibly Evidenced By: Elevated temperature; positive wound cultures; changes in wound drainage; signs and symptoms of hepatitis, bacterial endocarditis, or glomerulonephritis.

Desired Patient Outcome: Patient will be free of infection and complications related to the infection.

Interventions	Rationale
INDEPENDENT	
• Inspect injection sites frequently.	• Assesses signs of infection such as redness, swelling, warmth, and purulent drainage.
• Assess for spider angiomas and palmar erythema.	• Skin manifestations indicative of liver disease.
• Maintain isolation and aseptic technique.	• Reduces possibility of further infection and cross-contamination.
• Monitor for other signs and symptoms of infection.	• Increased temperature and heart rate, and skin changes may indicate the presence of infection.

Interventions	**Rationale**
• Assess for signs and symptoms of glomerulonephritis.	• Parenteral drug users with endocarditis, bacteremia, or other sources of infectious material can develop glomerulonephritis from septic emboli or from immune complex deposition.

COLLABORATIVE

• Obtain cultures of all purulent IV injection sites.	• Allows for specific identification and treatment of bacterial organisms.
• Administer antibiotics as ordered.	• Helps control infection and further contamination of adjacent tissue. Prevents systemic infection.
• Obtain serologic screening including hepatitis B surface antigen (HBsAg) and antibodies to both the surface protein (anti-HBs) and the viral core (anti-HB core).	• Provides for early detection and treatment of infectious hepatitis. If the results of these tests are negative, hepatitis B vaccine is given.
• Obtain HIV screen for all parenteral drug users after obtaining informed consent, and provide pre-test and post-test counseling.	• Patients who are actively using drugs intravenously are at high risk for acquired immunodeficiency syndrome (AIDS).

Nursing Diagnosis: Fear

May Be Related To:

• Disfigurement
• Death from the traumatic injury
• Isolation from others

Possibly Evidenced By: Verbalizations; apprehension; fearful; restlessness; insomnia; trembling; sympathetic stimulation.

Desired Patient Outcomes: The patient will experience minimal manifestations and verbalize fears and concerns.

Interventions	**Rationale**
INDEPENDENT	
• Use a firm, caring, receptive approach to provide patient with opportunity to discuss fears related to drug/alcohol dependency and current treatment.	• Some drug abusers (particularly those using benzodiazepine) are frequently poor "copers" and have turned to drugs to handle stress and anxiety. By allowing the patient to verbalize, the nurse can provide assistance in exploring nondrug options/alternatives for effective coping.
• Establish a straightforward, nonjudgmental, one-to-one relationship.	• Therapeutic communication focuses on increasing self-esteem, promoting self-care, maintaining confidentiality, confronting manipulative behavior, and teaching effective coping mechanisms.

Nursing Diagnosis: Fear
(*Continued*)

Interventions

- Offer the patient appropriate options and choices and incorporate into the plan of care interests, likes, and dislikes.

- Provide explanations and information about *all* care being given.

COLLABORATIVE

- Involve the entire burn team in the care of the patient.

- Administer haloperidol (Haldol) or diazepam (Valium) as ordered.

Rationale

- Some patients may feel psychologically immobilized following the injury. Reestablish sense of control over the environment within set limitation.

- Allows patient to understand treatment modalities and clarify any misconceptions the patient may be experiencing.

- Provides reinforcement and additional support for the patient and significant others, thereby reducing fears and anxiety.

- Reduces anxiety, confusion, and/or depression.

Nursing Diagnosis: Thought Processes (Alteration In)

May Be Related To:

- Intoxication or withdrawal from alcohol, including DTs
- Abrupt withdrawal from benzodiazepines (may cause a psychosis similar to DTs.)
- Hallucinations and suicidal behavior secondary to amphetamine and cocaine withdrawal.
- Altered perception and poor judgment secondary to marijuana use.
- Visual and auditory hallucinations as well as feelings of body image change and depersonalization secondary to PCP use.

Possibly Evidenced By: Hallucinations; delusions; altered sleep patterns; memory deficit; disorientation; and inability to follow or grasp ideas.

Desired Patient Outcome: The patient will verbalize appropriate ideas, awareness of surroundings, situation, and time orientation.

Interventions

INDEPENDENT

- Avoid whispering in areas out of the patient's sight, but within hearing range.
- Explain the care measures to be provided and the patient's responsibility regarding participation in care.
- Assess mental status, including mood and affect, frequently.

Rationale

- May precipitate or imitate auditory hallucinations thereby increasing anxiety.
- Promotes reality orientation; discourages hallucinations, delusions, and illusions.
- Manifestations of altered mood, affect, or level of consciousness may be chemical- or alcohol-related.

Interventions	Rationale
COLLABORATIVE	
• Treat underlying causes of hallucinations, DTs.	• Rules out and/or treat physiologic and psychologic problems.
• Administer medications as ordered, e.g., haloperidol (Haldol), diazepam (Valium).	• Reduces anxiety and agitation.
• Administer ammonium chloride.	• May be used to acidify the urine to enhance elimination of amphetamines.

Nursing Diagnosis: Family Process, Alteration In

(Refer to Chapter 7, page 97, for etiology, manifestations, desired patient outcomes, and interventions.)

Nursing Diagnosis: Coping, Ineffective, Individual/Family

(Refer to Chapter 7, page 92, for etiology, manifestations, desired patient outcomes, and interventions.)

Nursing Diagnosis: Sleep Pattern Disturbance

May Be Related To:

• Chemical abuse (particularly with the excessive use of stimulating agents)
• Delirium tremens.

Possibly Evidenced By: Verbalizations; interrupted sleep; changes in behavior and performance; irritability; disorientation; restlessness; and lethargy.

Desired Patient Outcomes: Patient will obtain adequate periods of sleep and rest.

Interventions	Rationale
INDEPENDENT	
• Provide quiet, comfortable atmosphere.	• Promotes restful sleep.
• Coordinate activities such as interviews and diagnostic studies to allow for at least 2-hour intervals of uninterrupted sleep.	• Decreases the patient's fatigue.
• Maintain optimal room temperature.	• Provides comfortable environment for sleep in the presence of hypermetabolic state and excessive body heat loss.

Nursing Diagnosis: Sleep Pattern Disturbance (*Continued*)

Interventions	Rationale
COLLABORATIVE	
• Administer diazepam (Valium) orally or IV and other sleep agents as ordered.	• Promotes sedation, prevents seizures and convulsions.

Nursing Diagnosis: Pain

(Refer to Chapter 9, page 169, for etiology, manifestations, desired patient outcomes, and interventions.)

Nursing Diagnosis: Nutrition (Alteration In), Less Than Body Requirements

May Be Related To:

- Decreased food consumption due to gastric irritation, anorexia, and caloric intake of alcohol rather than foods containing B vitamins and folic acid.
- Inadequate nutritional intake in chemical substance abusers. (On an active drug "run" [daily drug use], there is little time, money, or inclination for eating. Rapid and dramatic weight loss is particularly common with heavy cocaine use.)

Possibly Evidenced By: Weight loss, decreased plasma proteins, decreased albumin, decreased caloric intake, and decreased muscle mass.

Desired Patient Outcomes: Patient will achieve an adequate nutritional intake to meet the special metabolic needs of the alcoholic or substance abuser with a burn injury.

Interventions	Rationale
INDEPENDENT	
• Provide patient with small, frequent, high-protein, high-calorie, vitamin-enriched meals and snacks.	• In addition to meeting hypermetabolic needs, increased nutritional intake helps to deal with the excess hunger, which may exist when the effect of the drug is diminished.
• Instruct patient as to dietary needs.	• Increased understanding may lead to increased compliance and cooperation.
• Monitor daily calorie counts and weigh patient daily.	• Provides a guide to adequate calorie intake and progress of nutritional status.

Interventions	Rationale

COLLABORATIVE

- Consult dietitian and nutrition support service to help establish patient's nutritional needs.

- Administer antiemetics as ordered.
- Administer thiamine and folic acid.

- In addition to calculating nutritional needs for the burn injury, preburn nutritional status that has been affected by drug and alcohol use must also be considered.
- Relieves nausea and vomiting.
- Prevents or corrects nutritional deficiencies, and prevents Wernicke's encephalopathy which may develop if glucose is given to a patient low in thiamine and folic acid.

Nursing Diagnosis: Skin Integrity, Impairment Of

(Refer to Chapter 4, page 64, for etiology, manifestations, desired patient outcomes, and interventions.)

Nursing Diagnosis: Fluid Volume Deficit

May Be Related To:

- Alcohol ingestion
- Decreased fluid intake

(Refer to Chapter 9, page 165, for other etiologies, manifestations, desired patient outcomes, and interventions.)

Nursing Diagnosis: Impaired Mobility

May Be Related To:

- Imbalance secondary to effects of drugs used
- Imbalance secondary to effects of alcohol ingested

(Refer to Chapter 9, page 174, for other etiologies, manifestations, desired patient outcomes, and interventions.)

Nursing Diagnosis: Tissue Perfusion, Alteration In: Peripheral

May Be Related To:

• Effects of select drugs on the cardiovascular system

(Refer to Chapter 9, page 164, for other etiologies, manifestations, desired patient outcomes, and interventions.)

Nursing Diagnosis: Social Isolation

May Be Related To:

• Need to separate patient secondary to hallucinations
• Need to separate patient threatening harm to others.

(Refer to Chapter 7, page 90, for other etiologies, manifestations, desired patient outcomes, and interventions.)

Nursing Diagnosis: Post-Trauma Response

(Refer to Chapter 7, page 93, for etiology, manifestations, desired patient outcomes, and interventions.)

Nursing Diagnosis: Grieving

(Refer to Chapter 7, page 94, for etiologies, manifestations, desired patient outcomes, and interventions.)

Nursing Diagnosis: Adjustment, Impaired

(Refer to Chapter 7, page 95, for etiology, manifestations, desired patient outcomes, and interventions.)

Nursing Diagnosis: Anxiety

May Be Related To:

- Uncertainty of reaction to drug or alcohol withdrawal
- Uncertainty of ability to exist drug- or alcohol-free

(Refer to Chapter 7, page 98, for other etiologies, manifestations, desired patient outcomes, and interventions.)

Nursing Diagnosis: Powerlessness

May Be Related To:

- Hallucinations

(Refer to Chapter 7, page 96, for other etiologies, manifestations, desired patient outcomes, and interventions.)

Nursing Diagnosis: Parenting, Alteration In

(Refer to Chapter 7, page 105, for etiology, manifestations, desired patient outcomes, and interventions.)

Nursing Diagnosis: Self-Concept, Disturbance In

(Refer to Chapter 7, page 89, for etiology, manifestations, desired patient outcomes, and interventions.)

Nursing Diagnosis: Knowledge Deficit

(Refer to Chapter 9, page 176, for etiology, manifestations, desired patient outcomes, and interventions.)

REFERENCES

1. Brewer, C: Controlling the demon. Nursing Times 46:July 1986.
2. Nielsen, J, et al: Studies and parasuicide by burning. Journal of Burn Care and Rehabilitation 4:335, 1984.
3. Barillo, D, et al: Is ethanol the unknown toxin in smoke inhalation injury? Am Surg 52:641, 1986.
4. Ibid, p 335.
5. Birky, M, and Clarke, F: Inhalation of toxic products from fires. Bull NY Acad Med 10:997, 1981.
6. Cole, M, et al: Gasoline explosions, gasoling sniffing: An epidemic in young adolescents. Journal of Burn Care and Rehabilitation 6:532, 1986.
7. Ross, C: Gasoline sniffing and lead encephalopathy. Can Med Assoc J 12:1196, 1982.
8. Remington, G, and Hoffman, B: Gas sniffing as a form of substance abuse. Can J Psychiatr 29:31, 1984.
9. Cole et al, p 534.
10. Rottenburg, R: Cocaine: Chic, costly and what else? The Care Medic 1985 in "Patient Care" newsletter, September 15, 1980.
11. Lewis, D, and Senay, E: Treatment of drug and alcohol abuse. NIDA Medical Monograph Series, Rockville, MD, 1981.
12. Dyke, C, and Byck, R: Cocaine. Scientific American 128, March 1983.
13. Cohen, S, and Gallant, D: Diagnosis of drug and alcohol abuse. NIDA Medical Monograph Series, Rockville, MD, 1981.
14. Shapiro, J: The narcotic addict as a medical patient. Am J Med 45:555, 1968.
15. Mittleman, H, et al: Cocaine, American Journal of Nursing. 9:1092, 1984.
16. Wesson, D, and Jacoby, J: Medical treatment for complications of polydrug abuse. National Institute on Drug Abuse, Washington, DC, 1980.
17. Williams, A: Primary care of parenteral substance abusers. Nurse Practitioner 6:17, 1986.
18. Newton, M, et al: When the nurse suspects drug abuse. Plastic Surgical Nursing 113:115, 1986.
19. Ibid, p 118.

Chapter 17

ELIZABETH I. HELVIG AND
MELVA KRAVITZ

CARE OF THE DIABETIC PATIENT WITH BURNS

NURSING ASSESSMENT

Mortality

Diabetes mellitus has been diagnosed in 2 to 3 percent of the Western population.[1] Many more people are in a prediabetic state and will develop diabetes during times of acute illness or surgical stress. There are probably more than 10 million diabetics in the United States, with the number increasing rapidly due to improved diagnostic screening, an increased life span resulting in an increase in the number of elderly patients having diabetes, and improved care of the diabetic pregnant woman.[2] Diabetic patients who develop any additional medical condition have higher mortality and morbidity rates than do nondiabetics with the same medical condition. For example, the slightest wound in the foot of an insulin-dependent diabetic patient is a potentially major medical problem.[3] In a series of 155 patients ranging in age from 53 to 102 years (mean 80.8 years) with fractures of the upper end of the femur, the 15 diabetic patients had a mortality rate of 80 percent compared with a group mortality rate of 28.4 percent.[4] The healing rate is greatly prolonged in patients with diabetes, thus increasing the morbidity rate due to concomitant infections and prolonged hospitalizations. In burn patients with diabetes, the prolonged healing of both burn wound and donor sites become major obstacles to recovery.

Etiology

Diabetic patients have as a manifestation of their disease state an alteration in microcirculation. Macrovascular or macroangiopathic disease is one of the major complications of diabetes. Lipid deposition, medial calcification, and thickening of the basement membrane may lead to arterial insufficiency to the extremities. Neuropathy leads to peripheral nerve degeneration and decreased sensory receptor mechanisms. This combination of diminished blood supply to dissipate heat and decreased sensations to harmful stimuli leads the diabetic patient to injury that would be avoided in otherwise healthy patients. Scald burns to the lower extremities sustained during bathing or soaking the feet are often not recognized until several minutes have passed. Thus, in addition to the burn risk of the general population, diabetic patients sustain scald burns at an increased rate.

ANATOMIC/PHYSIOLOGIC CONSIDERATIONS

Hypermetabolism

Glucose kinetics are altered in all patients following major burn injury. Hyperglycemia is a common occurrence in critically ill patients with the elevation of fasting blood sugar above normal limits being related to the severity of the injury or the presence of systemic infection. Oral or intravenous (IV) glucose tolerance tests in patients following burn shock or systemic infection demonstrates prolonged elevations in blood glucose concentrations that are characteristic of the "diabetes of injury" or "stress diabetes." An increase in the flow of glucose through the extracellular fluid compartments in critically ill patients has been demonstrated in conjunction with a dampening of insulin inhibition of hepatic gluconeogenesis following injury.[5]

GLUCOSE INTOLERANCE

A massive catecholamine release, along with other anti-insulin hormones, is responsible for the characteristic glucose intolerance commonly experienced during the early postburn period.[6] Glucose disappearance is increased following injury in spite of persistent hyperglycemia. Glucose flow is related to the extent of body surface burn with return toward normal as burn wound closure is accomplished.[7] The tremendous autonomic efferent stimulation of a burn injury stimulates the catecholamine response that follows major burn injury. The fundamental hormonal effect of burn injury is a pronounced and sustained elevation of cortisol, growth hormone, catecholamines, and glucagon (stimulated by the catecholamines). During the initial stages of acute injury, insulin secretion appears to be inhibited, probably owing to the early predominance of epinephrine's alpha-adrenergic effects over its beta-adrenergic effects.[8] The tremendous catecholamine response that initially accompanies a major burn injury alters both serum glucose regulation and insulin flow.

INSULIN RESISTANCE

The initial response to burn injury, regulated primarily by norepinephrine, results in a marked elevation of serum glucose, diminution of insulin secretion, and a relative insulin resistance that gives rise to the "diabetes of injury."

Even patients with no underlying problem in serum glucose control often demonstrate markedly elevated serum glucose levels during the initial resuscitation phase following burn injury. Patients at this stage are usually unable to tolerate nutrition because of tremendous insulin resistance. Due to the gastric immobility that follows major burn injury, most of these patients do not receive enteral nutrition for the first 48 hours postinjury; in addition, the use of glucose-containing fluids for fluid resuscitation is contraindicated during the first 24 hours. The use of dextrose-containing resuscitation fluids is often associated with marked elevations in blood sugar, which may be dangerous to the patient. Although insulin is rarely required during the resuscitation period, it is occasionally necessary because of a marked elevation in serum glucose associated with glucosuria. During this critical time, IV insulin is probably the best choice since the uptake of subcutaneous and intramuscular insulin is variable and may not be efficacious.

Frequent monitoring of both the serum glucose level and the urine glucose excretion is essential. Whereas serum glucose levels in diabetic patients are often in the 200 to 300 mg/dl range, a finding of large amounts of sugar in the urine is an indication for the use of insulin. Because of the clinical finding of diuresis in the presence of glucosuria, evaluation of the adequacy of fluid resuscitation must be assessed using a variety of resuscitation criteria.

DIABETES OF TRAUMA

Trauma patients often present an abnormal metabolic picture that has been described as the "diabetes of trauma." This includes hyperglycemia and increased hepatic gluconeogenesis although insulin levels are normal or high. Additional changes include decreased glucose disposal rate, increased fractional removal rate of insulin and insulin resistance in peripheral tissues at the postreceptor level. Studies in normal individuals indicate a daily glucose requirement of 2 g/kg per day, but traumatized patients seem to require 2 to 4 g/kg per day.[9] The diabetes of injury may occur even when blood glucose concentrations are only minimally elevated.[10]

After the initial burn insult, catecholamine excretion continues to be very high but this appears to be regulated more by epinephrine. The hypermetabolic response to burn injury occurs soon after injury and is characterized by a very rapid increase in glucose turnover as well as increased anaerobic metabolism in the periphery with the Cori and alanine cycles performing a larger role in maintaining blood glucose levels. While serum glucose may be slightly elevated during this time, glucose flow is greatly enhanced and the glucose tolerance curve and response to insulin return toward normal.

During this period, nondiabetic patients are ordinarily able to tolerate large quantities of dextrose- and nondextrose-containing calories without marked abnormalities in their serum glucose. However, patients with underlying disorders in their glucose kinetics may react very differently. Those having mild or moderate diabetes may require greatly increased quantities of insulin as their need for glucose increases and their body becomes more active in gluconeogenesis. Blood glucose levels above 250 to 300 mg/dl should be controlled with IV insulin since subcutaneous insulin will not be absorbed at a therapeutic rate due to the edema and diminished peripheral capillary perfusion seen with major burn injury. On occasion, the administration of insulin via a continuous IV drip is indicated when blood glucose levels prove especially refractory to control. Patients whose metabolic needs are being met with tube feedings or IV hyperalimentation may prove to be very resistant indeed to the effects of insulin, sometimes requiring a decrease in their nutritional supplement before blood glucose levels can be brought under control.

As the burn wound heals and the metabolic rate gradually declines, serum glucose levels often become easier to control. The insulin requirement during the acute phase of the hypermetabolic response will gradually decline as the burn wound heals. Once wound closure is attained, insulin requirements return toward preburn requirements.

RISK VARIABLES

A number of patients who were not known previously to be diabetic will demonstrate marked resistance to insulin and require considerable insulin through the course of burn treatment. Such patients often remain diabetic and, especially in the elderly, are found to have been occult diabetics by history. These patients often demonstrate very high insulin requirements initially, which will taper as burn wound closure is accomplished. Diabetic patients who are doing reasonably well in the burn course and are stable with regard to their insulin requirements may suffer a worsening of their serum glucose control in the face of major metabolic stresses such as operative procedures, sepsis, or hypothermia. The presence of sudden marked elevations in serum glucose should suggest the possibility of such stress. In very elderly patients and infants, such increased stress may be heralded by a fall in blood glucose levels as well as in body temperature, as the catecholamine response decompensates and increased metabolic demands cannot be met.

SPECIAL NURSING CONSIDERATIONS

Wound Management

Wound management for the diabetic patient is usually conservative because healing of donor sites and partial-thickness burns is greatly prolonged. The burned extremity in a diabetic patient has compromised blood supply, which diminishes both the distribution of IV antibiotics and the absorption of topical antibiotics. The prolonged healing is a consequence of diminished circulation and cellular deprivation of nutrients and oxygen. Insulin-dependent peripheral use of glucose is of secondary importance in the metabolic picture after the first few days since glucose uptake in burn wounds, which is non−insulin dependent, proceeds at an accelerated rate in the presence of adequate perfusion.[11] Meticulous wound care accompanied by extremely gentle cleansing can promote healing over a prolonged period of time. Padding of the wound will decrease trauma to the healing wound but must be balanced with range of motion (ROM) exercises. Foot care for diabetic patients, whether the foot is burned or not, includes gentle cleansing and drying plus soft padding between the toes of patients on bedrest. Padding and cushioning of bony prominences to prevent further tissue destruction is essential.

Potential Complications

The patient's immune system is compromised by both the diabetes and the burn; therefore, the patient is at high risk for pneumonia, bladder infections, and thrombophlebitis. Patients are often heavily colonized with *Candida* at admission. Oral hygiene to prevent infection includes frequent gentle washes with diluted mouthwash and the frequent use of an oral antifungal medication such as nystatin (Mycostatin).

The acute phase of recovery in diabetic burn patients is greatly prolonged, and the survival rate is lower than in nondiabetic burn patients (see Table 17−1). The presence of epinephrine depresses insulin levels[12] and may convert the diabetic who was previously maintained on oral hypoglycemic agents to an insulin-dependent state. Patients who are maintained preburn on oral hypoglycemics may require transient insulin therapy during the acute states of adynamic ileus but may be able to change back to the oral agents once they are able to take an oral diet. Oral glucose stimulus leads to a much stronger insulin secretion than the IV administration of glucose as the beta-cells are stimulated by a variety of intestinal hormones such as gastrin, secretin, cholecystokinin, pancreozymin, and others.[13] Patients are at risk for diabetic ketoacidosis during sudden physiologic changes at times of high stress such as sepsis or perioperatively.[14] Acid-base imbalances occur and administration of bicarbonate should be considered when ventilatory compensation for metabolic acidosis is maximized and severe systemic acidosis persists despite adequate hydration and insulin therapy. Insulin promotes the intracellu-

TABLE 17 – 1. Frequent Complications in Diabetics Following Burn Injury

Progression to insulin-dependent state	Hypokalemia
Diabetic ketoacidosis	Hyponatremia
Sepsis	Infection
Acid-base imbalances	

lar entry of glucose and reduces fat metabolism, thereby diminishing the production of ketones. Oxidation of ketones generates bicarbonate and is therefore an exogenous source of base.[15] Considerable potassium is also lost during diabetic ketoacidosis and must be replaced while the patient is rehydrated with Ringer's lactate solution. Exchangeable body sodium content in metabolically stable diabetic patients may be as much as 10 to 15 percent above normal levels and may be reflected as hyponatremia unless treated in diabetic burn patients. In normotensive diabetic subjects, plasma volume is not significantly different from normal values; thus, the increased body sodium is accommodated in an expanded interstitial compartment of the extracellular fluid volume and/or there is an increase in intracellular sodium.[16]

Rehabilitation

The rehabilitation phase of healing is equally prolonged in diabetic burn patients. Skin breakdown, especially over bony prominences, is a frequent problem as is sheering trauma to healed areas. Maintenance on a diabetic diet and well-predicted insulin needs will reflect a control of the glucose-insulin balance and most diabetic patients will be discharged at or near preburn insulin requirements. The psychologic impact of burn scarring superimposed upon the altered body image diabetic patients already have has not been studied. The long-term incidence of scarring is high because the wounds take so long to heal. Even donor sites frequently develop extensive scarring in diabetic patients.

Both the morbidity and mortality rates for burn patients who were preburn insulin-dependent diabetics are high. Patients who develop the "diabetes of stress" tend to resolve the condition predischarge and do not appear to have an increased morbidity or mortality rate over the general population. Length of hospital stay is prolonged in diabetic patients, and the complication rate is higher. This is due, in part, to the obligatory conservative wound management made necessary by the diminished peripheral perfusion associated with the disease. Careful glucose monitoring and insulin regulation accompanied by meticulous wound care can support the healing process in burn patients who have previous diabetes mellitus.

NURSING CARE PLAN: CARE OF THE DIABETIC PATIENT WITH BURNS

Nursing Priorities

1. Maintain and promote effective oxygenation
2. Monitor and control serum glucose levels
3. Maintain a hemostatic balance in fluid and electrolytes
4. Minimize and control infection
5. Promote healing
6. Prevent complications
7. Initiate rehabilitative education
8. Promote functional return to community

Nursing Diagnosis: Breathing Patterns, Ineffective

May Be Related To:

- Metabolic acidosis secondary to breakdown of fatty acids.

Possibly Evidenced By:

- Kussmaul's respirations; acetone on breath; confusion.

Desired Patient Outcomes:

- Patient will not develop severe metabolic acidosis. Effective breathing patterns are maintained.

Interventions	Rationale
INDEPENDENT	

• Monitor for signs of acidotic state:
  ○ Confusion/mental changes
  ○ Acetone on breath
 	
  ○ Flushed face
  ○ Increased respiration
  ○ Abdominal pain (guarding and rebound/tenderness)
	• Provides a determination of acidosis.
	  ○ Due to decreased oxygenation
	  ○ Excretion of acetone through respiration
	  ○ Superficial vasodilitation
	  ○ To "blow off" excess pCO_2
	  ○ From decreased sodium or neuropathy (rule out ketoacidosis in the diabetic patient before doing laparotomy for abdominal pain)[17]

• Auscultate lungs and evaluate for signs of pulmonary edema during rehydration.	• Rehydration may quickly lead to overload in the patient with poor vascular tone.
COLLABORATIVE	
• Monitor urine and serum glucose and acetone.	• Excess counter-regulatory hormones (glucagon, growth, cortisol, and epinephrine) and decreased insulin promotes lipolysis and development of diabetic ketoacidosis.
• Monitor arterial blood gases (ABGs), paying special attention to pCO_2, pO_2, and pH.	• Changes in levels may indicate acidosis.
• Suction and administer oxygen as needed.	• Maintains effective oxygenation.
• Monitor patient for lactic acidosis.	• Lactic acid buildup interferes with production of acetoacetate (measured by laboratory tests) producing negative ketone laboratory tests. As lactic acidosis is corrected, ketones may increase significantly.[18]
• Bicarbonate may be given per physician order.	• Corrects acidosis.

Nursing Diagnosis: Fluid Volume Deficit

May Be Related To:

- Osmotic diuresis secondary to hyperglycemia.

Possibly Evidenced By: Decreased blood pressure; increased pulse; decreased or increased urine output; poor peripheral pulses; changes in electrolytes.

Desired Patient Outcomes: Patient will remain adequately hydrated or will be restored to adequate hydration with glucose and electrolytes within acceptable ranges.

Interventions

INDEPENDENT

- Monitor volume of urine output hourly or with each void. Measure specific gravity, sugar and acetone levels.

- Measure urine glucose on fresh urine obtained from second void or by needle aspiration from catheter.
- To be consistent, use same urine glucose measuring method.

- Monitor peripheral circulation and cerebral circulation. Explore complaints of weakness or dizziness for orthostatic hypotension. Compare supine, sitting, and standing blood pressures.

- Observe for signs of dehydration: excessive or reduced urine output, dry skin, poor skin turgor, dry mucous membranes, pleural friction rub, thirst.
- Monitor cardiac function, urine output, vital signs, and central venous pressure (CVP) for response to fluid therapy.
- Continually monitor neurologic status (coma score/level of consciousness) during rehydration.
- Monitor electrocardiogram (ECG), vital signs, and urine output during treatment of diabetic ketoacidosis; extra fluid may be required.

Rationale

- Large volumes of urine, exceptionally low specific gravity, and positive glucose in the urine are indicative of solute diuresis.
- Standing urine will not produce accurate glucose measurement.

- 1+ urine glucose with one brand may not be equivalent to 1+ with another brand.
- Diabetic neuropathy may effect autonomic nervous system (regulation of blood pressure and heart rate) resulting in a lowering of blood pressure when glucose levels decrease.[19] Episodes of dehydration may activate coagulation factors and lead to thrombosis or emboli.[20]
- Dehydration occurs with osmotic diuresis and disproportional fluid loss.

- Diuresis and hemoconcentration leads to decreased vascular volume and circulatory compromise.
- Cerebral edema may be a complication of fluid therapy following dehydration.

- Insulin administration facilitates movement of glucose and water intracellularly. A drop in vascular volume may develop, requiring fluid therapy to prevent shock.[21]

Nursing Diagnosis: Fluid Volume Deficit (*Continued*)

Interventions

COLLABORATIVE

- As per physician's orders, correct factors that may lead to hyperglycemia: infection, fever, inadequate insulin administration, decreased exercise, emotional crisis, open wounds, stress, increased or incorrect food intake.
- Positive urine glucose measurement should be followed by serum glucose measurement for more accurate glucose quantification.
- Monitor ECG and serum electrolytes — especially sodium, potassium, chloride, magnesium and phosphate, which may be lost through diuresis; continue to monitor during rehydration.
- When correcting hyperglycemia, evaluate glucose levels every 30 to 60 minutes. As per physician's order, change IV solution to one containing 5 percent glucose when serum values drop to about 250 mg/dl.

Rationale

- Hyperglycemia will occur with increased levels of glucagon, cortisol, epinephrine, and growth hormones. Underadministration of insulin and underutilization of calories (energy) will contribute to the condition.
- Serum glucose measurement is more precise and reliable than urine measurement.

- Serum levels may be decreased; decreased levels may not be apparent until rehydration, due to hemoconcentration secondary to dehydration.

- Avoid hypoglycemia rebound reaction when correcting hyperglycemia.

Nursing Diagnosis: Nutrition, Alteration In (Less Than Body Requirements)

May Be Related To:

- Hypermetabolic rate
- Inability to ingest or digest food
- Severe protein wasting from burn
- Inadequate "usable" nourishment to meet metabolic demands.

Possibly Evidenced By: Weight loss, decreased plasma proteins, decreased albumin, decreased caloric intake, decreased muscle mass, ketoacidosis.

Desired Patient Outcomes: Patient will remain in positive nitrogen balance, with glucose measurements remaining within established limits throughout hospitalization (150 to 250 mg/dl may be acceptable in the diabetic patient).

Interventions

INDEPENDENT

- Report failure to eat adequately at any meal, or unexpected interruptions in tube feeding.

Rationale

- Hypoglycemia may result: IV dextrose may need to be given.

Interventions	**Rationale**
• Recognize hypoglycemia by the presence of tremors, sweating, headache, hunger, rapid heart rate, blurred vision, unsteady gait, anxiety, hunger, fainting, tingling of tongue and lips.	• May be due to insulin reaction, lack of adequate food (carbohydrates) or lack of absorption of food that remains in the stomach, is lost through vomiting or is used up rapidly with unanticipated exercise.
• In long-term diabetics (more than 10 years' duration) hypoglycemia warning signs may be absent; recognition of hypoglycemia is by diminished cerebral function or confusion, decreased coordination, negativism, and coma.	• Neuropathies or decreased responsiveness to hormonal changes in the long-term diabetic may block the sympathetic responses to hypoglycemia.[23]

COLLABORATIVE

• Obtain diabetic and other nutritional history.	• Poorly controlled diabetes usually indicates poor nutritional status with reduced resistance to infection and poor wound healing.
• Administer insulin as per physician's order: gently mix but do not shake insulin vial. Draw up regular insulin first, then add longer-acting insulin. Double-check type of insulin and amount drawn up.	• Administration of high-protein, high-calorie diet must be balanced by insulin administration for utilization and maintenance of blood glucose level.
• Design an American Dietetic Association (ADA) diet that meets the patient's increased protein and calorie needs.	• Hypermetabolic needs will be met with a high-protein, high-calorie diet balanced with insulin intake.
• Provide a diabetic diet high in fiber.	• High-fiber diets may promote reduction in blood glucose, cholesterol, and triglyceride levels and promote gastrointestinal (GI) motility to decrease constipation.
• Administer thiamine as per physician order.	• Thiamine deficiency is common in poorly controlled insulin-dependent diabetics.
• Provide a diet low in saturated fatty acids and cholesterol.	• Minimizes cardiovascular complications of diabetes.
• Provide a diet with increased carbohydrate intake when patient experiences anorexia, nausea, vomiting, or limited oral intake.	• Carbohydrates most quickly elevate glucose levels.
• Provide a continuous enteral feeding to enable better glucose control (as per physician order). Selection of specific product used needs to take into consideration that commercial enteral diets vary widely in their carbohydrate contents.	• Constant infusion of enteral intake may improve tolerance of feedings and regulation of hormones.

Nursing Diagnosis: Nutrition, Alteration In (Less Than Body Requirements) (*Continued*)

Interventions

- Regulate serum glucose by close monitoring of glucose levels and the initiation of a sliding-scale insulin administration schedule or continuous insulin drip (as per physician order).
- Regulate serum pH; correct conditions contributing to alkalosis. Never administer insulin with alkaline substances.
- Regular insulin continuous IV infusion may be titrated based on serum glucose levels to maintain control (longer-acting insulins are never given IV).
- When administering insulin IV, double-check concentration of insulin, consider adding albumin to solution, and frequently check accuracy of infusion pump.

- Administer regular insulin with caution to patients with long-term, insulin-dependent diabetes.
- Therapy for hyperglycemia should be based on blood glucose levels; urine levels only gives approximations.[27]

Rationale

- Frequent glucose measurements and administration of regular insulin enables greater caloric intake while maintaining therapeutic serum glucose levels.

- Insulin is inactivated when the pH is higher than 7.5.[24]

- May be necessary for use of large quantities of nutrients.

- Insulin administration must be closely regulated. Insulin adheres to administration bag or bottle and tubing. Some suggest the addition of albumin to bind the insulin in solution.[25] Others feel that because the insulin is titrated to serum glucose, the relative concentration of the solution (how much is bound) is not significant as long as it is consistent.
- May have severe hypoglycemic (insulin) reaction to small amounts of regular insulin (5 to 10 units).[26]
- Many intensive care unit (ICU) drugs affect glomerular filtration of glucose, altering urine values either positively or negatively.

Nursing Diagnosis: Injury, Potential For Infection and Sepsis

May Be Related To:

- Diminished circulation secondary to vascular changes associated with diabetes.
- Growth of *Candida* or bacteria.
- Impaired immune competence

Possibly Evidenced By: Elevated temperature; positive cultures; changes in wound appearance.

Desired Patient Outcome: Patient's wounds will heal in a timely manner without development of complications.

Interventions

INDEPENDENT

- Maintain meticulous hygiene.

Rationale

- *Candida mycosis* is commonly found in sweaty areas on patients with diabetes.

Interventions	**Rationale**
• Turn every 1 to 2 hours.	• Minimizes skin breakdown and risk of pneumonia.
• Provide special attention to the diabetic's feet (burned or unburned). Evaluate for dry, scaly, hairless skin, and atrophy of tissue. Assess breaks in skin and toenail condition daily.	• Increased vascular disease leads to ischemia and diminished healing. Decreased sensation from peripheral neuropathy may be apparent. Gas gangrene may develop.
• Place patients with lower-extremity burns on bedrest with elevation of injury. Circulation distal to circumferential wraps should be assessed hourly to ensure adequate flow.	• Promote circulation by relieving pressure, minimizing edema, and paying close attention to the possibility of circulatory compromise.
• Maintain isolation technique for wounds.	• Infection coupled with poor peripheral circulation creates wounds resistant to treatment and healing.

COLLABORATIVE

• Remove Foley catheter as early as patient's condition allows. Monitor urine cultures for presence of bacteria and fungi; if present treat aggressively.	• The incidence of urinary tract infections in diabetic women is two to four times that of the general population.[28]
• Administer oral nystatin swish-and-swallow regimens and the addition of (Mycostatin) cream to topical antibiotics as indicated.	• *Candida albicans* is a common yeast skin infection in diabetics.
• Evaluate renal function prior to selection of antibiotic therapy.	• Impaired renal function due to neuropathy will inhibit excretion of certain antibiotics.
• Monitor aerobic and anaerobic cultures of wounds.	• Early detection and identification of organisms facilitates prompt treatment.
• Prevent hyperglycemia.	• Impairs leukocyte function; impairs lymphocyte and antibody formation.[29]
• Prevent ketoacidosis (refer to Nursing Interventions for Alteration in Nutrition, page 316).	• Ketoacidosis impairs phagocytosis and delays granulocyte activity.
• Monitor white blood cell (WBC) count.	• Leukocytosis may reflect hemoconcentration and stress or infection.

Nursing Diagnosis: Skin Integrity, Impairment Of

(Also refers to Chapter 4, p. 64, Skin Integrity, Impairment Of.)

May Be Related To:

• Impaired peripheral circulation and neuropathies, which may promote skin breakdown in the diabetic patient

Possibly Evidenced By: Delayed burn wound healing; unhealed donor sites; poor circulation.

Desired Patient Outcomes: Patient will not suffer any breakdown of unburned skin. Patient's skin will heal properly.

Nursing Diagnosis: Skin Integrity, Impairment Of (*Continued*)

Interventions	Rationale
INDEPENDENT	
• Monitor for any signs of tissue breakdown or infection (thrush, athlete's foot, sinusitis, carbuncles).	• Minimize potential of microorganism invasion. Allows for prompt treatment.
• Turn patient every 2 hours and pad bony prominences to minimize pressure areas.	• Skin of diabetic may be fragile; there may be decreased circulation to compromised areas.
• Observe for hypertrophy or atrophy of subcutaneous tissue; avoid these insulin administration sites.	• This local response to insulin is due to a variety of causes.
• Assure correct positioning and fit of splints.	• Improperly positioned splints may produce pressure areas.

Nursing Diagnosis: Urinary Elimination, Alteration In Pattern

May Be Related To:

• Polyuria secondary to solute diuresis.
• Urinary tract infections (UTIs) and paresis of the bladder

Desired Patient Outcomes: Patient will maintain bladder tone and remain free of UTIs.

Possibly Evidenced By: Polyuria; dysuria.

Interventions	Rationale
INDEPENDENT	
• Monitor frequency and volume of urine output.	• If bladder remains distended for prolonged periods, muscles will stretch and be slow to regain tone.
• Monitor blood urea nitrogen (BUN) and creatinine.	• Diabetes is the leading cause of renal failure; may be indicative of dehydration.
COLLABORATIVE	
• Discontinue Foley catheter as early as patient condition safely allows. Evaluate for bladder distention.	• Minimizes invasive procedures.
• Culture urine several times weekly. Observe for sediment, foul odor, cloudiness, or hematuria.	• Assesses for signs of UTI. Provides for prompt treatment.

Nursing Diagnosis: Bowel Elimination, Alteration In: Constipation

May Be Related To:

• Gastric atony.[30]

Possibly Evidenced By: Decreased frequency of elimination; hard, formed stools.

Desired Patient Outcomes: Patient will exhibit preinjury bowel patterns.

Interventions	Rationale
INDEPENDENT	
• Evaluate bowel elimination patterns; auscultate abdomen for presence, location, and characteristics of bowel sounds; evaluate character of stool.	• Severe constipation is a frequent complication of hospitalization in the diabetic population;[31] visceral neuropathy impairs colonic motility, resulting in atony and colon dilatation.
• Encourage increased oral fluid intake.	• Prevents hardening of stools; encourages gastric emptying.
COLLABORATIVE	
• Provide a high-fiber diet supplemented with Metamucil to promote GI function.	• High-fiber intake promotes GI motility.
• Check for fecal impaction in the absence of bowel movements.	• An enema may be indicated.

Nursing Diagnosis: Mobility, Impaired Physical

Also refer to Chapter 9, page 174, Mobility, Impaired Physical.)

May Be Related To:

• Muscle wasting and amputations.

Possibly Evidenced By: Inadequate ROM; limited mobility.

Desired Patient Outcomes: Patient will maintain adequate muscular and vascular tone.

Interventions	Rationale
INDEPENDENT	
• Develop a rehabilitation plan at the time of admission to minimize muscle wasting.	• Patient with lower extremity injuries may require prolonged bedrest.

Nursing Diagnosis: Mobility, Impaired Physical (*Continued*)

Interventions

- Assist patient from bedrest to ambulation. Check vital signs lying, sitting, and standing.
- Encourage Beurger exercises: In these exercises, the patient lies with legs elevated 30 to 60 degrees for 1 to 2 minutes, then sits with legs over the side of the bed for 3 to 4 minutes, then returns to supine position for about 4 minutes.
- Fit patient with shoes prior to ambulation.
- Ace-wrap legs toe to groin when dependent.

COLLABORATIVE

- Consult with physical therapist and occupational therapist.

Rationale

- Neuropathy may be mainfested by orthostatic hypotension.

- Beurger exercises are thought to improve extremity vasculature, muscle tone, and strength.

- Prevents injury to feet.

- Support to legs promotes vascular return.

- Allows for development of proper treatment plan.

Nursing Diagnosis: Self-Concept, Disturbance In Body Image

(Also refer to Chapter 7, page 89, Psychosocial Care.)

May Be Related To:

- Increased scaring secondary to prolonged (delayed) healing
- Amputations

Possibly Evidenced By: Verbalizations; preoccupation with scars; avoiding looking at wounds.

Desired Patient Outcomes: Patient will verbalize acceptance of self in situation.

Interventions

INDEPENDENT

- Encourage patient to voice concerns and thoughts; schedule time to listen to patient.
- Be reassuring, when reassurance is indicated.
- Set goals and praise achievements.

Rationale

- Verbalization aids in identification of issues that should be addressed by health care team.
- Fears may distort reality.

- Emphasizing the positive improves motivation and outlook.

Interventions	Rationale

COLLABORATIVE

- Continuously inform patient of medical status.
- Consistent information decreases anxiety and fears of "hidden" bad news.

Nursing Diagnosis: Pain

(Also refer to Chapter 9, p. 169, Pain.)

May Be Related To:

- Conservative treatment of burn injuries in the diabetic patient, resulting in prolonged healing time
- Donor sites' healing more slowly than in nondiabetics, resulting in prolonged hospitalization
- Peripheral neuropathies' altering the patient's perception of pain

Possibly Evidenced By: Verbalization, crying, increased vital signs, grimaces.

Desired Patient Outcomes: Patient will experience minimal pain throughout hospitalization.

Interventions	Rationale

INDEPENDENT

- Assess patient's ability to sense pain and reaction to pain.
- Teach relaxation and distraction methods of pain relief.

- Diabetic neuropathy may alter pain perception.
- Nonpharmacologic pain management methods may be effective in the diabetic patient.

COLLABORATIVE

- Administer medications for pain and sedation in low doses.

- Many diabetic patients are very sensitive to average doses.[32]

REFERENCES

1. Kleinberger, G: New aspects of parenteral nutrition with fat emulsions in injured patients. World J Surg 10:20, 1986.
2. Clark, AP: Diabetic ketacidosis. In Kenner, CV, Guzzetta, CE, and Dossey, BM (eds): Critical Care Nursing: Body–Mind–Spirit. Little, Brown & Co, Boston, 1985, p 943.
3. White, RR IV, et al: Management of wounds in the diabetic foot. Surg Clin North Am 64:735, 1984.
4. Davidson, TI and Bodey, WN: Factors influencing survival following fractures of the upper end of the femur. Injury 17:12, 1986.
5. Long, CL, et al: Carbohydrate metabolism in men: Effect of elective operations and major injury. J Appl Physiol 31:110, 1971.
6. Demling, RH: Fluid replacement in burned patients. Surg Clin North Am 67:15, 1987.
7. Wilmore, DW, Mason, AD Jr, and Pruitt, BA Jr: Insulin response to glucose in hypermetabolic burn patients. Ann Surg 183:314, 1976.

8. Pasulka, PS and Wachtel, TL: Nutritional considerations for the burned patient. Surg Clin North Am 67:109, 1987.
9. Nordenstrom, J: Parenteral nutrition in trauma: Glucose and lips. Acta Chir Scand (Suppl)522:195, 1985.
10. Michelsen, CB and Askanazi, J: The metabolioc response to injury: Mechanisms and clinical implications. J Bone Joint Surg 68A:782, 1986.
11. Baster, CR: Metabolism and nutrition in burned patients. Compr Ther 13:36, 1987.
12. Porte, D Jr, et al: The effect of epinephrine on immunoreactive insulin levels in man. J Clin Invest 45:228, 1966.
13. Grote, EH: The CNS control of glucose metabolism. Acta Neurochir (Suppl)31:1, 1981.
14. Porte, D Jr and Robertson, RP: Control of insulin secretion by catecholamines, stress and the sympathetic nervous system. Fed Proc 32:1792, 1973.
15. Latanzi, WE and Siegel, NJ: A practical guide to fluid and electrolyte therapy. Curr Probl Ped 16:7, 1986.
16. O'Hare, JP, et al: Impaired sodium excretion in response to volume expansion induced by water immersion in insulin-dependent diabetes mellitus. Clin Sci 71:403, 1986.
17. Rippe, JM, et al: Intensive Care Medicine. Little, Brown & Co, Boston, 1985, 784.
18. Clark, AP, p 95.
19. Rippe, JM, et al, p 782.
20. Rippe, JM, et al, p 792.
21. Rippe, JM, et al, p 791.
22. Rippe, JM, et al, p 781.
23. Marble, A, et al: Joslin's Diabetes Mellitus. Lea & Febiger, Philadelphia, 1985, p 400.
24. Clark, AP, p 957.
25. Clark, AP, p 952.
26. Rippe, JM, et al, p 785.
27. Rippe, JM, et al, p 784.
28. Marble, A, et al, p 740.
29. Rippe, JM, et al, p 782.
30. Marble, A, et al, p 716.
31. Marble, A, et al, p 716.
32. Marble, A, et al, p 715.

Chapter 18

ELIZABETH W. BAYLEY

CARE OF THE BURN PATIENT WITH AN INHALATION INJURY

NURSING ASSESSMENT

Mortality

Inhalation injuries are among the most devastating types of trauma resulting from exposure to fire and smoke. From 8000 to 12,000 people die annually in the United States from fire injuries.[1] Over half of these deaths—approximately 7000—results from inhalation injury.[2] In combination with major burns, inhalation injuries are often the lethal component of the total burn injury and present major problems in patient management. Inhalation injury increases mortality 30 to 40 percent when patients with cutaneous burns and inhalation injury are compared with patients with a similar amount of burn area and no inhalation injury component. Pulmonary pathology, primarily as a result of inhalation injury, now accounts for 20 to 84 percent of burn mortality.[3]

Aside from individuals who may have a concomitant inhalation injury, many individuals involved in fire scenarios have no cutaneous burns at all. In these patents, the total impact of the fire situation is manifested by the effects of inhalation injury. The majority of people who die from fire-related injuries fall into this category of smoke inhalation injury with no cutaneous burns.

This fact was first appreciated and reported in the medical literature after the experience at Massachusetts General Hospital with victims of the Coconut Grove fire in Boston in 1942. Many victims of that nightclub fire appeared to have only minimal cutaneous burns or other injuries and were managed accordingly. Subsequently, their conditions rapidly deteriorated and many died from respiratory problems that went unrecognized in the early hours postinjury. More recently, in the MGM Grand Hotel fire in Las Vegas in 1980, many bodies were discovered on the upper floors of the hotel, in rooms devoid of soot and remote from flames and heat. Sixty-four of 84 deaths were attributable to toxic gas inhalation.[4]

Etiology/Mechanisms of Injury

CARBON MONOXIDE POISONING

Of all types of inhalation injury associated with burn injury, carbon monoxide (CO) poisoning is the greatest killer at the scene of the accident. Carbon monoxide gas is a by-product of combustion. During fire and explosions, it is liberated into the air in large amounts during fires and explosions. This can cause the percentage of oxygen in a fire atmosphere to decrease from the usual 21 percent to less than 10 percent.[5] Other etiologies of CO poisoning include faulty furnaces and charcoal burners; use of gas and propane engines in an enclosed space; and automobile exhaust, inhaled either accidently or as a means of suicide.

LOWER AIRWAY INJURY

Injury to the lower airway is primarily a result of the effects of chemicals, rather than heat, on the respiratory passages. Because the specific heat of air is very low and the heat-exchanging mechanism of the upper respiratory tract is so efficient, even super-heated air is cooled considerably by the time it reaches the tracheobronchial tree. Steam, which has a heat-carrying capacity 4000 times that of hot air, is usually the only kind of injury that causes direct injury to the lung,[6] but this is very rare. Consequently, the lower respiratory tract and pulmonary parenchyma are spared thermal burns in most cases.

The mechanism of injury to the lower airway, therefore, is really in the category of *chemical* burn injury. The smoke from each fire is composed of a unique mixture of solid and liquid particles in gases. These gases, such as nitrous oxide and sulfur dioxide, combine with lung water to generate corrosive acids and alkalis. For example, hydrogen chloride, a strong acid, is liberated in great quantities by the combustion of polyvinyl-chloride, a synthetic material widely used in home furnishings and construction. When burned, it releases 40 percent of its volume as hydrochloric acid. Like other plastics, polyvinylchloride releases very dense smoke at relatively low temperatures (200 to 300°C).[7] In addition to causing intense mucosal burns of the respiratory tract, hydro-chloric acid may adsorb onto small carbon particles, and this can be inhaled as far as the alveoli.

Another toxic agent is phosgene, a lipid component of smoke that penetrates the tracheobronchial tree and may produce full-thickness mucous membrane loss. It also can adsorb into carbon particles, causing alveolar destruction. Exposure to aldehydes, again produced through burning wood furniture and wallpaper, causes protein denaturation and subsequent cellular damage.[8]

UPPER AIRWAY INJURY

Direct heat can cause injury to the structures of the upper airway including the oral cavity, the nasopharynx, pharynx, and vocal cords. Frequently, in conjunction with the heat, there are also chemical burns of these structures from the highly toxic gases produced by the fire.

A blast of hot air causes a reflex closure of the epiglottis and cords, preventing damage to the airway. When the intake of hot air is steady and sustained, it is very effectively cooled by the moist air already within the respiratory tract, as mentioned earlier. Although air is a very poor conductor of heat, some hot air does reach the upper airway, where it causes an inflammatory response that may lead to the very dangerous occurrence of airway obstruction.

Lung excursion and compliance may become restricted as a result of cutaneous burns and inhalation of smoke and subsequent fluid therapy. In patients who have circumferential full-thickness burns of the chest, the progressive development of edema over time causes the skin to become inelastic and constricting. This produces a tourniquet effect around the thorax and decreases chest excursion and the ability to breathe with an adequate tidal volume.

A restrictive abnormality also occurs in patients with large cutaneous burns following resuscitation with large amounts of crystalloid fluid. The lungs are not exempt from the generalized edema that occurs in body tissue after a major burn, including tissues that is removed from the wound site. As lung water increases, a noncardiogenic pulmonary edema occurs and lung compliance is decreased.

A by-product of the effect of chemical irritants from smoke on the respiratory passages is increased extravasation of fluid into the pulmonary parenchyma. This also restricts lung function by decreasing compliance. This noncardiogenic pulmonary edema causes progressive pulmonary failure which is resistant to many current pulmonary therapies.[9]

ANATOMIC/PHYSIOLOGIC CONSIDERATIONS

Carbon Monoxide Poisoning

For many years, emphasis has been placed on carboxyhemaglobin levels in determining the impact of carbon monoxide poisoning. The CO molecule has a great affinity for hemoglobin — an affinity that is 250 times greater than that for oxygen.[10] Therefore, carbon monoxide preferentially ties up hemoglobin sites and prevents oxygen from attaching. The amount of hemoglobin available for carrying oxygen is decreased and, as a result, the blood oxygen content and oxygen saturation are reduced.

More recent evidence, however, attributes the toxic action of carbon monoxide to its effect on the cytochrome system and respiration at the cellular level.[11] Carbon monoxide directly inhibits the action of the cellular cytochrome system by binding to these iron-containing proteins. It directly inhibits cellular respiration by competing with oxygen receptors on the cytochrome chain.

Carbon monoxide causes hemoglobin to bind to oxygen with abnormal tenacity, so that the oxyhemoglobin dissociation curve progressively shifts to the left. Thus, oxygen tension in the tissues must decrease to very low levels before appreciable amounts of oxygen are released from hemoglobin and made available to the tissues. It has been demonstrated that a high level of dissolved CO must be present in the blood for CO to block cellular respiration. On the other hand, a high carboxyhemoglobin level with little dissolved carbon monoxide in the plasma will result in relatively few toxic symptoms.

An important thing to remember is that carboxyhemoglobin levels often do not correlate with clinical findings. The effects of acute CO poisoning vary depending on the CO concentration in the environment, the activity level of the victim, and the duration of exposure. Also, the nurse must be aware that since blood samples for carboxyhemoglobin levels are usually drawn in the hospital after resuscitation with oxygen at the scene and during transport, they do not reflect accurately the maximum or initial level of exposure.

Lower Airway Injury

A number of specific physiologic and pathologic events occur when someone inhales smoke. Within moments of exposure, movement of cilia lining the respiratory tract ceases, resulting in impaired clearance of mucus and debris. Blood flow increases to the tracheobronchial tree as part of the inflammatory response, resulting in congestion and edema. At the level of the alveoli, almost instantaneous inactivation of preformed surfactant occurs, thereby contributing to atelectasis.[12]

Another consequence of the inhalation of toxic gases is bronchospasm due to direct irritation of airways or to neural reflexes. The initial symptom complex comprises bronchospasm, bronchiolar edema, and impaired airway flow, leading to a decrease in dynamic compliance. Also contributing to decreased dynamic compliance is edema of the smaller airways, which results in increased airway resistance.

At this time the individual may produce carbonaceous sputum as well as increased mucus in response to the chemical irritants. Inspissated mucous plugs form in the small airways, resulting in distal airway obstruction. Lower airway obstruction results in air-trapping and, as expected, ventilation perfusion inequality.

The lining of the epithelium of the trachea and bronchi undergo necrosis with shedding and formation of psuedomembranes, causing partial or complete obstruction of the small airways. Type I alveolar cells are damaged and the alveolar basement membrane is exposed. Fibrin, proteinaceous material, and cell debris-hyaline membranes are formed. A marked polymorphonuclear leukocyte infiltration takes place and intra-alveolar edema and hemorrhages occur.[13-15]

There is increased microvascular permeability in bronchial and pulmonary microvascular beds. An increase in pulmonary capillary permeability, with resultant outpouring of fluid into the lung interstitium, also has been observed. The fluid that leaks out of the vessels into the lung parenchyma is exactly the same kind of fluid as plasma.

It is believed that increase in fluid formation is the pathogenic mechanism for the progressive pulmonary failure that occurs 48 to 72 hours postinjury. After several days, bacterial invasion may supervene, leading to purulent bronchitis or bronchopneumonia. A long-term effect of smoke inhalation on the lower airways is fibrosis.

"The degree and type of anatomic and physiologic alterations caused by a toxic gas are determined by a number of factors:

1. The physical environment in which the exposure occurs. Closed spaces or poorly ventilated areas are most often the site of severe inhalation injury.
2. The irritating properties of the gas. Symptoms of irritation such as eye and nasal burning sometimes can alert the victim and avert prolonged exposure. However, some gases, such as hydrogen cyanide and phosgene have pleasant odors (sweet almond and new mown hay, respectively) which encourages victims to inhale deeply, unaware of their lethal toxicity.
3. The depth and rate of the victim's breathing.
4. The victims' susceptibility. For example, smokers have subclinical damage of the lung epithelium, which lowers their resistance to toxic gases.
5. The concentration of toxic gases and duration of exposure by water-soluble gases that dissolve in the mucus of nasopharynx, larynx, and trachea (e.g., sulfur dioxide, ammonia, and chlorine). Water-insoluble gases, such as nitrous oxide and phosgene injure the small airways and alveoli."[16]

Upper Airway Injury

The inflammatory response to heat injury to the upper airway is manifested by erythema and blistering of the buccal and pharyngeal mucosa, edema of the uvula, and laryngeal spasm. Singed nasal hairs and nares, sore throat, dysphagia, and hoarseness may be present. However, it is essential to appreciate that a significant number of patients who are later found to have inhalation injury may have none of these obvious signs. As many as one third have no facial burns and half never produce carbonaceous sputum. Only by means of fiberoptic bronchoscopy can upper airway injury be completely recognized or excluded with certainty.

The edema that results from thermal and chemical assault may progress to obstruction of the airway in from 30 minutes to 48 hours after injury. If securing the airway by insertion of an artificial airway is postponed until clinical signs of airway and pulmonary involvement become manifest, the presence of massive face and neck tissue edema in patients who have concomitant cutaneous burns (Color Plate 42) may change that rather simple maneuver into an unachievable task with disastrous outcome.[17] At best, a tracheostomy will have to be performed when an endotracheal tube placed earlier would have sufficed. In patients with inhalation injury without cutaneous burns, intrinsic edema can also compromise the airway both quickly and insidiously.

Restrictive Defects

Restrictions on lung excursion due to circumferential thoracic cutaneous burns are caused primarily by the inability of the patient to move successfully against the pressure and decreased elasticity of the edematous overlying skin. Hence, tidal volume decreases and respirations increase in rate and decrease in depth. Fluid in the lung parenchyma, caused by the inflammatory response to toxic chemical irritants in the airways, reduces the ability for oxygen and carbon dioxide to be exchanged at the alveolar-pulmonary capillary interface. Decreased PaO_2 and increased retention of CO result and lead to eventual respiratory acidosis and tissue hypoxia. The pathophysiologic changes resulting from smoke in inhalation injury are summarized in Figure 18–1.

RISK VARIABLES

Persons in a fire in an enclosed space are at high risk for inhalation of products of combustion. This in turn puts them at high risk for CO poisoning, lower and upper airway trauma, and consequences of restrictive defects which develop as a part of the body's response to heat and chemical assault. The elderly tend to sustain inhalation injury more often than younger individuals, and when they do, they have a much greater chance of succumbing to that injury than do younger persons.[18]

Very small children are frequently victims of CO poisoning. With fear and confusion in a fire situation, they may try to hide from the flames and smoke, seeking refuge in a bathroom or closet or other small place where they feel safe. Children are particularly susceptible to the effects of hypoxia, which can quickly result in cerebral edema and respiratory arrest.

Other individuals at great risk for inhalation injury are those trapped in a burning building or vehicle because of their injuries or prior disease. Immobility prevents them from moving away from the smoke produced by the fire. Persons with chronic lung disease and those with a history of smoking may also be less able to respond to therapy and thus have a higher risk of prolonged morbidity or mortality related to inhalation injury.

Pathophysiologic changes resulting from the components of smoke inhalation injury

Component	Pathologic changes	Physiologic changes
Carbon monoxide-cyanide toxicity (onset of symptoms immediate)	Binding hemoglobin by carbon monoxide; binding of cytochrome system by cyanide and carbon monoxide	Decreased oxygen saturation (normal PaO_2; impaired delivery and utilization of oxygen; lactic acidosis
Upper airway injury from heat (onset of symptoms after 18–24 hr)	Laryngotracheal mucosal edema; possible obstruction of upper airways with secondary atelectasis	Obstruction-induced hypoventilation; atelectasis; increased shunt; hypoxemia
Lung damage from acids and aldehydes (onset of symptoms both early and delayed)	1. Possibly immediate broncho-constriction and bronchorrhea; early onset of chemical irritation of airways	Decrease in dynamic compliance and functional residual capacity; increasing ventilation-perfusion mismatch and atelectasis; increased work in breathing
	2. Early impairment of mucociliary action; decreased clearance of mucus	
	3. Delayed inflammatory response; neutrophil, macrophage products; proteases; oxygen radicals; arachidonic acid metabolites	"High-protein" edema in severe cases; secondary hypovolemia with decreased oxygen delivery; increasing shunt; hypoxemia, edema, and consolidation
	4. Bronchiolar edema; surfactant denaturation and increased protein permeability in severe cases	
	5. Mucopurulent secretions after 2–4 days; mucosal slough and bronchiolar obstruction; bacterial colonization; impaired clearance	Infection-induced ventilatory abnormalities; superimposed sepsis syndrome
	Bronchopneumonia after 3–14 days; death in 5%–8% of patients without burns and in > 50% with major burns	

FIGURE 18–1. Pathophysiologic changes resulting from the components of smoke inhalation injury. (From Demling, RH: Smoke Inhalation Injury, Postgraduate Medicine, 82(1):64, with permission.)

NURSING ASSESSMENT PRIORITIES

History

A cardinal concept in the assessment of victims of inhalation injury is the fact that *pulmonary abnormalities are not always apparent.*[19] Therefore, a complete history of the fire situation and the patient's health care background is an essential component of adequate care. Because symptoms of inhalation injury may be delayed for as long as 8 to 24 hours or more after injury, a complete and fairly detailed history of the accident involving potential smoke inhalation is taken as soon as possible after the injury. The information, obtained from the patient or first responders (such as family members, fire fighters, or paramedics), includes (1) a description of the physical environment of the fire incident (i.e., whether it was an enclosed smoke-filled area; a large, well-ventilated area; or out of doors); (2) the type of burning material; (3) the length of time the patient was in the smokey area; (4) the condition of the patient when rescued is also ascertained.

In the emergency department (ED), the nurse also obtains information on treatment given including how long the patient has been receiving oxygen. History of other illnesses, particularly those that compromise the pulmonary system, current medications, and allergies must also be determined.

Physical Assessment

In general, the earlier the onset of symptoms of inhalation injury, the more severe the injury is likely to be. Since CO is one fraction of the gaseous fraction of smoke, patients suffering from smoke inhalation almost always have some degree of CO poisoning. The initial symptoms of toxicity can be confused easily with those of other disorders, and a high index of suspicion is necessary to diagnose correctly many of the accidental exposures. Because there is no method of measuring CO at the cytochrome level, the neurologic examination remains the primary method of assessment. Due to their high metabolic rates, the central nervous system (CNS) and the heart are the most susceptible to CO toxicity and are therefore the areas that offer major cues.

Neurologic signs and symptoms include fatigue, dizziness, ataxia, headache, confusion, combativeness, seizures, hallucinations, and coma. Evaluation of the cardiac system may reveal tachycardias and dysrhythmias and such ischemic changes as depressed ST segments, primarily in leads II, V_5, and V_6, can be seen. Victims with coronary artery disease are at greater risk of developing angina and myocardial infarction. It should also be noted that the cherry-red skin color described in some texts is seen infrequently and thus is unreliable.

Respiratory manifestations that develop in response to other components of smoke inhalation include tachypnea, cough, hoarseness, stridor, dyspnea, retractions, wheezing, sooty sputum, chest pain or tightness, rales, and rhonchi. Cutaneous burns of the face and neck, burned or sooty nares and nasal vibrissae, erythema and blisters of the lips, buccal and pharyngeal mucosa, and edema of these areas may also be noted. These signs and symptoms are summarized in Table 18–1.

Diagnostic Studies

Numerous laboratory and other diagnostic measures can help in making an early diagnosis of smoke inhalation and the extent of the damage. Arterial blood gases (ABGs) typically are normal initially; perhaps a mild hypoxia or an increased alveolar-arterial gradient is apparent. Keep in mind that lethal upper airway obstruction may occur

TABLE 18–1. Signs and Symptoms of Carbon Monoxide Toxicity

Neurologic Manifestations	Cardiac Manifestations	Respiratory Manifestations
Fatigue	Tachycardia	Tachypnea
Vertigo	Dysrhythmias	cough
Ataxia	Depressed ST segment	Hoarseness
Headache	Angina	Stridor
Confusion		Dyspnea
Combativeness		Retractions
Seizures		Wheezing
Hallucinations		Sooty sputum
Coma		Chest pain
		Tightness in chest
		Rales
		Rhonchi
		Facial burns
		Neck burns

without any change in ABGs. However, these values do provide important baseline information. Abnormal ABGs are suspicious of an injury to the tracheobronchial tree or lower airways. As with most other data, the trends with serial ABGs are watched carefully.

A carboxyhemoglobin level is obtained in all victims from a fire environment or in other instances where unconsciousness has mysteriously occurred in a closed space. Normal CO levels vary from 0 to 15 percent, with smokers commonly having the latter levels. Levels approaching 50 to 60 percent are considered lethal but may be rapidly lowered with oxygen therapy.[20] A low carboxyhemoglobin level does not mean that inhalation injury has not occurred. However, an elevated carboxyhemoglobin level indicates that inhalation of combustion products has indeed occurred, and exposure to other toxic gases may then be presumed.

Fiberoptic bronchoscopy (Color Plate 43) is the only method that accurately evaluates upper airway trauma by allowing direct visualization.[21] In burn centers this method is a common procedure early postinjury whenever inhalation injury is suspected. Preparation of the patient includes ensuring that the stomach is empty, intravenous (IV) sedation, preparation for emergency intubation, and topical anesthesia for the nasal and posterior pharyngeal and later, bronchial region. In 10 minutes or less it is possible to carefully inspect the upper and lower airways, noting any evidence of edema, erythema, ulceration, or soot deposits. With an outer diameter of 6.0 mm and suction channel within, this invasive tool also allows removal of secretions for culture and Gram's stain.

Although airway injury is now reliably diagnosed by fiberoptic bronchoscopy, the early diagnosis of parenchymal injury is not easily made. Therefore, a chest x-ray is an essential diagnostic tool in early care. The initial film usually appears normal but provides the necessary baseline for later comparisons.

In a study of 56 patients with significant smoke inhalation at the New York Hospital–Cornell University Hospital, signs of alveolar and interstitial edema were observed on chest x-ray within the first 24 hours in the majority.[22] In addition to the usual presentation of pulmonary edema, subtle radiographic findings of interstitial edema such as perivascular fuzziness and peribronchial "cuffing" or thickening were observed.

Pulmonary function studies can also assist in the diagnosis of inhalation injury. Spirometry provides a sensitive noninvasive test for the presence of inhalation injury to the lower tracheobronchial tree. Normal spirometry probably excludes significant injury to the lower respiratory tract because derangement of the forced expiratory volume and flow and forced vital capacity occur early.

Spirometry can be performed on admission and every 4 hours thereafter. Reliable data are best obtained from a cooperative patient without severe facial burns. Progressive deterioration in spirometric parameters is diagnostic of smoke inhalation injury. This tool is also useful in evaluating resolution of pulmonary injury and in documenting permanent lung damage, resulting from inhalation injury.

Another pulmonary function test in common use for the victim of suspected inhalation injury involves graphing maximal inspiratory and expiratory curves on the same graph, producing what are called "flow volume loops."[24] Evaluation of these loops allows the physician to distinguish between restrictive and obstructive conditions and between extrathoracic and intrathoracic airway obstructions.[25]

Another objective test for the diagnosis of inhalation injury is the xenon 133 lung scan. In this procedure, radioactive xenon 133 is administered intravenously and followed by serial scintiphotographs, which permits evaluation of the components of respiration including ventilation abnormalities associated with airway damage. Since xenon 133 is poorly soluble in water, it is excreted almost entirely into the alveolae during its first passage through the lung. Serial scanning through the lung shows that normal wash-out of this isotope takes less than 90 seconds; in those patients with airway damage, however, wash-out is delayed and also asymmetrical.[26] Bronchial spasm or obstruction, airway edema, mucosal sloughing, and bronchial casts will all delay isotope clearance. This test is extremely accurate except in patients with previous underlying lung disease, but is not universally available because xenon has a short half-life.

MEDICAL MANAGEMENT

Prophylactic Intubation

Control of the upper airway is achieved by either endotracheal intubation or tracheostomy at the first sign of impending airway obstruction.[27] This includes patients who present with stridor or severe dyspnea in the emergency department. Other universally agreed upon criteria for early intubation are found in Table 18–2.

Others with more liberal criteria for early intubation, prophylactically intubate all patients with a clinical diagnosis of inhalation injury, to aid in humidification, pulmonary toilet, and prophylactic provision of positive pressure.

Most physicians prefer the nasotracheal approach, using as large a tube as possible (8.0 mm) to permit adequate suction.[29] The intubation may be done using the fiberoptic bronchoscope or with a rigid bronchoscope and Magill forceps. A high-volume, low-

TABLE 18–2. Common Criteria for Intubation
with Inhalation Injury[28]

Smoke inhalation accompanied by coma
Respiratory depression
Posterior pharyngeal swelling
Nasolabial full-thickness burns
Circumferential neck burns
Burns of the upper airway confirmed by fiberoptic bronchoscopy

TABLE 18–3. Comparison of Nasotracheal Intubation and Tracheostomy

	Advantages	Disadvantages
Nasotracheal	Nonoperative placement Tube easily removed Decreased bacterial contamination of lungs Less traumatic with burns of neck	Difficult to keep tube secured Materials used to secure the tube need to be modified with changes in edema Subglottic stenosis Vocal cord damage Damage to nasal cartilage
Tracheostomy	Pulmonary toilet facilitated Increased patient comfort Oral alimentation easier	Risk of greater tracheal injury Erosion of innominate artery

pressure cuff is advocated with pressure adjusted to minimal leak and kept below 25 cm H_2O if possible.

In many patients, once edema decreases, extubation can be done within a few days postinjury. However, others are in for a long bout with an artificial airway. When that is predicted to be the case, whether long-term nasotracheal intubation or early tracheostomy is the treatment of choice is unclear. A comparison is found in Table 18–3.

With nasotracheal intubation, advantages include nonoperative placement, ability to remove the tube easily if no longer necessary, a longer and less direct route for bacterial contamination of the lungs, and the advantage with patients who have neck burns of not having to cut through the burns or interfere with burn care of the neck.[30] Keeping the tube in place can be a problem for patients with facial burns. Double-backed tape and some manufactured devices specifically for that purpose may be useful if care is taken to check for proper fit, which changes as edema increases and decreases. Endotracheal tubes can also be wired to the teeth to allow proper position.

Because the patient who is intubated will temporarily lose the ability to communicate vocally, the nurse attempts to allow the patient to talk to the family before intubation. If not a true emergency, the intubation can often wait a few minutes. Such patient advocacy may be much appreciated by both patient and family as the length of intubation is initially unknown and it may be weeks before normal communication can be re-established.

With a tracheostomy, pulmonary toilet, the comfort of the patient, and oral alimentation are all facilitated,[31] but both methods of providing an artificial airway can cause potential complications. With nasotracheal intubation, these include the development of subglottic stenosis, vocal cord damage, and necrosis of nasal cartilage, especially if there are cutaneous burns of the nares. With tracheostomy, tracheal ulceration and stenosis may also occur. Excessive cuff pressures can result in tracheoesophageal fistulas or erosion of the innominate artery with life-threatening hemorrhage.

Those who have studied these problems and made comparisons between the two method seem to favor long-term nasotracheal intubation. With tracheostomy tubes, the contact area between cuff and tracheal wall may be smaller that with an endotracheal tube, but the pressure per unit airway area necessary to achieve an adequate seal may be considerably higher and cause greater tracheal injury than the endotracheal tube. Generally, the longer the period of intubation, the greater the likelihood of airway sequelae.

Continuous Positive Airway Pressure (CPAP)

It has been observed that insertion of an artificial airway in burn patients with inhalation injury often precipitates almost intractable noncardiogenic pulmonary edema, decreased lung compliance, and decreased lung volume. The presence of a tracheal tube in patients with a decreased pulmonary volume prevents the individual from being able to increase airway pressure by approximating the vocal cords during expiration and may cause alveolar collapse at the end of expiration.

It is postulated that CPAP restores the glottic mechanism of maintaining intrapulmonary pressure, which is eliminated by tracheal intubation. Decreased morbidity and increased survival have been documented, as CPAP improves oxygenation and pulmonary measurements without any of the detrimental effects seen with mechanical ventilation and positive end-expiratory pressure (PEEP).[32]

Humidified Oxygen

Until the carboxyhemoglobin is known, administration of 100 percent oxygen by tight-fitting nonrebreathing face mask is done at the scene (Color Plate 44) of the fire on the assumption that CO was inhaled. The half-life of carboxyhemoglobin declines from 250 minutes in a person breathing room air, to 40 to 60 minutes in one breathing 100 percent oxygen. Hypoxia due to oxygen depletion in the fire atmosphere may be corrected by the time the patient arrives in the ED. For patients with chronic obstructive pulmonary disease (COPD), it is recommended that 24 percent to 28 percent oxygen be given.

Humidification of inspired air has been used since the Coconut Grove fire when steam kettle and steam room heaters resulted in improvements in patient comfort and breathing. Once CO levels have been brought down (hopefully within an hour or so) the patient can usually be managed on low-flow humidified oxygen.

Pharmacologic Management

There are several pharmacologic agents that can be useful in the management of the patient with inhalation injury. Intravenous bronchodilators such as aminophylline can provide dramatic relief from the acute irritating effects of combustion by-products on the tracheobronchial tree.

Steroids, however, are a subject of great debate. Theoretical benefits include a reduction in mucosal edema and bronchospasm and maintenance of surfactant function. In two noteworthy studies of their use in patients with cutaneous burns and inhalation injury, Pruitt[33] could demonstrate no advantage. However, in a randomized prospective trial Moylan and Alexander[34] documented a fourfold increase in mortality in the steroid-treated group presumably secondary to steroid immunosuppression and decreased tracheobronchial clearance mechanisms.

The response to steroid treatment following isolated smoke inhalation injury (that is, no cutaneous burns) had not been studied in human beings until the MGM Grand and Hilton Hotel fires in Las Vegas.[35] Victims were triaged randomly to one of four local hospitals. The therapeutic approach in all four was essentially the same and included oxygen therapy coupled with appropriate supportive care (chest physical therapy, sputum induction, and ventilatory support). However, in two institutions physicians were instructed by pulmonary consultants to administer steroids (approximately 10 mg dexamethasone equivalent every 6 hours for 48 hours). In the other two institutions the patients did not receive steroids.

The only statistically significant difference in the characteristics of the steroid and nonsteroid group was age, with the nonsteroid treated group averaging 6 years older than the steroid-treated group. In this study, there were no detectable differences in outcome with respect to morbidity and mortality. There may still be physicians who advocate an early single large IV bolus or either methylprednisolone or dexamethasone in hopes of preventing or a least decreasing some of the tracheobronchial inflammatory response.

Prophylactic use of antibiotics has been shown to be of no benefit and only leads to development of resistant strains of bacteria.[36] In instances of clinical signs of pneumonia, which may appear within a few short days of inhalation injury, particularly in patients with concomitant cutaneous burns, empirical choices for treatment prior to culture results usually include coverage of penicillin-resistant *Staphylococcus aureus* in the first few days postinjury and of gram-negative organisms—especially *Pseudomonas*—in subsequent days. Sputum cultures are obtained every 2 days to assess the need for antibiotic intervention.

One other pharmacologic agent noted in the literature is the use of nebulized heparin to increase expectoration of proteinaceous material resulting from severe lower airway injury.

Also in the category of pharmacologic agents, fluid therapy is considered for patients with inhalation injury. This has been studied primarily in patients with concomitant cutaneous burns, who have massive fluid needs based on the physiology of burn shock and evaporative losses from the burn wound. Traditionally, fluid therapy in patients with combined burns and inhalation injury has been kept to a minimum, to minimize pulmonary edema. This practice has been questioned and studied in recent years in animal models. These studies have shown that fluid resuscitation appropriate to the animal's other needs (i.e., maintenance of cardiac output and pulmonary capillary wedge pressure) results in decreased formation of lung water, has no adverse effect on pulmonary histology, and actually improves survival.[37] Fluid overload, however, must be avoided.

Physiotherapy

There is universal agreement that postural drainage, the encouragement of coughing and deep breathing, and incentive spirometry are useful adjuncts in the treatment of inhalation injury. Figure 18–2 depicts the sequence of management noted earlier.

Mechanical Ventilation

Patients with lower airway injury are followed with serial ABGs. If progressive respiratory insufficiency ensues and cannot be corrected by increasing the oxygen flow rate, then intubation and the use of a volume ventilator may be necessary. Hypoxemia usually results from ventilation perfusion abnormalities.[38] Relatively large tidal volumes (10 to 15 ml per kg) are used to prevent atelectasis. High fractions of inspired oxygen (FIO_2) may be necessary initially with the goal of achieving oxyhemoglobin saturation greater than 90 percent. Mixed venous and arterial oxygen should be monitored to determine the adequacy of the FIO_2.

PEEP improves the ventilation of poorly ventilated or nonventilated segments of lung and prevents alveolar collapse.[39] The goal in using PEEP is to improve oxygenation so that an FIO_2 of 0.5 or less is adequate. Recommendations resulting from a study of 84 patients with inhalation injury at Cook County Hospital included treating alveolar hypoventilation with the least number of mechanical breaths per minute needed to augment the patient's spontaneous breaths and maintain normal pCO_2 using intermittent mandatory ventilation.[40]

Ventilatory support is withdrawn only if the patient is stable, adequately nourished, and has sufficient muscular strength. Standard criteria include:

FIO_2 of 0.4 or less
Tidal volume greater than 5 ml per kg
Static compliance greater than 10 ml per kg

If patient has been exposed to smoke

Assume carbon monoxide-cyanide toxicity
Administer 90%-100% oxygen by face mask if
patient is awake or by endotracheal tube if
patient is obtunded

Maintain high fractional inspired-oxygen
concentration until CNS symptoms resolve
and carboxyhemoglobin level is <10%

Access for adequacy of airway
Take history and make physical examination

Examine airway with laryngoscope and
bronchofibroscope

If airway is even moderately damaged
Insert endotracheal tube, give humidified
oxygen, and maintain pulmonary toilet

If lower airway is injured
Maintain pulmonary toilet, use suction

Administer bronchodilators

Use positive airway pressure if acute
respiratory failure is likely (positive
end-expiratory pressure after 12-24 hr)

Restore and maintain fluid balance

Avoid steroids and prophylactic antibiotics

If lower airway is not injured
Maintain airway until edema
resolves (2-4 days)

Observe patient for airway
infection (eg, bronchitis,
pneumonia)

If condition worsens (4-10 days)
Continue pulmonary toilet to
prevent obstruction of upper and
lower airways, shunt, and
nosocomial infection

Add antibiotics at first evidence
of airway infection

If condition resolves
Maintain careful surveillance
for nosocomial infection for
next 7-10 days

FIGURE 18-2. Sequence of management for patients with smoke inhalation injury. (From Demling, RH: Smoke Inhalation Injury, Postgraduate Medicine, 82(1):64, with permission.)

Negative inspiratory force greater than 30 cm H_2O
Resting minute volume less than 10 liters per minute
Maximum voluntary ventilation more than twice minute volume[41]

Hyperbaric Oxygen (HBO)

There are now more than 100 HBO facilities in the United States.[42] However, controversy exists concerning if and when HBO is needed in the treatment of CO poisoning. If carboxyhemoglobin levels are very high or the patient's clinical manifestations suggest severe CO inhalation, HBO therapy should probably be considered. Hyperbaric therapists suggest that those with CO levels greater than 20 percent, a history of loss of consciousness, persistent neurologic deficits and cardiac abnormalities should be referred to hyperbaric therapy. They advocate that any patient exhibiting neurologic symptoms other than mild headache and nausea should be treated with HBO.[43]

Others would suggest that patients with carboxyhemoglobin greater than 40 percent need HBO because this level represents a significant exposure and the risk of secondary complications is increased.[44] Certainly any patient who receives 100 percent oxygen for several hours with minimal neurologic improvement, even though CO levels return to normal, should be recommended for HBO. Therapy with HBO effectively displaces CO from hemoglobin, myoglobin, and cytochrome systems. It improves neurologic status by maintaining viability of neurons in the ischemic brain until circulation is restored by reducing cerebral edema which occurs secondary to diffuse anoxia and CO poisoning. The high tissue oxygen levels achieved by HBO may clear the tissues of residual carbon monoxide and result in clinical improvement.

HBO not only enhances CO elimination but appears to decrease the incidence of neurologic sequelae. HBO at three atmospheres absolute reduces carboxyhemoglobin half-life to 23 minutes and immediately dissolves enough oxygen into the plasma (approximately 6.4 volumes percent) to meet the body's metabolic needs, even in the absence of functioning hemoglobin.[45]

SEQUELAE OF INHALATION INJURY

If individuals survive the critical phase following severe inhalation injury, during which pulmonary edema and bronchopneumonia may result in respiratory insufficiency, they will proceed into a repair phase that lasts many weeks. Friable granulation tissue in the airway may cause hemoptysis. As new respiratory epithelium develops, the cells do not have normal function. There is decreased airway size because of the cuboidal nature of the cells and excessive mucus production is present. Cilia activity is decreased. Alveoli continue too show emphysematous characteristics and the patient may have a persistent cough due to airway irritation. In some patients chronic lung disease results.

Bronchial stenosis, bronchial obliterans, and bronchiectasis, due to the destruction of airway tissue and chronic pooling of secretions with low grade infection, can occur. Chronic bronchitis is common. Tracheal stenosis and the need for serial dilation may also occur. The lung parenchyma itself may undergo fibrotic changes. Often there will be a general decrease in pulmonary reserve as reflected in pulmonary function studies.

Long-term effects of inhalation injury also relate to the effects of CO poisoning. Predominant among these are neurologic sequelae particularly in those who do not receive hyperbaric oxygenation. These are manifested by personality changes and memory impairment.

NURSING CARE PLAN: CARE OF THE BURN PATIENT WITH AN INHALATION INJURY

1. Maintain patent airway
2. Promote effective breathing pattern
3. Maintain adequate ventilation
4. Promote adequate tissue oxygenation

Nursing Diagnosis: Airway Clearance, Ineffective, Potential For

May Be Related To:

- Excessive or thick secretions
- Decreased compliance
- Edema of upper and lower airway secondary to thermal and chemical injury to tissues lining the airway with resultant inflammatory response and fluid shifts

Possibly Evidenced By: Erythema and blisters of buccal mucosa and pharynx; carbonaceous sputum, wheezing or rhonchi, cough, increased respiratory rate, sore throat, hoarseness, stridor.

Desired Patient Outcomes: Patient will demonstrate the following:

- Clear breath sounds on auscultation
- Respiratory rate and depth within normal limits
- Pulmonary function parameters within normal limits
- Chest x-ray unremarkable for signs of atelectasis or pneumonia
- Minimal respiratory secretions that are colorless, thin, and readily expectorated

Interventions	Rationale
INDEPENDENT	
• Position head in slight hyperextension to afford optimal airway during initial first aid.	• Reduces airway obstruction and opens airway for maximal function.
• Maintain adequate pulmonary toilet. Suction gently as needed using aseptic technique.	• Clears airway; prevents injury to irritated tissues; reduces opportunistic infection.
• Encourage patient to turn, deep-breathe, and cough frequently. Use incentive spirometry and hyperinflations frequently.	• Keeps pulmonary secretions mobile and promotes drainage. Promotes alveolar inflation and function.
• Assess breath sounds and note changes after coughing and suctioning.	• Evaluates response to treatment and provides early indication of airway congestion or obstruction.
• Provide postural drainage and chest physiotherapy.	• Mobilizes secretions and prevents stasis of mucus in portions of the lungs and bronchi that can result in bronchial or lobar pneumonia.

Nursing Diagnosis: Airway Clearance, Ineffective, Potential For (*Continued*)

Interventions	Rationale
• Keep intubation equipment at bedside and be alert for signs of respiratory obstruction.	• Respiratory obstruction can occur suddenly and may result in respiratory and cardiac arrest if not treated immediately.
• Inspect secretions for evidence of carbon particles and sloughed tissue.	• Indicates severity of inhalation injury and need for extreme caution in suctioning and intubation procedures.
• Monitor rate, depth, quality of respirations, and response to respiratory therapy including mechanical ventilation.	• Provides evaluation of patient response to progressive effects of inhalation injury and effects of therapy.
• Maintain adequate hydration.	• Keep secretions thin and enables patient to cough secretions up; facilitates suctioning.
• Monitor for signs of infection: fever, change in sputum, chest pain, vital sign change, pathogens in sputum.	• Enables prompt treatment of major complication of inhalation injury—pneumonia.

COLLABORATIVE

Interventions	Rationale
• Administer bronchodilators; antibiotics.	• Dilates airway by relaxing bronchial muscles; reduces growth of bacteria in compromised host.
• Assist with intubation as needed.	• Provides artificial airway.
• Provide oxygen and adequate humidification.	• Promotes adequate tissue oxygenation; humidification required to counter drying effects of oxygen on respiratory tissues.
• Provide mechanical ventilation, CPAP, and PEEP, as required.	• Counteracts effect of circumferential chest burns, which decrease chest excursion, and counteracts lung edema, which decreases compliance; keeps alveoli inflated to afford optimal oxygen and carbon dioxide exchange.
• Assist with bronchoscopy, suction, and obtaining specimens.	• Provides diagnostic information required for adequate treatment; removes debris, which could obstruct airway.
• Monitor serial chest x-rays.	• Provides indication of progression of effects of inhalation injury and response to therapy.
• Monitor serial ABGs and carboxyhemoglobin level.	• Provides indication of development of respiratory acidosis and tissue hypoxemia and/or CO poisoning.
• Assess readiness for extubation.	• Resolution of airway edema, adequate levels of tissue oxygenation, and adequate pulmonary function remove need for artificial airway which can result in complications when prolonged.

Nursing Diagnosis: Breathing Pattern, Ineffective, Potential For

May Be Related To:

- Hypoxia
- Obstructed airway
- Restrictive defects resulting from CO poisoning, thermal and chemical irritation of airways with edema
- Edema from circumferential full-thickness burns of the chest
- Pulmonary edema

Desired Patient Outcomes: Patient will demonstrate the following:

- Effective breathing pattern established with normal rate, depth, and rhythm
- Symptoms of hypoxia absent
- ABGs within normal limits

Interventions	Rationale
INDEPENDENT	
• Auscultate chest frequently.	• Determines character of breath sounds.
• Assess breathing pattern for tachypnea, use of accessory muscles, stridor, or other abnormal pattern.	• May indicate progressive hypoxemia, impending respiratory obstruction, or effects of CO poisoning.
• Monitor respiratory rate, depth, or tidal volume, compliance.	• Evaluates progressions of respiratory effects of smoke inhalation and concomitant cutaneous burns, which affect chest excursion and lung compliance.
• Elevate head of bed to semi-Fowler's position.	• Improves chest excursion and tidal volume. Provides optimal inspirations. Decreases the work of breathing compared with other positions.
• Coach patient in developing functional breathing pattern.	• Promotes slower, deeper breathing and reduces the effects of anxiety on respirations.
• Encourage deep-breathing, coughing; suction as needed.	• Promotes slower, deeper breathing and reduces the effects of anxiety on respirations. Clears airway when patient cannot adequately do so.
• Ensure that chest dressings are not constrictive.	• Affords maximal chest excursion; edema from chest burns can cause progressive skin tightness, which causes tourniquet-like effect; circumferential chest dressings can add to this effect if too tight.
• Provide psychologic support; teach relaxation techniques.	• Hypoxia and breathlessness cause great psychologic distress and resultant anxiety counters therapeutic goals, including effective breathing patterns or weaning from mechanical ventilation.
• Provide pain relief after assessing carefully to differentiate pain and hypoxia.	• Pain increases metabolic stress and fosters more rapid, shallow respirations which are less effective than the normal breathing patterns seen in comfortable patients.

Nursing Diagnosis: Breathing Pattern, Ineffective, Potential For (*Continued*)

Interventions	Rationale
COLLABORATIVE	
• Monitor ABGs.	• Determine progression of hypoxemia and need for or response to therapy.
• Administer humidified oxygen as needed.	• Improves tissue oxygenation and reduces anxiety associated with tissue hypoxia.
• Provide mechanical ventilation and give muscle relaxants as prescribed.	• Mechanical ventilation allows control of patient breathing to meet therapeutic goals; muscle relaxation may be required to achieve optimal synchrony of patient and machine to provide optimal tissue oxygenation.
• Monitor serial ABGs.	• Inadequate ventilation results in decreased pO_2, and increased pCO_2 over time.
• Provide mechanical ventilation, CPAP, and PEEP as needed.	• Provides control of ventilation to deliver preset tidal volume, FIO_2, rate to afford optimal oxygen to alveoli; counters problems of decreased compliance and chest construction.
• Prepare patient for escharotomy (Color Plate 45) and assist surgeon as needed.	• Incision through full-thickness burns of chest along longitudinal lines allows improved chest wall excursion.
• Monitor for readiness to wean from mechanical ventilation; encourage gradual independence from mechanical ventilator; continue to monitor closely.	• As pulmonary parameters approach normal and lung compliance and chest wall restriction decrease, patient may be ready to breathe unassisted. Process must be gradual, according to defined protocols, taking into consideration psychologic dependence on ventilator and patient's physiologic response to weaning.

Nursing Diagnosis: Gas Exchange, Impaired

May Be Related To:

- Decreased blood oxygen content.
- Airway obstruction.
- Impaired alveolar function secondary to CO poisoning, thermal and chemical injury to respiratory passages.
- Pulmonary edema

Possibly Evidenced By: Decreased pO_2, increased pCO_2, increased respiratory rate, cyanosis, shortness of breath, confusion, restlessness.

Desired Patient Outcomes: The patient will experience carboxyhemoglobin level within normal limits; be free of symptoms of respiratory distress, and have ABGs within normal limits, normal neurologic status, normal cardiac rate and rhythm, and adequate tissue oxygenation.

Interventions	**Rationale**
INDEPENDENT	
• Monitor respiratory rate, rhythm, depth, signs of hypoxemia and hypoxia continuously.	• Respiratory rate increases and depth may alter as patient attempts to take in more oxygen for exchange at alveolar and tissue level.
• Assess neurologic and cardiac status.	• These tissues are very oxygen dependent and are first to show signs of inadequate oxygenation. May be manifested by mental confusion, irritability, lethargy, somnolence; increased cardiac rate, dysrhythmias.
• Assess breath sounds.	• Auscultation of chest permits detection of presence of secretions that block exchange of oxygen and carbon dioxide.
• Encourage patient to cough secretions out; suction as needed to maintain patent airway.	• Removes secretions that form barriers to oxygen and carbon dioxide exchange.
• Monitor intake and output; avoid fluid overload.	• Prevents pulmonary edema, which decreases ability of oxygen and carbon dioxide to exchange at alveolar level.
• Encourage deep-breathing, use of incentive spirometry, hyperinflation hourly.	• Maintains optimal alveolar function, thus affording optimal exchange of oxygen and carbon dioxide.
• Provide adequate rest.	• Decreases metabolic rate and oxygen consumption by muscles, therefore allowing more oxygen to be available for vital organ function.
COLLABORATIVE	
• Provide humidified 100 percent oxygen until CO level is known; adjust accordingly; adjust for COPD patient as prescribed.	• Decreases half-life of CO rapidly in case of suspected CO poisoning; oxygen can be toxic if given at 100 percent for too long; a high oxygen concentration will alter COPD patient's usual compensatory mechanisms and decrease stimulus to breathe.
• Administer bronchial dilators as prescribed.	• Opens airways by relaxing muscles and facilitates oxygen and carbon dioxide entry and exit.
• Use sedation and analgesia judiciously to reduce metabolic rate and oxygen consumption without causing respiratory depression.	• Anxiety and pain increase metabolic rate and tissue oxygen consumption; overzealous use may decrease CNS respiratory drive.

Nursing Diagnosis: Gas Exchange, Impaired (*Continued*)

Interventions	Rationale
• Prepare patient for treatment with hyperbaric oxygenation according to specific protocols.	• Hyperbaric oxygen effectively displaces CO from hemoglobin, myoglobin, and cytochrome systems. The pressures used and the flammability of the oxygen are two of several factors that require specific interventions prior to the treatment to reduce risk of patient injury.

Nursing Diagnosis: Skin Integrity, Impairment Of

(Refer to Chapter 4, page 64, for etiology, manifestations, desired patient outcomes, and interventions.)

Nursing Diagnosis: Infection, Potential For

(Refer to Chapter 9, page 171, for etiology, manifestations, desired patient outcomes, and interventions.)

Nursing Diagnosis: Pain

(Refer to Chapter 9, page 169, for etiology, manifestations, desired patient outcomes, and interventions.)

Nursing Diagnosis: Tissue Perfusion, Alteration In: Cardiopulmonary

May Be Related To:

• Upper airway trauma secondary to inhalation injury
• Lower airway trauma secondary to inhalation injury

Possibly Evidenced By: Dyspnea, tachypnea, stridor, use of accessory muscles, cyanosis, confusion, abnormal ABG values, and adventitious breath sounds.

Desired Patient Outcomes: Patient will have normal breath sounds, ABG results within normal limits, and demonstrate normal breathing patterns.

(Refer to interventions under Nursing Diagnoses of Airway Clearance, Ineffective; Gas Exchange, Impaired; and Breathing Patterns, Ineffective page 339, 341, and 342.)

Nursing Diagnosis: Nutrition, Alteration In, Less Than Body Requirements

(Refer to Chapter 9, page 172, for etiology, manifestations, desired patient outcomes, and interventions.)

Nursing Diagnosis: Fluid-Volume Deficit

(Refer to Chapter 9, page 165, for etiology, manifestations, desired patient outcomes, and interventions.)

Nursing Diagnosis: Social Isolation

(Refer to Chapter 7, page 90, for etiology, manifestations, desired patient outcomes, and interventions.)

Nursing Diagnosis: Coping, Ineffective Family/Individual

(Refer to Chapter 7, page 92, for etiology, manifestations, desired patient outcomes, and interventions.)

Nursing Diagnosis: Post-Trauma Response

(Refer to Chapter 7, page 93, for etiology, manifestations, desired patient outcomes, and interventions.)

Nursing Diagnosis: Anxiety

May Be Related To:

• Uncertainty about future ability to live independently

(Refer to Chapter 7, page 98, for other etiologies, manifestations, desired patient outcomes, and interventions.)

Nursing Diagnosis: Grieving

(Refer to Chapter 7, page 94, for etiology, manifestations, desired patient outcomes, and interventions.)

Nursing Diagnosis: Fear

(Refer to Chapter 7, page 175, for etiology, manifestations, desired patient outcomes, and interventions.)

Nursing Diagnosis: Adjustment, Impaired

(Refer to Chapter 7, page 95, for etiology, manifestations, desired patient outcomes, and interventions.)

Nursing Diagnosis: Powerlessness

(Refer to Chapter 7, page 96, for etiology, manifestations, desired patient outcomes, and interventions.)

Nursing Diagnosis: Family Process, Alteration In

(Refer to Chapter 7, page 97, for etiology, manifestations, desired patient outcomes, and interventions.)

Nursing Diagnosis: Self-Concept, Disturbance In

(Refer to Chapter 7, page 89, for etiology, manifestations, desired patient outcomes, and interventions.)

Nursing Diagnosis: Knowledge Deficit

(Refer to Chapter 8, page 176, for etiology, manifestations, desired patient outcomes, and interventions.)

REFERENCES

1. Dyess, DL: Inhalation injuries. Current Concepts. Trauma Care 8:4, 1985.
2. Calahane, M and Demling, RH: Early respiratory abnormalities from smoke inhalation. JAMA 251:771, 1984.
3. Herndon, DN, Thompson, PB, and Traber, DL: Pulmonary injury in burned patients. In Proceedings of the Symposium: Respiratory Care of the Burned Patient, 2. American Burn Association, Orlando, FL, March 27, 1985.
4. Dyess, p. 4.
5. Dyess, p. 6.
6. Peters, WJ: Inhalation injury caused by the products of combustion. CMAJ 125:249, 1981.
7. Cohen, MA and Guzzardi, LJ: Inhalation of products of combustion. Ann Emerg Med 12:628, 1983.
8. Calahane and Demling, p 772.
9. Texidor, HS: Pulmonary complications in burn patients. J Can Radiol Assoc 34:264, 1983.
10. Peters, p 250.
11. Norkool, DM: Treatment of acute carbon monoxide poisoning with hyperbaric oxygen: A review of 115 cases. Ann Emerg Med 14:1168, 1985.
12. Cohen and Guzzardi, p 629.
13. Herndon et al, p 10.
14. Treat, RC: Inhalation injuries. In Hummel, RP: Clinical Burn Thrapy. John Wright–PSG, Boston, 1982.
15. Peters, p 250.
16. Dyess, p 4.
17. Venus, B, et al: Prophylactic intubation and continuous positive airway pressure in the management of inhalation injury in burn victims. Crit Care Med 9:519, 1981.
18. Thompson, PB, et al: Effect on mortality of inhalation injury. J Trauma 26:163, 1986.
19. University of Texas, Biomedical Communications Department: Inhalation Injury (Slide Tape Program). Health Sciences Center, University of Texas, Dallas.
20. Vermeer, M: Carbon monoxide poisoning. J Emerg Nurs 8;217, 1982.
21. Cohen and Buzzardi, p 630.
22. Texidor, HS et al: Smoke Inhalation: Radiologic manifestations. Radiology 149:383, 1983.
23. Cohen and Buzzardi, p 630.
24. Kryger, M, et al: Diagnosis of obstruction of the upper and central airways. Am J Med 61:85, 1976.
25. Miller, RD and Hyatt, RE: Evaluation of obstructing lesions of the trachea and larynx by flow volume loops. Am Rev Respir Dis 108:475, 1973.
26. Moylan, JA: Smoke inhalation and burn injury. Surg Clin North Am 60:1533, 1980.
27. Herndon et al, p 15.
28. Bartlett, RH, et al: Acute management of the upper airway in facial burns. Arch Surg 111:744, 1976.
29. Cohen and Guzzardi, p 630.
30. Herndon et al, p 15.
31. Herndon et al, p 15.
32. Venus et al, p 522.
33. Artz, CP, Moncrief, JA, and Pruitt, BA: Burns: A Team Approach. WB Saunders, Philadelphia, 1979, p 101.
34. Moylan, JA and Alexander, LG: Diagnosis and treatment of inhalation injury. World J Surg 2:185, 1978.
35. Robinson, NB, et al: Steroid therapy following isolated smoke inhalation injury. J Trauma 22:876, 1982.
36. Dyess, p 7.
37. Herndon et al, p 17.
38. Dyess, p 8.
39. Ibid.
40. Venus et al, p 520.
41. Dyess, p 8.
42. Myers, RA and Schnitzer, BM: Hyperbaric oxygen use. Postgrad Med 76:83, 1984.
43. Norkool, p 1170.
44. Norkool, p 1170.
45. Norkool, p 1170.

BIBLIOGRAPHY

Brandenburg, J: Inhalation injury: Carbon monoxide poisoning. Am J Nurs 80:98, 1980.

Budassi, SA: Smoke inhalation. J Emerg Nurs 8:156, 1982.

Clark, CJ, et al: Respiratory injury in the burned patient: The role of flexible bronchoscopy. Anaesthesia 38:35, 1983.

Fein, A, Leff, A, and Hopewell, PC: Pathophysiology and management of the complications resulting from fire and the inhaled products of combustion: A review of the literature. Crit Care Med 8:94, 1980.

Gaston, SF and Schumann, LL: Inhalation injury: Smoke inhalation. Am J Nurs 80:85, 1980.

Hart, GB, et al: Treatment of smoke inhalation by hyperbaric oxygen. J Emerg Med 3:211, 1985.

Heimbach, DM: Smoke inhalation: Current concepts. Top Emerg Med 3:75, 1981.

Judkins, KC and Brander, WL: Respiratory injury in children: The histology of healing. Burns 12:357, 1986.

Lund, T, et al: Upper airway sequelae in burn patients requiring endotracheal intubation or tracheostomy. Ann Surg 201:374, 1985.

Madden, MR, Finkelstein, JL, and Goodwin, CW: Respiratory care of the burn patient. Clin Plast Surg 13:29, 1986.

Robertson, C: A review of the use of corticoosteroids in the management of pulmonary injuries and insults. Arch Emerg Med 2:59, 1985.

Robinson, L and Miller, RH: Smoke inhalation injuries. Am J Otolaryngol 7:375, 1986.

Sataloff, DM and Sataloff, RT: Tracheotomy and inhalation injury. Head Neck Surg 6:1024, 1984.

Stephenson, BA: Smoke inhalation: The invisible injury. RN 47:36, 1984.

Surveyor, JA: Smoke inhalation injuries. Heart Lung 9:825, 1980.

Wooldridge-King, M: Nursing considerations of the burned patient during the emergent period. Heart Lung 11:353, 1982.

CARE OF THE BURN PATIENT IN ACUTE CARE SETTINGS

Chapter 19

LISA MARIE BERNARDO

CARE OF THE BURN PATIENT IN THE EMERGENCY DEPARTMENT: TRIAGE AND TRANSFER

The immediate care of the burn-injured person makes a critical difference in the person's course of hospitalization. Prompt emergency treatment, which includes stopping the burning process, establishing an airway, restoring breathing and circulation, initiating fluid resuscitation, and providing emotional support, plays a crucial role in the patient's outcome.

The emergency nurse treats the injured person, as well as that person's family, by helping them through their grief, loss, and pain. Surviving a burn injury is a very harrowing experience. Emotional support must be readily available for all parties involved, including the prehospital personnel.

The purpose of this chapter is to identify the steps in the resuscitation process, to understand the criteria for transferring injured persons to burn centers, and to provide suggestions for emotional support to the burn patient and the family.

NURSING ASSESSMENT PRIOR TO ARRIVAL

Individual Patient/Paramedic Notification

The preparation for the burned person begins before the patient arrives in the emergency department (ED). After the paramedics or firefighters treat the person in the field,[1] they notify the ED of the patient's age, sex, history, vital signs, head-to-toe assessment, and estimated time of arrival at the hospital. Depending on the patient's degree of injury, the nurse prepares a trauma room (for moderate or major burns) or a surgical room (for minor burns). The equipment needed is for intubation/oxygenation, cardiac and blood pressure monitoring, intravenous (IV) access and blood collection, and gastric and bladder decompression. External heat sources and sterile dressing supplies are also prepared. The trauma team (if the hospital is a trauma center) or other personnel, such as anesthetists, social workers, or burn personnel (if the hospital has such a unit) are notified of the patient's condition and estimated time of arrival.

Multiple Patients/Paramedic Notification

In the event of a multicasualty situation in which more than three people with significant injuries present to the ED at the same time, the hospital disaster plan may need to be activated. With situations involving radiation or hazardous materials exposure, measures must be instituted to protect the staff. Ideally, specially designated facilities must treat this type of emergency, and patients should be diverted to that institution.

Individual Patient/No Notification

When a burn-injured person arrives by private vehicle without advance notification, it is the triage nurse's responsibility to assess and evaluate the patient and the injury. The nurse assesses the patient's airway, breathing, circulation, and extent of injury and informs the Emergency Department physician of the assessment.

Multiple Patients/No Notification

In the unfortunate event of one's own employees being burned or if multiple individuals arrive without warning, the triage nurse assesses each patient's airway, breathing, circulation, and extent of injury. Additional ED medical and nursing assistance is requested and a disaster plan may need to be activated.

NURSING ASSESSMENT UPON PATIENT ARRIVAL

It is important to remember that nonburn trauma accompanies about one third of major burn admissions.[2] While the burn and the trauma are medically treated separately, the nurse treats the patient as a whole person. Therefore, the nurse must perform a thorough head-to-toe assessment on every burn-injured patient, being aware of the possibility of associated trauma relative to the mechanism of burn injury. The nursing assessment of the burn-injured patient, the same as for any trauma patient, begins with the primary survey. This involves assessing the patient's airway, breathing, and circulatory status (ABCs). However, with the burned patient, stopping the burning process supercedes the primary survey. The nurse cannot treat the person without stopping this process, to prevent further harm to the patient and to protect the nurse. When stopping the burning process in flame, scald, electrical, and chemical burns, all clothing and jewelry are removed. The nurse also assesses for heat dissipation from the skin by holding a hand over the burned area; if heat is being given off, the burning process is still in progress and must be stopped. Cooling the skin with copious amounts of sterile room-temperature water or saline is one method to use with flame or scald burns.

The airway is assessed for patency; if the airway needs to be opened, the jaw-thrust or chin-lift maneuver is used. This is done if a cervical spine injury is suspected due to an explosion, fall from a height, unrestrained or restrained motor vehicle passenger or pedestrian accident, electrical high-voltage shock, or lightning strike. The cervical spine must be immobilized with a rigid collar, cervical immobilization device (CID), and long back board. These measures can be used even if the neck is burned until the cervical spine is cleared by anterior-posterior (AP) and lateral cervical x-rays. However, if cervical immobilization must continue, frequent assessment of the neck must be done to prevent airway compromise from edema and the collar itself.

Breathing is assessed by the "look, listen, and feel" method for air exchange at the patient's head; next the carotid pulse is palpated (the brachial pulse can be palpated in the child). As the collar is applied, the neck is checked for jugular vein distention (JVD) and tracheal deviation. The chest is auscultated for bilateral breath sounds and adventitious sounds, as well as for symmetry and equal expansion. Because of the potential for eschar constriction (or flail chest, tension pneumothorax, and hemopneumothorax in the multiple trauma patient), the chest must be periodically reassessed for changes. The apical heart rate is auscultated for rhythm, rate, and clarity.

After the primary survey, the abdomen is assessed for distention, tenderness, and pain. The pelvis is assessed for intactness, and the extremities for deformities, movement, sensation, and pulses. Finally, the patient must be log-rolled and the posterior areas checked for further burns, impaled objects, bruises, tenderness, and so on. Throughout the assessment, the nurse evaluates the patient's neurologic status; this includes calculating the Glasgow Coma Scale and ascertaining level of consciousness. The nurse obtains the history of the injury, pain, alcohol or drug use, current medications, allergies, and past medical history. During this interaction, the nurse may be able to understand if the patient was burned as a suicide attempt or an abusive event.

The burn injury is assessed last; this consists of determining the percentage, depth, and area of the burn injury. With electrical burns, entrance and exit wounds must be identified. The "Rule of Nines" (for adults) and the Lund and Browder chart (for children) are two formulas for estimating the percentage of burn injury. One easy rule to remember is that the patient's closed palm represents approximately 1 percent of his or her body surface area.[3] Depth of the burn is determined by first-, second-, or third-degree classification. The outcome of the assessment is the mild, moderate, and major classifications (refer to Table 19–1). During the assessment process, external heat sources are utilized for temperature maintenance. Injury history includes the mechanism of injury, time of injury, length of contact with burn agent, efforts to stop the burning process, and location of injury (i.e., indoors or outdoors).

After the head-to-toe assessment and the designation of minor, moderate, and major burns (only a few minutes), the resuscitation measures are initiated. Continual reassessment every 15 minutes while the patient is in the Emergency Department is essential. Lifesaving interventions begin with endotracheal intubation and the provision of high-flow supplemental oxygen. Fluid resuscitation, using large-bore (at least 16-gauge) peripheral catheters, is initiated in burns greater than 20 percent TBSA[4,5] in adults and 10 to 15 percent TBSA in children or the elderly.[6] Lactated Ringer's is the solution of choice, and it is administered according to fluid resuscitation formulas as selected by the ED physician (refer to Chapter 9, Table 9–5). Fluid resuscitation formulas are merely a guide to resuscitation; fluid administration should be based on the patient's vital signs, urine output, and overall condition.[7] A Foley catheter is inserted to measure urine output and to ensure adequate fluid resuscitation. Also, a nasogastric tube is inserted and connected to low intermittent suction to decompress the stomach with burns more than 25 percent TBSA,[8] as paralytic ileus follows a burn injury. Emotional support is provided to the patient throughout the resuscitative event by speaking calmly, explaining all procedures, and touching the patient gently in unburned areas. During this time, transfer to a burn center is arranged by the referring and admitting physicians. If the hospital has a burn unit these nurses are involved from the time of arrival in the ED. All patient records must be copied and sent with the patient to the referring facility. Qualified personnel must accompany the patient, relative to the patient's needs. This

TABLE 19-1. Severity of Burn Injury

Category	Description	Disposition
Major burns	Adults with >25% TBSA; children under 10 and adults over 40 with 20% TBSA	Stabilize in emergency department (ED)
	Full-thickness burns of ≥10% TBSA	Transfer to specialized burn center
	All burns involving face, eyes, ears, hands, feet, or perineum that are likely to result in functional or cosmetic impairment	
	All high-voltage, electrical burns	
	All burn injuries complicated by inhalation injury or trauma	
Moderate burns	Partial- and full-thickness injury of 15–25% TBSA in adults *or* 10–20% in children <10 years and adults >40 years	Treat in ED; admit to hospital
	<10% of full-thickness burns that do not present serious threat of functional or cosmetic impairment of eyes, ears, hands, face, feet, or perineum	
Minor burns	<15% TBSA in adults; 10% TBSA in children and elderly	Treat in ED, can be admitted to hospital or discharged to home for subsequent followup
	<2% full-thickness injury without cosmetic or functional risk to eyes, ears, face, hands, feet, or perineum	

From American Burn Association: Guidelines for service standards and severity classifications in the treatment of burn injury. Bull Am Coll Surg 69:24, 1984, with permission.

may include any or all of the following: physician (emergency, critical care), anesthetist, nurse (emergency, transport), paramedic and respiratory therapist. If air or land transport is utilized by an outside agency the patient is prepared for transfer. A complete report is given to the transport team. The team may elect to perform additional stabilization procedures that were not done in the ED such as endotracheal intubation, intravenous line placement, or escharotomy. During transport, the patient's vital signs, level of consciousness, fluid management, and urine output are continuously monitored. Upon arrival, the transport team gives a report to the receiving team and delivers the referring hospital's records.

For minor burns, while the same head-to-toe assessment is performed, the outcome is different. Again, treating the patient's burns include treating the whole patient. Followup is determined by the patient's age, areas burned, compliance with dressing changes, and distance from the hospital. Any questions concerning compliance with dressing change, followup ED return, and medication administration warrant further investigation before the patient leaves the department. Admission to the hospital may be elected to ensure compliance with medical treatments.

NURSING CARE PLAN: CARE OF THE BURN PATIENT IN THE EMERGENCY DEPARTMENT

Nursing Priorities

1. Stop the burning process
2. Maintain patent airway and cervical spine control
3. Manage associated life-threatening injuries
4. Maintain homeostatic balance in fluid and electrolytes
5. Minimize pain and suffering
6. Assess neurologic status
7. Assess musculoskeletal status
8. Assess gastrointestinal and genitourinary status
9. Minimize and control bacterial contamination
10. Provide an appropriate knowledge base to patient and family
11. Maintain holistic approach to nursing care
12. Prepare for transfer or transport

Nursing Diagnosis: Injury, Potential

May Be Related To:

- A continuing burning process (it must be stopped in order to prevent further damage to patient and to promote safety for the rescuer)

Possibly Evidenced By: Smoldering skin; smoldering clothes.

Desired Patient Outcomes: No further damage to the patient as manifested by the termination of heat dissipation from areas of injury, smothering of flames, removal of electricity or chemical, and removal from radiation. Safety to the rescuer as manifested by freedom from injury.

Interventions	Rationale
INDEPENDENT	
• Extinguish burning process	
Flame	
○ Have person stop, drop, and roll: roll the person in a blanket or rug, run cool water over burn or cover burn with moist towels to stop burning process.	○ Extinguishes flames by smothering them; water disperses heat and helps to alleviate pain.
Scald	
○ Apply cool, moist towels; run cool water over burn area; do not apply ice directly to the skin. If burn area is greater than 15 to 20 percent TBSA, apply cool water with caution.[9]	○ Stops burning process by dispersing heat, relieves pain; ice causes further tissue damage; cooling measures can drop the body temperature in burns of this percentage and ventricular fibrillation may result.[10]

Nursing Diagnosis: Injury, Potential (Continued)

Interventions	Rationale

Electrical

○ Home: Do not touch person; turn off power at fuse box.

○ Stops the flow of electricity.

○ Outdoors/High Tension: Do not touch person; wait for help.

○ Person may still be in contact with electricity; very dangerous, wait for expert help.

Chemical

○ Remove clothing; it is desirable to wear a heavy rubber gown, rubber gloves, and safety goggles.[11] If clothing is heavily coated with dry chemical, brush chemical off first. This is best done in the field or in a decontamination or isolation room in the ED. (Refer to hazardous materials management guidelines at the hospital.)

○ Prevents contamination of rescuer; if clothing is not removed, greater injury occurs by increased tissue loss. Brushing chemicals limits amount of contamination to skin during clothing removal.

○ Brush dry chemicals from skin.

○ Water may cause a chemical reaction and further injury. Most dry chemicals are activated with water.

○ Place patient in a decontamination shower; if home, use a garden hose. Shower or flush injury site with water for 15 to 30 minutes prior to transport.[12] If no life-threatening injuries are present, shower or flush longer if injured person continues to complain of burning or itching, or if blisters continue to form. Double-bag contaminated clothing.

○ Decreases the concentration of the chemical and removes it from the wound. This decreases the rate and amount of reaction between the chemical and skin.[13] Continuous, copious washing with tepid water helps to minimize the burn depth; the duration of lavage is related to the chemical concentration, length of exposure time, and amount of chemical on the skin.[14]

○ Avoid the use of neutralizing agents.

○ Wastes time; also, specific neutralizing agents may, through a chemical reaction, generate more heat, thereby causing more tissue necrosis.[15,16]

• For all burns:

○ Provide an external heat source in moderate to severe burns (in-ceiling warmer lights, space blankets).

○ Helps patient retain body heat; excessive chilling and shivering causes more energy to be used, precipitating metabolic acidosis and possible cardiac arrhythmias.

○ Remove all clothing and jewelry.

○ Due to edema formation, constricting articles can impair circulation.

○ Use clean or sterile gloves, linen, and so on, when treating patient.

○ Prevents infection. If sterile articles are not available, use clean ones. Do not waste time trying to find sterile materials. Covering the patient with clean

Interventions	Rationale

sheets or sterile dressings also decreases the air current over the burn and minimizes the pain.[17]

COLLABORATIVE

- Any attempt to stop the burning process can be performed with another rescuer.

- Basic first aid is every team member's responsibility.

Nursing Diagnosis: Airway Clearance, Ineffective

May Be Related To:

- **Flame injury:** With a flame burn in an enclosed space, noxious fumes (including CO) are inhaled, causing an inhalation injury.
- **Scald injury:** With a steam burn to the face and neck area, inhalation injury is suspected. Also, the resultant edema and possibly a constrictive injury from circumferential third-degree burns to the chest may inhibit respiratory efforts. Observe for direct tissue injury (redness, inflammation, blisters).
- **Chemical injury:** Chemical burns can cause an inhalation injury from the chemical reactions in the tissues of the oral structures. Ingested chemicals (corrosives) can cause airway injury if aspiration occurs. Oral burns and resultant edema may impede the flow of air to the trachea.
- **Electrical injury:** Cardiopulmonary arrest can occur with high-voltage electrical injury or lightning strike. Electrical burns of the oral cavity can impede the flow of air to the trachea.

Possibly Evidenced By: Steam burns on face; carbonaceous sputum; soot in mouth; harsh cough; redness, inflammation; blisters in oral cavity; restricted chest expansion; stridor; singed nasal hairs; nasal flaring; use of accessory respiratory muscles.

Desired Patient Outcomes: The patient will maintain a patent airway and demonstrate adequate air exchange as manifested by pink skin and mucous membranes, equal and bilateral breath sounds, and equal and bilateral chest expansion.

Interventions	Rationale

INDEPENDENT

- Maintain open airway:
- The airway is opened by the jaw-thrust or chin-lift maneuver. A hard cervical collar is applied to maintain alignment if a cervical spine injury is suspected.
- Nasopharyngeal or oral pharyngeal airway devices should be inserted with caution in the patient with extensive oral burns caused by chemicals or flames.

- In the burn-injured patient, cervical spine injuries are suspected with falls, explosions, and electrical contact or lightning strikes.
- Manipulation with these devices may further injure the damaged tissues.

Nursing Diagnosis: Airway Clearance, Ineffective (*Continued*)

Interventions	Rationale
○ Assess for blisters inside the patient's mouth.	• Blisters indicate a risk for airway obstruction.[18] Although upper airway obstruction from laryngeal edema may not occur for 12 to 24 hours postinjury,[19] it is prudent to control the airway early in treatment.

COLLABORATIVE

• Provide supplemental oxygen at 100 percent as orddered during transfer and prior to intubation via humidified face mask or bag valve device.	• Helps to prevent hypoxia.
• Obtain arterial blood gases (ABGs) and carboxyhemoglobin on arrival in ED.	• Assess for impaired gas exchange and CO poisoning.
• Prepare for endotracheal intubation:	
○ Prepare equipment for endotracheal intubation. Ensure the proper functioning of all equipment (larygoscope blades and handles, suction). Draw up medications for rapid sequence intubation.	○ Prevents delay in treatment.
○ Ventilate patient with 100 percent oxygen via bag valve device and reservoir for at least 1 minute prior to intubation attempt.	○ Helps to prevent hypoxia.
○ Auscultate for breath sounds in all lobes, at the sternal notch, and at the epigastrium. Observe for equality and symmetry in chest expansion.	○ Ensures proper placement of endotracheal tube.
○ Secure endotracheal tube.	○ May be difficult with severe facial burns. Consider using commercially available endotracheal tube securing devices, or use two tracheostomy ties; tie each securely around tube. Have one set of ties above ears and one set below ears. Other methods are suggested in the literature.[20] This is especially important if patient will be transported to another facility.
○ Obtain a portable chest x-ray.	○ To check tube placement in trachea.
• Administer humidified oxygen, encourage coughing and deep breathing; perform nasotracheal suctioning after normal saline instillation; prepare for bronchoscopy by pulmonary physicians.	• Endotracheal lavage encourages clearance of carbonaceous material from upper airways; assesses extent of airway damage.

Nursing Diagnosis: Gas Exchange, Impaired

May Be Related To:

- Edema of alveolar capillary membranes secondary to inhaled particulates
- Fluid accumulation in the lungs secondary to excessive fluid resuscitation[21]
- High-voltage electrical shock

Possibly Evidenced By: Dyspnea, increased cough, rales, rhonchi, decreased PaO_2, restlessness, confusion, cyanosis, increased $PaCO_2$.

Desired Patient Outcomes: The patient will demonstrate adequate ventilation as manifested by clear and equal breath sounds, symmetrical chest expansion, no signs or symptoms of respiratory distress (nasal flaring, accessory muscle use, retractions), and normal laboratory values.

Interventions	Rationale
INDEPENDENT	
• Assess respiratory status:	
○ Auscultate breath sounds in all anterior and posterior lobes bilaterally every 15 minutes, or as patient condition warrants, to detect any changes and overt complications. Listen for rhonchi, rales, wheezing, or absent breath sounds. Observe for symmetrical chest expansion. Observe for signs and symptoms of a pneumothorax, hemopneumothorax or tension pneumothorax.	○ Detects any changes and overt complications; with incomplete chest expansion or circumferential chest burns, one lung may not properly aerate due to constriction of the chest wall. Also with suspected multiple trauma, a flail chest may be present. These multiple fractures can cause a pneumothorax or a hemopneumothorax, manifested by absent breath sounds on the affected side. Tracheal deviation, away from the affected side, is a sign to look for in a tension pneumothorax. Circumferential burns cause a bilateral decrease in lung expansion evidenced by a decreased volume of air flow, rapid shallow respirations, and signs and symptoms of hypoxia.
• Observe for upper airway and lower airway respiratory difficulty.	• Upper airway involvement includes stridor, whereas lower airway involvement includes nasal flaring, retractions (substernal, supraclavicular and infraclavicular and intercostal), and wheezing.
• Administer 100 percent oxygen by tight-fitting face mask for the breathing patient. If hypoxemia (PaO_2 less than 60 mmHg) or hypercarbia (PaO_2 more than 55 mmHg) is present after oxygen therapy is initiated, endotracheal intubation is performed.[22]	• Provides oxygen to alveoli for adequate gas exchange.

Nursing Diagnosis: Gas Exchange, Impaired (Continued)

Interventions	Rationale
• Assist with ventilations in the non-breathing patient using a bag valve device and 100 percent oxygen. Intubate and begin mechanical ventilation.	• Provides oxygen to the alveoli for adequate gas exchange.
• Observe for headache, dizziness, nausea, pink–cherry red skin and mucous membrane color, tachycardia and tachypnea.[23]	• Signs and symptoms of CO poisoning.
• Elevate head of bed.	• The head of bed is elevated in patients *without* history of multiple trauma who are in respiratory distress. If cervical spine injuries are suspected, the patient must remain immobilized in a hard collar and cervical immobilization device on a long backboard and kept flat until the cervical spine series is read as negative.
• Suction oral or endotracheal secretions; use saline instillation if carbon material present.	• Maintains airway patency; allows for adequate gas exchange; normal sterile saline instillation facilitates removal of carbonaceous material, thereby limiting the degree of chemical irritation and lung injury.

COLLABORATIVE

• Assist in obtaining ABGs and carboxyhemoglobin levels.	• Results determine ventilatory capabilities and guide changes in oxygen therapy.
• Assist in obtaining portable chest x-ray.	• Shows atelectasis, pneumothorax, endotracheal tube placement.
• Assist with escharotomy to chest.	• Escharotomy relieves constriction to chest wall and allows for adequate lung expansion.

Nursing Diagnosis: Fluid Volume Deficit, Potential

May Be Related To:

• Circulating fluid deficit secondary to capillary leakage into the interstitial spaces

Possibly Evidenced By: Electrolyte imbalances, metabolic acidosis, hypovolemia, decreased urine output, decreased central venous pressure, decreased pulmonary artery pressure, weight loss, decreasing mental status, decreased blood pressure and increased pulse.

Desired Patient Outcomes: Patient will maintain adequate fluid volume and systemic perfusion as manifested by stable vital signs and a urine output of 0.5 to 1.0 ml/kg per hour in the child;[24] 50 ml/hr in the adult; with conducted electrical injury, aim for 70 to 100 ml/hr.[25]

Interventions	Rationale
INDEPENDENT	
• Monitor vital signs and hemodynamic parameters at least every 15 minutes: auscultate apical pulse; palpate peripheral pulses; check nail beds.	• Pulse rate and blood pressure measurement reflect need for fluid resuscitation. Signs of hypovolemic shock may indicate internal bleeding from a chest, abdominal, or pelvic/femur injury in the multiple trauma patient. Apical heart rate is auscultated for clarity, rhythm, and murmurs. Peripheral pulses are measured for amplitude and equality. If peripheral pulses cannot be palpated, a Doppler device is used; escharotomies should be considered. Nail beds are checked for briskness of capillary refill and color.
• Measure blood pressure in either the upper or the lower extremities. The cuff can be placed directly over a burn or a 4 × 4 inch gauze pad can be placed on the extremity prior to the cuff application.[26] Do not apply the cuff to an amputated extremity or to an extremity with a circumferential burn or vascular impairment.	• Applying a cuff to an amputated extremity or an extremity with a circumferential burn or vascular impairment will give inaccurate readings and will further impair circulation.
• Apply cardiac monitor leads and electrodes. Electrodes can be placed over burned skin if necessary. Alternate placement areas may be used, such as the shoulders or forehead.	• Serves as a monitor for tachycardia (decreased oxygen to cells, stress, fear, cold); ectopic beats (stress, decreased oxygen); pacer spikes (implanted pacemaker); bradycardia (sign of impending arrest in children); ventricular fibrillation (metabolic acidosis); asystole (cardiac arrest).
• Obtain 12-lead ECG in patients with electrical burns.	• Provides a record of myocardial activity postinjury.
• Monitor urine output for volume, specific gravity, and hemachromogens.	• Decreased urine output and specific gravity are an early indication of fluid volume deficit. Hemachromogens released by red blood cells (RBC) muscle tissue injury leads to tubular necrosis if not recognized or treated with aggressive fluid resuscitation.[27]

Nursing Diagnosis: Fluid Volume Deficit, Potential (*Continued*)

Interventions	Rationale

COLLABORATIVE

- Assist in insertion of two large-bore peripheral lines, preferably in the upper extremities.

- Needed for venous access to obtain blood specimens (complete blood count/differential, electrolytes, prothrombin time/partial thrombin time, blood urea nitrogen, glucose, creatinine; type and cross-match, other studies such as ETOH/drug screen) and begin fluid resuscitation. Upper extremities are preferred to the lower extremities because of the high incidence of phlebitis and septic phlebitis in saphenous veins.[28] IV lines can be started in burned areas. If possible, do not start in a circumferentially burned extremity or one that is vascularly impaired.

- Assist with infusion of IV solutions for fluid resuscitation (refer to Chapter 9, Table 9–3). Number the IV bags as they are infused.

- Lactated Ringer's solution is the crystalloid of choice for fluid resuscitation. Various formulas for fluid resuscitation exist. More common formulas for adults include 2 to 3 ml/kg per percent TBSA for burned adults (revised Brooke, 1979) or 4 ml/kg per percent TBSA (Baxter) over 24 hours. One half of the total amount of fluid is administered in the first 8 hours (from the time of injury); the second half is administered over the next 16 hours. IV bags are numbered to keep an accurate account of fluid infusions. Colloids may be administered with some formulas; however, the use of colloids in the first 24 hours postinjury is controversial at this time.

- Prepare for insertion of a central venous line. A cutdown kit is prepared and the proper-sized catheters are obtained. Potential sites for insertion are the saphenous, femoral, antecubital, subclavian, and external jugular veins. Intraosseous infusions may be attempted in the pediatric patient via the unburned tibia.

- If the burn-injury is very extensive and no peripheral sites can be accessed, a central line is inserted. This serves as a guide for fluid replacement and hemodynamic status.

- Explain to the patient what will happen.

- Helps to alleviate anxiety.

- Assist in dressing the site with an occlusive dressing following insertion.

- Prevents infection; prevents dislodgement.

- Monitor placement of the jugular or subclavian line with an x-ray.

- All catheters are checked for patency prior to fluid infusion.

Nursing Diagnosis: Pain

(Refer to Chapter 9, page 169, for etiology, manifestations, desired patient outcomes, and interventions.)

Nursing Diagnosis: Sensory-Perceptual Alteration

May Be Related To:

- A concomitant head injury
- Alterations in fluid and electrolyte balances
- Hypoxia

Possibly Evidenced By: Altered level of consciousness; altered communication patterns; motor uncoordination; disorientation.

Desired Patient Outcomes: Patient will maintain normal neurologic functioning as manifested by being awake, alert, oriented; patient has intact reflexes and moves all extremities purposefully and spontaneously.

Interventions	Rationale
INDEPENDENT	
• Perform a neurologic assessment at least every hour. Level of consciousness is assessed by asking name, place, time, history of injury, what was done prior to patient's arrival in the emergency department, past medical history, and allergies. Ask patient about pain and ability to move. Test motor and sensory function, strength, and pupil size. Feel and observe scalp and skull for additional burns, lacerations, or uneven contour.	• Provides baseline information about patient.
• Observe for cerebrospinal fluid (CSF) or blood from nose and ears.	• In the multiple trauma patient, this would indicate a basilar skull fracture.
• Explain procedures in terms patient can understand.	• Provides patient with reassurance.
• Observe for emotional response; patient may have anger, guilt, denial, fear, pain, hostility, combative behavior.	• Provides clues to patient's affect and may indicate changes in neurologic state.
• Observe for seizure activity. If a seizure occurs, open the airway, provide suction and oxygen, and log-roll patient onto side.	• Following a lightning or electrical injury, a seizure may occur.

Nursing Diagnosis: Sensory-Perceptual Alteration (*Continued*)

Interventions	Rationale
COLLABORATIVE	
• Administer IV pain medication as ordered in severe burns; oral pain medication in minor burns; consider nitrous oxide in patients without head or inhalation injuries.	• If adequate respiratory and neurologic functioning are present, IV pain medications are administered. The most common is morphine sulfate 3 to 5 mg IV (adults), titrated to the desired analgesic effect every 20 to 40 minutes.[29] Do not give medications intramuscularly (IM) to avoid deposition of the medication into a nonperfused area.[30] IV administration ensures a uniform, timely distribution throughout the body.[31] Do not give narcotics to a patient with agitation or anxiety until hypoxemia or hypovolemia are ruled out.[32] Also, hemodynamic instability during resuscitation results in variable absorption, which may cause drug accumulation and later sudden absorption into the circulation, causing fatal apnea.[33]
• Administer anticonvulsant medications as ordered.	• Prevents/controls seizure activity.

Nursing Diagnosis: Injury, Potential For Musculoskeletal Impairment

May Be Related To:

• Concomitant fractures and dislocations secondary to cause of injury

Possibly Evidenced By: Deformities, dislocations, changes in peripheral pulses, impaired mobility, pain, and tenderness.

Desired Patient Outcomes: Patient will maintain musculoskeletal integrity, as manifested by symmetrical mobility and sensation.

Interventions	Rationale
INDEPENDENT	
• Assess peripheral circulation every hour or more frequently if circulatory impairment is appreciated.	• Changes in peripheral pulses are an indication of further damage. Early assessment prevents further trauma and/or allows for prompt treatment.

Interventions	**Rationale**

- Assess musculoskeletal functioning.

- Immobilize spine.
- Maintain proper body alignment.
- Encourage movement of extremities if no fractures. Elevate burned extremities on pillows or blankets.
- Cover open fractures with a sterile dressing.

- Fractures or dislocations from electrical or lightning injuries are suspected with pain, deformity, and asymmetrical movement.
- Prevents spinal cord damage.
- Prevents contractures.
- Movement also assists in maintaining function. Elevation improves circulation.
- Casts cannot be placed on a burned area due to potential necrosis and no freedom of dressing change.

COLLABORATIVE

- Assist in splinting. If burned extremities are fractured, dress skin and splint with a molded splint (Jones dressing).
- Assist with escharotomy (refer to Chapter 4): Prepare equipment (scalpel, bovie, if available). Explain procedure to patient; premedicate as ordered. Tissue pressures may be obtained before the escharotomy. Pressures even slightly over 40 mmHg may cause permanent nerve and muscle damage.[39]
- Apply dressings following the escharotomy: apply a topical antimicrobial agent. Monitor sites for evidence of bleeding during first few hours after procedure.
- Position extremities above the level of the heart following the escharotomy. Monitor extremities for adequate circulation every 2 hours until edema begins to subside (48 to 72 hours postburn).

- Maintains proper body alignment.

- Circumferential burns to the extremities impede circulation, movement, and sensation. Preparation provides for a better, less painful procedure.

- Assists in preventing infection. Bleeding needs to be monitored to prevent further fluid loss.

- Elevation minimizes edema and promotes better circulation.

Nursing Diagnosis: Skin Integrity, Impairment Of

May Be Related To:

- Burn injury

Possibly Evidenced By: Disrupted skin layers; changes in wound: drainage, odor, color, tenderness, swelling.

Desired Patient Outcomes: The patient's burned areas will heal and will not become infected. Body temperature and adequate perfusion will be maintained at a normal level.

Nursing Diagnosis: Skin Integrity, Impairment Of (*Continued*)

Interventions	Rationale
INDEPENDENT	
• Use clean, sterile equipment when caring for patient.	• Prevents further contamination of wound.
• Wash hands before and after caring for patient.	• Prevents spread of infection.
• Dress all invasive sites and burn wound with sterile dressings.	• Prevents organisms from entering body through catheter site; limits contamination of burn wound.
• Use sterile technique in all patient care.	• Prevents spread of infection.
COLLABORATIVE	
• Apply ordered antimicrobial agents (refer to Chapter 4, page 44).	• If small surface areas are involved, the antimicrobial agent is applied to the cleaned area. In large surface area burns, antimicrobial agents are not used in the emergency setting. The burn unit team will only have to remove the agent to reassess the patient's injury.
• Clean and assist debridement of burned area.	• In minor burns, the area may be cleaned with a mild soap and water.[40] If blisters are present, the decision to break or leave them intact depends on the preference of the physician. If the blisters have already broken, the loose, dead skin may be debrided gently with sterile scissors and forceps; some burn units leave the dead skin on the wound unless there is evidence of purulence. Hair in the burned area may be shaved. The color of the burned area, as well as the presence of intact eschar, pain, sensation, and bleeding are all noted. In moderate or major burns, the area may or may not be cleaned, depending on the patient's condition. This is because Airway, Breathing, and Circulatory support (ABCs) are the priorities. A wound of this magnitude is better left for the burn team to treat. However, one exception is chemical burns, wherein the liquid chemical is flushed with copious amounts of sterile saline or, in the case of dry chemical, is brushed off (refer to Chapter 3).
• Apply sterile dressings.	• In minor burns, a light dressing of 2 × 2 inch and 4 × 4 inch gauze pads and gauze rolls are used. Cotton-filled dress-

Intervention	**Rationale**
	ing materials should not be used, as they do not permit drainage. Digits are wrapped separately, and axilla burns are dressed so that the burn surfaces do not touch. Contractures will occur if two skin surfaces touch. Always refer burns of the face, eyes, ears, hands, feet, and perineum to the burn or plastic surgical care team.
• Adequate supplies for home dressing changes must be ordered by the physician or given to the patient and family prior to discharge from the ED (refer to Chapter 8).	• Improper dressing materials will cause further skin damage.
• In moderate burns, dry sterile dressings are the choice.	• Wet dressings may further decrease the patient's temperature. In the extensively burned patient, ABCs are the priority; covering the patient with a sterile, clean sheet and space blanket to keep the patient warm is recommended.
• Administer tetanus toxoid IM. If patient has had previous immunization, administer tetanus toxoid if toxoid has not been given in the past 5 years. If patient has never been immunized, administer human tetanus–immune globulin and toxoid.[41] Do not administer both in the same site. In children age 7 or older administer Td (tetanus-diphtheria toxoid). In children younger than age 7, DTP should be used; if pertussis vaccine is contraindicated, use DT (diphtheria-tetanus toxoids).[42]	• Prevents tetanus. Administering both globulin and toxoid in same site will cause them to bind, which prevents immunization. Td provides adequate diphtheria immunity.
• Assist in documentation of involved areas and treatment on patient's chart (refer to Chapter 2 for estimation of percentage and depth). Photograph any burns, especially with suspected abuse, that will be treated on an outpatient basis.	• Supplies a record of ED care.

Nursing Diagnosis: Knowledge Deficit: Burn Injury

(Also refer to Chapter 9, p. 176.)

May Be Related To:

- Lack of knowledge of the healing process
- Lack of knowledge about scar tissue, swelling, exercise, splints, pain, and pressure garments
- Lack of knowledge about nutritional needs, potential for fluid deficit, and alteration of gastrointestinal function

Nursing Diagnosis: Knowledge Deficit: Burn Injury (*Continued*)

Possibly Evidenced By: Verbalizations, inability to answer questions and/or perform return demonstration.

Desired Patient Outcomes: Patient and family are able to verbalize knowledge and perform return demonstrations correctly.

Interventions	Rationale

INDEPENDENT

- Assess patient's and family's need for education.

- Affords nurse the opportunity to determine the best method for patient and family teaching.

- Teach patient and family how to clean and dress wound for outpatient treatment.

- Prevents infection and complications.

- Teach patient and family how and when to administer antibiotics and pain medications for outpatient treatment.

- Promotes patient comfort; prevents infection.

- Explain and demonstrate to patient and family the use of splints and proper range of motion (ROM) exercises.

- Promotes cooperation. Prevents contractures.

- Explain states of wound healing. Provide information regarding increased fluid and nutritional needs and potential for fluid deficit and gastrointestinal distress. Instruct patient and family to monitor the aforementioned for 24 to 48 hours, and to report if urine output is decreased and/or if nausea and vomiting occur.

- Facilitates participation and compliance. Allows for early detection of complications.

- Provide information about local support groups.

- Provides for additional resources.

- Demonstrate to patient and family ways to promote comfort (e.g., relaxation tapes, guided imagery).

- Gives alternatives other than pain medication.

COLLABORATIVE

- Give written discharge instructions and followup care.

- Physician may have specific times or days for patient to return for wound checks.

- Have patient and family sign written instructions; retain one copy for emergency record.

- Documents that information was given; patient and family have copy to refer to at home.

- Give patient and family a phone number to call and a person to contact.

- Provides continuity of care.

- Consult social services if there is any doubt about patient's and family's ability to comply with instructions or to obtain supplies.

- Any doubts about compliance must be cleared *before* the patient and family are discharged. This prevents future problems with infection, scarring, and so on.

Intervention	**Rationale**
	If the circumstances surrounding the burn injury are suspicious of abuse or suicide, the patient must be evaluated by social worker or psychiatry/mental health care worker prior to discharge. This may prevent another abusive situation. If it is recommended that the patient should not be discharged, admission to the hospital is warranted for patient safety.
• Initiate crisis intervention for the family of the severely burned patient.	• Having social service, pastoral service, and other health care professionals support the family is essential. It is helpful if the family is given the name of a contact person at the receiving burn unit to help them prioritize their needs.
• Allow the family to see the patient prior to transport.	• If the patient dies, the family may regret not having said goodbye.

Nursing Diagnosis:
Grieving, Dysfunctional

May Be Related To:

- The family experiencing sudden death in the ED. This type of loss is especially traumatic because it is unexpected. The deceased and family may have argued previous to the accident, or suicide or abuse/neglect is suspected (as when an unattended child burns down the house); in such situations additional shock, anger, and denial are experienced. Anger may be directed at staff for "not doing everything" to save the deceased.

Possibly Evidenced By: Verbalizations, denial of loss, anger, crying, alterations in concentration.

Desired Patient Outcomes: The family will develop a realistic understanding of trauma event and loss of loved one as manifested by saying goodbye and appropriate use of supportive services.

Interventions	**Rationale**
INDEPENDENT	
• Notify family of patient's arrival in ED. Simple statements to reflect the need for their presence are best. Encourage family not to hurry but to safely get to the ED.	• Allows for safe arrival of family.

Nursing Diagnosis: Grieving, Dysfunctional (*Continued*)

Interventions

- Prepare patient for family viewing:
  - Wrap child in blanket, exposing unburned areas as appropriate, and dim the lights. Cover adult with blanket and expose an unburned hand. Dim the lights. Keep endotracheal tubes and IV lines in place for coroner as required.
- Inform family of patient's death.

- Allow family to be with patient.
- Prepare family and room:

  - Provide seats. Have room cleaned prior to their arrival. Allow parents to hold child, tell them child will feel heavier. Have family supports be in room. Have social and religious services available. Family may want last rites, baptism or other religious service performed; ask the family their wishes instead of automatically assuming they want a religious counselor. Allow adequate viewing time (keep within 1 hour). Other immediate family may want to see patient. Patient may be moved to a quiet, private location prior to family's arrival. Ask about funeral director; find one family member to help with this. Reassure family that patient did not suffer and that everything possible was done for him or her.
- Initiate contact to Compassionate Friends or other community support groups. Followup social service support must also be arranged, usually 1 week following the incident.
- Prepare body for funeral director, coroner, and morgue in accordance with hospital policies on postmortem care.

- Save clothing for evidence.

Rationale

- Allows for appropriate viewing since burns cause disfigurement. All burn accidents are coroner cases.

- Best if heard from physician because this gives a sense of finality and belief that everything possible was done.
- Assists in grieving process.
- Adequate preparations help to lessen this traumatic situation.

- Allows family to deal with grief and death rituals in own way; assists family to deal with stress of current situation.

- Some states have autopsy requirements on all patients who die within 24 hours of admission or following trauma. The body is prepared in the usual manner.
- In the case of a suspicious death (arson, suicide, abuse) clothing is saved in paper bags and signed over to the appropriate authorities.

Nursing Diagnosis: Knowledge Deficit: Safety

May Be Related To:

- Lack of education regarding safety

Possibly Evidenced By: Verbalizations, repeated injuries.

Desired Patient Outcomes: Patient will be absent of further injury as manifested by no repeat burn incidents.

Interventions

INDEPENDENT

- Assess patient's and family's understanding of burn injury process.
- Teach simple burn safety relative to patient/family age, developmental level, and comprehension ability (refer to Chapter 23).
- Plan a community-school prevention program with ED nurses.

Rationale

- Provides information on how to teach burn prevention.
- Greater chance for success in patient/family understanding of burn prevention.

- Increases greater awareness of burn prevention.

Nursing Diagnosis: Injury (During Transport), Potential For

May Be Related To:

- Discharge from the ED to home
- Interdepartment transfer from ED to inpatient unit
- Interhospital transfer from ED to burn/trauma center
- Special considerations during air transport

Possibly Evidenced By: Hemodynamic nonstabilization of patient; incomplete ED records.

Desired Patient Outcomes: Patient transferred safely, as manifested by airway patency, respiratory sufficiency, hemodynamic stability, and completed records.

Interventions

INDEPENDENT

Discharge to Home

- Refer to Knowledge Deficit: Burn Injury, page 121.

Interdepartment Transfer

- Ensure patency of airway and respiratory adjuncts, IV lines, nasogastric tube, Foley catheter, and external heat source.

Rationale

- Decreases chances of dislodgment during transfer process.

Nursing Diagnosis: Injury (During Transport), Potential For (*Continued*)

Interventions	Rationale
• Ensure that receiving unit is notified and prepared for patient.	• Allows for smooth transfer.
• Complete all ED flow sheets, with particular attention to intake and output totals.	• Promotes continuation of resuscitation process.
• Prepare and bring appropriate equipment during the transfer, such as intubation equipment, oxygen tank, IV catheters and fluids, blankets, medications, and so on (Table 19–2).	• Provides a backup in case of accidental dislodgment.
• Allow family to visit with patient prior to transfer.	• The receiving unit will be busy admitting the patient, and the family will have an additional wait until a visit is possible; allays some anxiety in the family if they are allowed to visit (or at least see) the patient, in case the patient should expire before they can visit in the receiving unit.

Interhospital Transfer From Emergency Department to Burn/Trauma Center:

COLLABORATIVE

• Assist ED physician or trauma surgeon in contacting the receiving burn/trauma center.	• Begins transfer process.
• Assist physician/surgeon to contact a transport service (air or ground transport) if receiving institution does not provide this service.	• Allows transport team to prepare for drive or flight.

INDEPENDENT

• Complete ED flow sheet and photocopy for receiving facility (Fig. 19–1.)	• Allows for a record of treatment to accompany patient.
• Allow family to visit with patient prior to leaving the ED.	• Family may not have the opportunity to visit the patient in the receiving facility, or patient may expire prior to the family's arrival. Allows family to see that the patient is being cared for by competent, caring personnel.
• Ensure adequacy of personnel and equipment to meet patient's needs.	• At times, the patient may be transported with a ground ambulance and no advanced life support personnel (emergency medical technicians). It may be the hospital's responsibility to supply advanced life support personnel to ac-

TABLE 19–2. E.D. Supplies for Burn Care*

Topical Antimicrobial Agents
   povidone-iodine solution
   povidone-iodine ointment
   Silvadene cream
   Neosporin ointment
   Xeroform gauze
Pharmaceuticals
   Analgesics (narcotic, nonnarcotic)
   Tetanus toxoid
      Dt
      Td
      Hypertet
      Tetanus toxoid booster
   D_5LR, LR, and so on
Dressing Supplies
   Gauze rolls
   Sterile gauze pads
      2×2s
      4×4s
   Porous tape
   Stockinette
   Sterile gloves
   Sterile towels, drapes, sheets
   Sterile H_2O/saline
   Sterile instrument sets
      Cutdown trays
      Suture sets
      Scalpels/blades (for escharotomies)
      Razors
   Eye-care equipment
      Fluorescein
      Slit-lamp
Other Capabilities
   In-ceiling warmer/heat lamps
   Ventilator
   Decontamination area
      Shower
      Double-bags for disposal of clothing, and
         so on
      Room ventilation
   12-Lead ECG machine
   Doppler device
   Automatic blood pressure measuring device
   Wall chart for burn care (can be obtained
      from the local burn center)

*This is in addition to the standard emergency equipment for airway management, fluid resuscitation, drug administration, and the like.

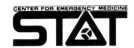

SPECIALIZED TREATMENT AND TRANSPORT

PRE-TRANSPORT WORKSHEET

Call 800-MED-STAT (633-7828)

Or if outside of Pennsylvania

412-647-STAT (647-7828)

(Please complete only relevant portions)

Patient Information
Please use addressograph plate

BRIEF HISTORY:

PAST HISTORY: COPD _____
Cardiac _____ Diabetes _____
Hypertension _____ Seizures _____
CVA _____ ETOH _____
Last Meal _____ Other _____

PHYSICAL EXAM (as indicated):

HEENT—

Lungs—

Heart—

Abdomen—

Neuro—

Extremities—

MEDICATIONS (dose, route & time):

VITAL SIGNS					
Time					
Pulse					
B/P					
Resp					
Level of Consciousness					

INTAKE/OUTPUT (for past 24 hours)

PO—   Urine—
Crystalloid—   NG Tube—
Colloid—   Estimated
Whole Blood—   Blood Loss—
PRBC   FFP—   Platelets—

IV#	SITE	GAUGE	FLUID	RATE
1				
2				
3				
4				

ALLERGIES: MAST SUIT: Time Applied—

LAB WORK:

EKG—

Chest X-ray—

Cervical Spine—

Other X-rays—

Ventilator:

Endo-tube Size—
FI02—
Rate—
Tidal Vol—
IMV/AC—
CPAP/PEEP—

Lytes:

Date/Time—
Na—
K—
Cl—
C02—
Gluc—
BUN—
Creat—
Calcium—

ABG's:		
Time—		
FI02—		
pH—		
p02—		
pC02—		
%Sat—		
HC03—		

CBC:

Date—
H/H—
WBC—
Platelets—
Protime—
PTT—
Blood Type—

FIGURE 19-1. Pretransport and transport records on the burned patient must be completed before departure from the emergency department. (Records reproduced by permission from STAT [Specialized Treatment and Transport], Center for Emergency Medicine of Western Pennsylvania, Pittsburgh, PA. Forms developed by Karen M. Klein, RN, MSN.)

STAT
TRANSPORT RECORD
412-647-7828

CENTER FOR EMERGENCY MEDICINE OF WESTERN PENNSYLVANIA

MO.	DAY	YEAR	TRANSPORT NUMBER	GEOGRPHICAL SITE CODE (SCENE)

PATIENT NAME:

SEX M-F	AGE	(CIRCLE ONE) Y M D	PATIENT PICK'D UP	IF HSP	TEAM: PIC/DRIVER		No.

LOCATION

| DATE OF BIRTH | | | 1. HOSPITAL | 4. RESIDENCE | MD |
| MO | DAY | YEAR | A. ED / B. CR. CARE | 6. AIRPORT / 7. ABORT | |

DESTINATION

MED. REC. No.

C. NEO / D. FLOOR / E. OR / F. CATH LAB / G. OTHER   8. OTHER / 9. SCENE

E.T.S.:
E.T.S.:

PT. CLASS.		TRAUMA SCORE	INIT.	FINAL	GLASGOW COMA	INIT.	FINAL	MECH. INJ.	PATIENT TAKEN TO	IF HSP	OTHER

INCIDENT LOCATION (SCENE)	A-SYMPTOMS/INJURY TYPE	CASE SEVERITY	PATIENT STATUS DURING TRANSPORT	MEDICAL COMMAND:

BEFORE TRANSPORT | DURING TRANSPORT

1. MOTOR VEHICLE   5. MINE
2. HOME   6. STREET
3. COMMERCIAL   7. FARM
4. FACTORY/INDUSTRY   8. OTHER

✓ IF ACCIDENT ☐

B-ANATOMICAL INJURY SITE

CASE SEVERITY
1. MINOR
2. MODERATE
3. SEVERE
4. LIFE THREAT
5. D.O.A.
6. CTB
TIME _____

PATIENT STATUS DURING TRANSPORT
1. IMPROVED
2. UNCHG'D. STABLE
3. UNCHG'D. UNSTABLE
4. WORSENED
5. EXPIRED ENROUTE
6. NOT TRANSPORTED

MEDICAL COMMAND:
1. TELEPHONE
2. PROTOCOL   5. RADIO
4. MD. AT SCENE   8. MD. ON BOARD

ARR. AT PT.	LV. WITH PT.

ALLERGIES

PATIENT'S MEDICATIONS

MEDICATIONS/IVS/BEFORE TRANSPORT

	INTAKE: BEFORE	DURING TRANS.	OUTPUT: BEFORE	DURING TRANS.
CRYSTALLOIDS			EBL	
COLLOIDS			UO-	
OTHER			OTHER	
TOTAL			TOTAL	

LABS	HGB	HCT	WBC	NA	K	CL	CO₂	GLUC	pH	SAT	pO₂	pCO₂	HCO₃	%O₂	MISC.

HX. PX. PROGRESS:

_____ (20) _____ (26) _____ (07) _____ (51) _____ (35)
MONITOR / ___02 @ _____ VIA ___ / _____ STIFF COLLAR / ___ C.I.D. (TAPE & BAGS) / _____ STRETCHER

MILITARY TIME	PULSE S W	R	RESP. R I AND SR	BP SYST DIAST.	MONITOR	CODE	AIDS & DRUGS/FLUIDS	CODE	ROUTE	COMMENTS	PROTOCOL

TRANSPORT   Page _____ of _____   SIGNATURES _____ /

STAT FORM — 4

FIGURE 19-1. *Continued.*

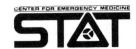

ESTIMATION of PERCENT of BURN

PLEASE SHADE BURNED AREAS

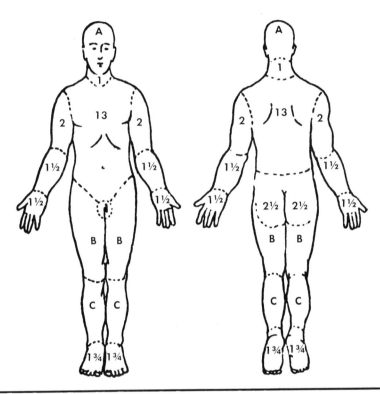

Relative Percentage of Areas Affected by Growth

	—Age in Years—					
	0	1	5	15	10	ADULT
A—½ of head	9½	8½	6½	5½	4½	3½
B—½ of one thigh	2¾	3¼	4	4¼	4½	4¾
C—½ of one leg	2½	2½	2¾	3	3¼	3½

Total Per Cent Burned_____2°+ _____3°= _____

FIGURE 19–1. *Continued.*

Intervention	Rationale
	company the patient, such as an ED nurse, paramedic, physician, respiratory therapist, and anesthetist (if airway compromise is anticipated or the patient is intubated). The same equipment needed for interdepartmental transfer must be obtained for this type of transport.
• When the transport team arrives (ground or air), a complete report is given, including copies of the ED flow sheet and any x-rays or diagnostic tests that were done.	• Provides for continuity of care.

Special Considerations for Air Transport

Intervention	Rationale
• Flight nurse receives report from ED nurse. The flight team (composed of a combination of nurse/physician/paramedic) may elect to perform stabilizing procedures not already completed by the ED team.	• The space inside of a helicopter is very limited. Therefore, maneuvering to perform stabilizing procedures, such as endotracheal intubation or IV insertion, may be extremely difficult. The flight team wants to ensure that the patient is stable enough to be flown.
• The flight nurse assesses the patient from head to toe and assures the proper functioning of all invasive and adjunct equipment (Fig. 19–2).	• Promotes safety; ensures patency while being transferred.

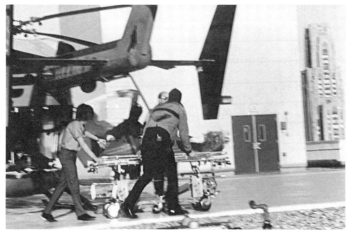

FIGURE 19-2. The flight team continuously monitors the burned patient until arrival at the burn/trauma center. (Photo courtesy of STAT [Specialized Treatment and Transport], Center for Emergency Medicine of Western Pennsylvania, Pittsburgh, PA.)

Nursing Diagnosis: Injury (During Transport), Potential For (*Continued*)

Interventions	Rationale
• During flight, the nurse monitors the patient's vital signs and ensures proper body temperature by keeping the patient covered.	• In the patient with serious burns, low cabin humidity coupled with the flight altitude and the "greenhouse effect" on warm sunny days increases the patient's evaporative fluid loss. Fluid replacement should be adjusted accordingly, using blood pressure and urine output as guides.[43]
• The flight nurse reassures the patient during the flight.	• The patient may be afraid during transport in the helicopter. Emotional support helps to calm the patient thereby decreasing his or her stress.

Nursing Diagnosis: Infection, Potential For

(Refer to Chapter 9, page 171, for etiology, manifestations, desired patient outcomes, and interventions.)

Nursing Diagnosis: Tissue Perfusion, Alteration in

(Refer to Chapter 9, page 164, for etiology, manifestations, desired patient outcomes, and interventions.)

Nursing Diagnosis: Post-Trauma Response

(Refer to Chapter 7, page 93, for etiology, manifestations, desired patient outcomes, and interventions.)

Nursing Diagnosis: Fear

(Refer to Chapter 7, page 175, for etiology, manifestations, desired patient outcomes, and interventions.)

Nursing Diagnosis: Adjustment, Impaired

(Refer to Chapter 7, page 95, for etiology, manifestations, desired patient outcomes, and interventions.)

Nursing Diagnosis: Powerlessness

(Refer to Chapter 7, page 96, for etiology, manifestations, desired patient outcomes, and interventions.)

Nursing Diagnosis: Anxiety

(Refer to Chapter 7, page 98, for etiology, manifestations, desired patient outcomes, and interventions.)

Nursing Diagnosis: Self-Concept, Disturbance In

(Refer to Chapter 7, page 89, for etiology, manifestations, desired patient outcomes, and interventions.)

Nursing Diagnosis: Coping, Possible Ineffective

(Refer to Chapter 7, page 92, for etiology, manifestations, desired patient outcomes, and interventions.)

REFERENCES

1. Edlich, RF, et al: Firefighter's guide to emergency rescue and care of the victim burned in structural fire. Journal of Burn Care and Rehabilitation 43:367, 1983.
2. Nordberg, M: Questions and controversies in burn care. Emerg Med Serv 17:25, 1988.
3. American College of Surgeons Committee on Trauma: Burns ATLS Course Student Manual. American College of Surgeons, Chicago, IL, 1985, p 156.
4. Ibid, p 155.
5. Bunkis, J and Walton, RL: Burns. In Trunkey, DD and Lewis, FR (eds): Current Therapy of Trauma, ed 2. BC Decker, Philadelphia, 1986, p 381.
6. Ibid, p 381.
7. American College of Surgeons Committee on Trauma, p 157.
8. Ibid, p 158.
9. Moylan, JA: First aid and transportation of burned patients. In Artz, C, Moncrief, J, and Pruitt, B (eds): Burns: A Team Approach. WB Saunders, Philadelphia, 1979, p 152.

10. Ibid, p 152.
11. Klein, DG and O'Malley, P: Topical injury from chemical agents: Initial treatment. Heart Lung, 16:52, 1987.
12. American College of Surgeons Committee on Trauma, p 159.
13. Luterman, A, Fields, C, and Curreri, PW: Treatment of chemical burns. Emerg Med Serv 17:37, 1988.
14. Klein and O'Malley, p 52.
15. Moylan, p 151.
16. McManus, WF: Immediate emergency department care. In Artz, C, Moncrief, J, and Pruitt, B (eds): Burns: A Team Approach. WB Saunders, Philadelphia, 1979, p 163.
17. Moylan, p 152.
18. Nordberg, p 27.
19. Moylan, p 152.
20. Gordon, MD (ed): Anchoring endotracheal tubes on patients with facial burns. Journal of Burn Care and Rehabilitation 8:233, 1987.
21. Bayley, EW and Smith, GA: The three degrees of burn care. Nursing 87, 17:38, 1987.
22. Bunkis and Walton, p 380.
23. Moylan, p 152.
24. Helvig, B: Trauma to the integument: Burns. In Howell, E, Widra, L, and Hill, MG: Comprehensive Trauma Nursing: Theory and Practice. Scott, Foresman/Little, Brown, College Division, Glenview, IL, 1988, p 390.
25. McManus, p 163.
26. Emergency Nurses Reference Library: Burns. Nursing 85 Books. Springhouse Corp, Springhouse, PA, 1985, p 661.
27. McManus, p 164.
28. American College of Surgeons Committee on Trauma, p 155.
29. Budassi, SB, Marvin, JA, and Jimmerson, CL: Manual of Clinical Trauma Care: The First Hour. CV Mosby, St Louis, 1989, p 295.
30. Hammond, JS and Ward, CG: Complications of the burn injury. Crit Care Clin 1:175, 1987.
31. Budassi, S and Barber, J: Mosby's Manual of Emergency Care: Practices and Procedures, ed 2. CV Mosby, St Louis, 1984, p 533.
32. McManus, p 162.
33. Bunkis and Walton, p 386.
34. McManus, p 161.
35. American College of Surgeons Committee on Trauma, p 159.
36. Ibid, p 159.
37. Emergency Nurse's Reference Library, p 667.
38. American College of Surgeons Committee on Trauma, p 158.
39. Bayley and Smith, p 38.
40. McManus, p 159.
41. Ibid, p 160.
42. Committee on Infectious Diseases, American Academy of Pediatrics: Repair of the Committee on Infectious Diseases, ed 21. American Academy of Pediatrics, Elk Grove Village, 1988, pp 411–412.
43. STAT Flight Manual: STAT (Specialized Transport and Treatment) Center for Emergency Medicine of Western PA, 1984. Revised 1988.

BIBLIOGRAPHY

Cloutier, L and Dziekan, F: Burns. In Cosgriff, J and Anderson, D: The Practice of Emergency Care, ed 2. JB Lippincott, Philadelphia, 1984.
Fonger, L: Emergency! First aid for burns. Nursing 82, 9:69, 1982.
Groves, M: Burns. In Strange, J: Shock-Trauma Care Plans. Springhouse Corp, Springhouse, PA, 1987.
Hayter, J: Emergency nursing care of the burned patient. Nurs Clin North Am 13:223, 1978.
Jacobs, L and Bennett, B: Emergency Patient Care: Prehospital Ground and Air Procedures. MacMillan, New York, 1983.
Jacoby, F: Nursing Care of the Patient with Burns, ed 2. CV Mosby, St Louis, 1976.
Mikhail, JN: Acute burn care: An update. J Emerg Nurs 14:9, 1988.

Chapter 20

PATRICIA SMITH-REGOJO

CARE OF THE BURN PATIENT IN THE OPERATING ROOM

Excision and skin grafting are required for the survival of the burned patient if he or she has a full-thickness burn or infected partial-thickness burn. Proper debridement and wound coverage become necessary for decreasing the chance of infection, promoting rehabilitation, shortening the hospital stay, and returning the patient to society. Frequent surgical interventions in a short period of time are a common sequela for the patient with a burn injury. Reconstructive surgery for the purpose of restoring function and aesthetics is also of great importance for the patient in the rehabilitative phase of burn care.

The operating room nurse is a valuable member of the burn team and must possess the skill and knowledge of working with a highly technical and precise team. Therefore, the nurse who cares for the burned patient must be able to identify the risks involved, recognize potential threats to safety, and take proper interventions to alleviate danger and promote life during the entire operative procedure.

PREPARING THE PATIENT FOR SURGERY

Success of the operative procedure depends on the readiness of the patient. Preoperative teaching by the nurse caring for the patient or the nurse from the operating room helps lessen the anxiety the patient may experience from fear and lack of knowledge. Subjects in the teaching plan include, but are not limited to, reasons for surgery; definition of the type of surgery such as wound debridement, skin grafting, contracture release, or reconstructive work; preparation for surgery; expectations upon arrival to the operating room and recovery room; and postoperative regimens. Also included are respiratory exercises with return demonstration, circulatory exercises while immobilized, and comfort measures. The nurse must remember to guide the explanations according to appropriateness for the age and condition of the patient. Pictures, pamph-

381

lets, and tours of the operating room are means of teaching and preparing the patient and or family. Since many burn patients require frequent operating room visits, reinforcement of what has been taught is necessary for each procedure. Instruction must meet the patient's needs and level of understanding. Documentation of preoperative teaching should be included in the nursing record.

CHOICE OF ANESTHESIA

Anesthesia preparedness and selection is another vital aspect of care for the burn patient going to surgery. Since burns do not discriminate in their location, they can pose unique problems for the anesthesiologist and the burn team. Prior to surgery a complete assessment of the patient's medical and surgical history and physical examination by the anesthesiologist or nurse anesthetist are necessary so that the management of anesthesia will be safe and efficient. Certain key factors determine the choice of anesthesia particular to the burn patient.

Location and Size of Burn Injury

During the first phase of burn care, edema of the face, lips, tongue, oropharynx, and larynx threaten proper airway maintenance and make intubation particularly difficult. In the acute phase, scar tissue in the respiratory tract and contraction formation in the mouth and neck region will again challenge airway maintenance during surgery. A precautionary plan of anesthesia is important. Frequently, the use of the fiberoptic bronchoscope is used for intubation purposes.

Use of Fiberoptic Bronchoscopy for Intubation

As soon as the patient arrives in the operating room and is placed on the table, proper monitoring equipment is secured to the patient including the ECG leads for cardiac monitoring, blood pressure cuff for continuous pressure readings, pulse oximeter to reflect oxygen saturation, temperature probe, and stethoscope. All equipment, including the fiberoptic bronchoscope and ventilator, are checked for safety and function prior to the patient's entry.

Generally, a small dose of sedation is administered to the patient to help relieve anxiety. During the entire procedure, explanations are given to the patient for reassurance and understanding.

The nasal passage is preferred for better security and maintenance of the endotracheal tube during the operative procedure, but there are times the oral route must be used secondary to extensive damage or difficulty passing the endotracheal tube. After sedation takes place, the proper-sized endotracheal tube is placed over the fiberoptic bronchoscope tube. The lighted fiberoptic bronchoscope is passed through the upper airway. To reduce coughing and gagging, the epiglottis and vocal cords are sprayed with a topical anesthetic. Afterwards, the endotracheal tube is slipped off the fiberoptic bronchoscope tube into the visualized trachea and advanced as necessary. To confirm placement of the endotracheal tube, the anesthesiologist will auscultate for spontaneous respirations. The fiberoptic bronchoscope is removed and the patient is attached to the ventilator after the endotracheal tube is secure in place. The patient is now ready to be induced with general anesthesia.

Condition and Age of the Burn Patient

Burns can inflict at any time and to any person. The condition and the age of the patient will determine the choice of anesthesia, fluid resuscitation needs, and length of the procedure. The pulmonary or cardiac status of an elderly burn patient may not withstand the length of the procedure or the fluids required for the procedure. Various other factors are also considered. Is the burn patient already intubated and maintained on high peak pressures? Is the operating room equipped to maintain as safe and efficient care as the intensive care unit (ICU)? Is emergency treatment readily available? Is there other trauma involved that may complicate the surgery? Is the resuscitative period over for the patient, and how well is the burn patient diuresing?

Type of Surgical Procedure and Technique Used

The type of surgery the burn patient will undergo and the particular technique used will determine the length of the procedure, estimated amount of blood loss, fluid replacement, and recovery period. The location of the surgery will determine the position of the patient, such as prone or supine, resulting in special arrangements for anesthesia induction and maintenance. It is crucial for the surgical team to map out what will be done prior to surgery so that the anesthesiologist can be well prepared and surprises kept to a minimum. Communication is vital at this time.

Current Medications

The nurse determines what narcotics, sedatives, and tranquilizers the patient has been receiving. The patient's last dose will determine the need for preoperative sedation. Since most acute care burn patients are receiving some sort of narcotizing agent around the clock, preoperative medication is not needed, but proper documentation will alert the anesthesiologist to the need for any supplemental doses.

The anesthesiologist will also determine if the patient should receive his or her current maintenance medication either with small sips of water at a scheduled time or intravenously prior to surgery.

Often the patient will receive additional doses of antibiotics preoperatively or intraoperatively as ordered by the surgeon. Some medications potentiate the effects of anesthesia. The medication administration record must accompany the burn patient to the operating room so that the burn team will be aware of all medications administered.

PREPARATION OF THE OPERATING ROOM

The operating room must be completely prepared before the patient arrives. This will enable the circulating nurse to accompany the patient or greet the patient and to remain with the patient until the procedure commences.

A good rapport with the surgical team is vital for facilitating the flow of the procedure. Preparedness is the key. Special attention to room arrangement plays an important factor for the burn patient. The operating room nurses or a separate team should be educated in all aspects of burn care so there is complete understanding of the physiologic and psychologic changes the patient experiences.

The surgical suite should be equipped to accommodate the needs of the burn patient. Many operating rooms have special burn carts for dressing supplies, irrigating set-ups, and instruments that can be wheeled to various suites. Other hospitals have specialized burn operating rooms where all the equipment is housed in one place and not removed except for cleaning.

Lighting in the operating room must be bright, without casting shadows. An efficient lighting apparatus enables the team to visualize the depth of the wound and adjust the light when necessary under sterile conditions.

One of the most essential components of room preparation is temperature control. Since the nature of the burn injury facilitates hypothermia, the operating room temperature should be no less than 76°F. The higher temperature can make it uncomfortable for the surgical team but is necessary for the safety and ability of the patient.

The operating room nurse is responsible for maintaining the patient's temperature. A warming blanket is placed on the operating table since much of the patient is exposed during the procedure. The rest of the patient's body is covered with warmed sterile blankets. Heat lamps (portable or mounted in the ceiling) are used for extra warmth. All fluids that will come in contact with the patient are warmed including prep solutions and irrigating solutions. Blood and intravenous (IV) fluids are administered through blood warmers. Traffic in and out of the operating room is kept to a minimum to keep drafts away from the patient. Doors are kept closed at all times.

When the procedure consists of double teaming, arrangement of the workspace for the entire surgical team is designed carefully. Double teaming is often performed for patients with a large burn injury. One team excises and prepares the burn wound for skin grafting while the other team procures the skin from a donor site. The number of trips to the operating room and the length of time under general anesthesia is reduced with double teaming. The operating room nurse is directly accountable for coordinating both surgical teams and simultaneously meeting the patient's needs.

TRANSPORTING THE BURN PATIENT TO THE OPERATING ROOM

Burn patients vary in their capacity for enduring a trip to the operating room. Intensive care patients can be so critical that a ride through a hallway or in an elevator could be lethal. Most patients are transported to the operating room in the usual manner as any other surgical patient. But a critically ill burn patient might require a trial period of manual respiration for 10 minutes with the Ambu bag to see if he or she can sustain that amount of time off a ventilator to be transported to the operating room. Some health care workers question this procedure and the scheduling of surgery at such a critical time, but the surgery itself will be an attempt to save the patient's life and is crucial for survival.

At the time of transport the preoperative checklist will be completed and the patient will be ready so that there are no delays. A patient who is quite stable can easily be transported to surgery via a stretcher with the assistance of the operating room transportation aid. A nurse does not need to accompany the patient. On the other hand, a critical burn patient will need the help of many. The patient might have to be transferred in his or her own bed. At least five people will be needed to push the bed with all the added equipment. The nurse taking care of the patient and the nurse from the operating room will be in charge of facilitating the movement and monitoring all hemodynamics. One person, preferably the anesthesiologist or respiratory technician, will be in charge of bagging and monitoring the respiratory status of the patient. The surgeon or someone else from the medical team will be on transport to assist with monitoring the patient, in addition to other ancillary help, to enable a quick and stable ride. Emergency drugs and all monitoring equipment should be visible and easily accessible during transport. All burn patients regardless of stability are covered with extra warm blankets to keep their body temperature within safe limits. Any splints needed for the operative area will also accompany the patient to the operating room.

OPERATIVE PROCEDURES

Wound Excision

The practice of early excision and skin grafting is becoming more popular. Multiple studies have shown that early excision and grafting reduces both the length of hospitalization and the cost, lessens the amount of pain and anguish the patient experiences, decreases the amount of infections and complications, speeds recovery, and returns the patient to a functional capacity in a shorter period of time. Today, small percent burns —less than 5 percent—can be excised and skin grafted in one-day surgery centers.

Two types of wound excision are performed, depending on the type of wound and the amount of burn to be excised. They are tangential excision and fascial excision. Tangenital excision sequentially shaves the wound until a viable bleeding bed has been reached. There is much blood loss with tangenital excision. Fascial excision requires removing the wound all the way to the subcutaneous tissue and fat, and is used for full-thickness injuries such as contact burns, electrical injuries, and prolonged chemical burns. Advantages and disadvantages of both procedures are listed in Table 20–1.

Skin Grafting and Donor Sites

Skin grafting is the process of taking unburned skin from one area of the body and placing it over the excised burn wound. Skin grafting promotes healing and reduces the size of the wound, which in turn decreases the hypermetabolic demands that are put on the body after a burn injury. When the skin is taken directly from the patient the procedure is called autografting. Autografting is the most optimal form of skin grafting because the patient is using his/her own skin. For many patients the selection of the donor site is as crucial as the burn wound itself. For others, there is no choice of selection because of the extent of the injury and threat to life.

Donor sites for autografting are selected on the basis of priority with regard to the amount of skin needed, availability, and cosmetic results. For example, a patient with a

TABLE 20–1. Burn Wound Debridement—Tangential Versus Fascial Excision

Advantages	Disadvantages
Tangential Excision (Sequential)	
Less cosmetic defects	Greater blood loss
Need for less operating room time	Need experienced surgical team
	Risk graft "take" because of questionable dermal bed
	Might lead to fascial excision
Fascial Excision	
Less blood loss with more control	Greater cosmetic defect
Graft bed more reliable	Need for longer operating room time
Less experience needed	Difficult graft "take" over joints
Used for large life-threatening burns	Possible loss or damage to tendons, ligaments, or superficial nerves

small burn on the abdomen will have a donor site next to the wound to keep the injury in the same proximity since donor sites have the ability to scar. Yet, a person with a large percent of his/her body surface area injured might only possess the scalp for a donor site. Donor sites can be used again but each "take" is thinner. Each site requires 7 to 14 days for healing.

If possible, donor sites should be mapped out prior to surgery so that the entire surgical team will be aware of the preparations needed for positioning the patient and excising the wounds. A donor site prep will be ordered the evening before surgery or the day of surgery. The area is scrubbed with povidone-iodine (Betadine), shaved, and wrapped in a sterile towel. There is still controversy as to whether to shave an area hours before surgery because of the chance of opening the skin to wound infections.

The type of skin graft obtained is also based on priority of need, availability, and cosmetic result. Larger burns are grafted with meshed skin that takes the shape of a lattice window. The meshing allows the surgeons to cover a large-area burn wound with a small piece of skin by stretching it and securing it in place with sutures or staples. The surgeon will procure the skin from the donor site by using an instrument called a dermatome (Fig. 20–1). Dermatomes can be operated manually or electrically. There are different sizes of dermatomes for specific grafting purposes. The skin is shaved in various widths and thickness from the donor site (Fig. 20–2). It is the responsibility of the scrub nurse to mesh the skin that has been harvested. The graft is placed on plastic carriers with the epidermis side up. The scrub nurse must have a full understanding of the workings of the mesher and be able to complete the work quickly and accurately. The carrier is rolled through the mesher while small holes are cut into the piece of skin (Fig. 20–3). The small holes form the lattice shaping and enable the graft to be stretched. Skin grafts can be meshed in different sizes to accommodate special needs such as size and location of the wound (Color Plate 46).

Grafts that are not meshed are called sheet grafts. Sheet grafts are used in areas where cosmetic defects and scarring are the main issues of healing. Faces, hands, upper chests, breasts, and small burns are grafted with sheet grafts. Sheet grafts are held in place with Steri-strips or small cosmetic sutures.

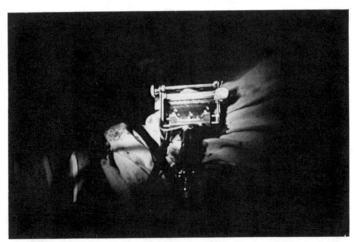

FIGURE 20–1. The electric dermatone is used to harvest skin for an autograft. (Photo courtesy of D. Hensell, St. Agnes Medical Center Burn Treatment Center, Philadelphia, PA.)

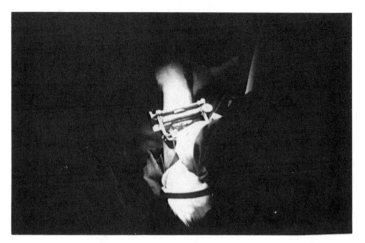

FIGURE 20-2. The electric dermatone is used to shave grafted skin in different widths and sizes. (Photo courtesy of D. Hensell, St. Agnes Medical Center Burn Treatment Center, Philadelphia, PA.)

Wound Coverage

It is vital to the success of the graft to keep the graft immobilized. After securing the grafts a bulky dressing is placed on the wound. Each burn unit differs in their approach to wound dressing. It is generally physician preference, but the nurse must be aware of the type of dressing used so that he or she will be completely prepared to dress the wound, especially if more than one burn surgeon practices in the center.

Not all wounds are grafted. Some might only be excised to rid the injury of bacteria containing eschar and to decrease the size of the wound. At this time there may be no or limited donor sites present to use. If autografting is unavailable, the surgeon can elect to use homograft (cadaver skin) or heterograft (pig skin). Varieties of biosynthetic dressings for wound coverage are becoming popular. Dressings are generally left in place over the graft 2 to 5 days postoperatively to ensure a good take.

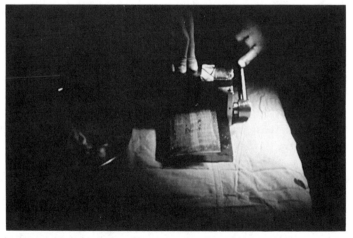

FIGURE 20-3. The graft is placed on a plastic carrier and rolled through the mesher by the scrub nurse. (Photo courtesy of D. Hensell, St. Agnes Medical Center Burn Treatment Center, Philadelphia, PA.)

TABLE 20-2. Coverage for Donor Sites

| Product | Special Considerations | |
	Advantages	Disadvantages
Scarlet Red	Easy to apply Cost-effective Long shelf-life Healing 7-14 days	Falls off easily unless stapled Can stain linen Becomes tight as it dries Need to expose to heat lamp to dry
Op-Site	Less painful Healing 7-14 days Easy to remove Easy to observe wound Long shelf-life Cost-effective	Need intact border to adhere Edges have tendency to roll; difficult to apply Fluid collects under dressing, leaks with ambulation if not aspirated
Biobrane	Less painful Healing 7-14 days Long shelf-life	Expensive Needs to be stapled or sutured with pressure dressing first 24 hours Collection of exudate under dressing Delayed wound separation
Xeroform	Similar to Scarlet Red Easy to apply Less expensive Long shelf-life	Becomes tight as it dries.

Donor sites are treated similarly to a partial-thickness wound and can be dressed in a number of ways. There are many products available for donor site coverage (Color Plate 47). The most common are listed in Table 20-2.

NURSING ASSESSMENT

Upon arrival in the operating room, the nurse must quickly assess and prepare the patient for surgery. A head-to-toe assessment is necessary for obtaining pertinent baseline information before the start of the procedure. It is imperative that the nursing preoperative checklist is completed and signed prior to transport. When the patient enters the operating room area the following tasks must be performed: the nurse verifies patient identification by comparing the medical record number on the chart with the identification band of the patient, and if possible, asks the patient if the name is correct. The chart is examined for an operative permit and blood consent. Since burn patients can have multiple surgeries, it is important to have the correct permit available and signed by the appropriate people. The chart is also examined for the history and physical, noting allergies, past surgeries, and any medical problems.

Neurologic System

The patient's response to stimulus, pupil reactions, awareness, communication, and orientation is documented. The patient's neurologic status will change drastically during the length of the surgical procedure secondary to the affects of anesthesia and possible hypothermia. It is important to have pertinent baseline information before starting the surgical procedure.

Cardiovascular System

Recorded preoperative vital signs are noted and the anesthesiologist is assisted in obtaining a set of vital signs prior to anesthesia. This can be done while the patient is initially placed on all the monitoring equipment. The latest blood work for hemoglobin, hematocrit, clotting studies, and electrolytes is evaluated. It is verified that blood is available in the operating room and the blood is checked (including comparison of donor number, patient identification number, blood type, and expiration date), and is made ready to be hung. Because of excessive bleeding during wound debridement at least two or more units of packed red blood cells are available.

Intravenous fluids are documented including the amount and type. If no intravenous line is present, areas of access are noted. A large-gauge catheter is used for fluid and blood administration so that there is no chance of dislodging the IV line after the patient is placed in the operative position. Peripheral pulses are palpated or a Doppler device is used if necessary. Multiple dressings and excessive edema make it difficult to assess the burn patient for proper circulation. All nail polish is removed, if this has not been done already, in order to have an access to assess for capillary refill and tissue perfusion. Additional dressings are also removed. The ECG is evaluated and any dysrhythmias are documented prior to surgery.

Respiratory System

The lungs are auscultated for adventitious sounds, and the latest chest x-ray and arterial blood gases (ABGS) are evaluated if indicated. Physician orders for oxygen therapy and/or ventilator settings are verified. Patients are assessed for edema or obstruction secondary to an inhalation injury, circumferential burn, or excessive hypertrophic scarring that will make oxygenation and intubation difficult. If present the fiberoptic bronchoscope is made available for intubation. The nurse assesses for the presence of excessive secretions due to inhalation injury and/or pulmonary edema. Suction equipment is maintained for proper function and accessibility. Color, amount, and consistency of secretions are assessed and documented.

Gastrointestinal System

The burn patient should have nothing by mouth (NPO) at least 6 to 8 hours prior to surgery, to prevent vomiting and aspiration of stomach contents. If a nasogastric tube is present, the anesthesiologist is consulted as to whether it should be placed to suction. The abdomen is inspected and auscultated for bowel sounds. Bowel sounds might be absent due to an paralytic ileus, which is common in burns grater than 20 percent total body surface area (TBSA).

Genitourinary System

Intake and output (I&O) 24 hours preoperatively is assessed to establish information regarding fluid balance. The nurse also checks the time the patient last voided. A Foley catheter is inserted, if ordered, and may be accomplished after the patient is under anesthesia, to avoid undue anxiety and discomfort for the patient. For an accurate output record, the Foley bag should be emptied prior to the procedure. It is verified that the Foley catheter can drain adequately after the patient is placed in the operative position.

Muscular/Skeletal System

The patient is assessed and the chart reviewed for any injuries prior to placing the patient in the operative position. Fractures are aligned and immobilized according to physician orders. The nurse considers the approximate length of the procedure, making sure alignment will not cause any neurovascular compromise. Areas of excessive pressure are padded. Patient movement prior to anesthesia is noted. Also the nurse checks splinted areas for pressure points and protects these points accordingly.

Integumentary System

The nurse reviews the physician orders for preparing the donor site prior to surgery. Since removing dressings and preparing the operative areas are painful and uncomfortable procedures for the patient, the nurse waits until the anesthesiologist has anesthetized the patient to perform those duties. Old dressings are removed and discarded since they are considered contaminants. Only the dressings from the areas to be operated on are removed to prevent exposure and spread of infection.

Psychologic/Social Considerations

Patients are assessed for their knowledge of the operation. The chart is consulted for documentation of preoperative teaching. All procedures are explained and all questions answered to help decrease anxiety that will make induction of anesthesia difficult. The patient is never left alone. It is validated that the family members have a place to stay and that updates will be communicated to them during and after the procedure.

REPORTING TO THE RECOVERY ROOM

The operating room nurse has been with the patient from the beginning of surgery to the end. He or she has had the ability to observe the procedure from the surgical and anesthesiology aspects and can report significant information to the recovery nurse.

Patients who can easily be reversed and extubated in the operating room or are stable enough will go directly to the recovery room. Critical patients and those requiring extensive respiratory care will return to the intensive care unit (ICU). Regardless of where the patient goes, recovery is the same, except the anesthesiologist may elect not to reverse the critical care patient immediately after surgery.

Toward the end of the surgical procedure the nurse calls the recovery room or ICU to let the other nurses know the approximate time of arrival and any equipment they will need to care for the patient. A quick status report can be given if the operating room nurse has the time. Otherwise, a full report can be given upon arrival to the designated area.

The anesthesiologist usually reports the respiratory care of the patient during surgery including additional sedation preoperatively and intraoperatively: anesthetizing procedure, fluid therapy, and blood loss or replacement. Depending on the institution, the surgeon or the anesthesiologist will determine what type of ventilator settings and respiratory care the patient will require postoperatively. Significant data that the operating room nurse will report include; the type and location of the procedure performed; length of the procedure; status of the patient during and after the procedure; medications given preoperatively, intraoperatively, and postoperatively; complications; and specific instructions regarding dressings, splints, and positioning.

The operating room nurse must be fully prepared to care for the "specialty" patient who is undergoing a surgical procedure. The burn patient is no exception. Patients with a burn injury pose exceptional problems in the operating room. Quick and accurate assessment skills of the professional nurse will identify the risks involved and maintain the safety of a burn patient. In addition, interventions can be implemented to promote stability and lessen the chance of surgical complications.

NURSING CARE PLAN: CARE OF THE BURN PATIENT IN THE OPERATING ROOM

Nursing Priorities

1. Maintain patent airway and adequate ventilation.
2. Maintain hemodynamic stability.
3. Prevent hypothermia.
4. Minimize and control bacterial contamination.
5. Maintain holistic approach in meeting psychosocial needs of patient and significant others.

Nursing Diagnosis: Breathing Pattern, Ineffective

May Be Related To:

- Hypertrophic scarring causing stricture formation
- Respiratory depression secondary to the use of narcotics or antibiotics along with anesthetic agents

Possibly Evidenced By: Difficult intubation, hoarseness, stridor, wheezing, cyanosis, cough, and circumferential chest burns (altered chest excursion).

Desired Patient Outcomes: Patient will experience a patient airway; an effective breathing pattern will be maintained.

Interventions	Rationale
INDEPENDENT	
• Assess and record breath sounds preoperatively: review patient record for respiratory status.	• Baseline information is necessary to recognize deviations.
• Maintain a current knowledge base regarding the anesthetic agents used including preoperative medications, induction, and reversal therapy.	• Knowledge of the anesthetic agents will enable the nurse to be prepared for untoward reactions and necessary interventions (Table 20–3).
• Be able to recognize the different stages of anesthesia.	• Knowledge of the different stages will enable the practitioner to know when it is safe for the surgical procedure to be performed, when danger is imminent, and what interventions are necessary for treatment (Table 20–4).

TABLE 20-3. Common Anesthetic Agents
Used With Burn Patients

Medication	Classification	Usage	Adverse Actions
Nitrous oxide	Inhalation anesthetic	Produces analgesia; used as a vehicle for other anesthetics; reduces amount of inhalation anesthetic used	Cardiac depression
Isoflurane	Inhalation anesthetic	Nonirritating to the respiratory tract; muscle relaxant	Strong odor, cardiac depression
Enflurane (Ethrane)	Inhalation anesthetic	Same as isoflurane; bronchodilation	Cardiac depression, hypotension, coughing/ laryngospasm
Halothane	Inhalation anesthetic	Nonpotent, nonirritating to the respiratory tract; bronchodilation; decreases postoperative nausea and vomiting, no need to use high concentration	Cardiac depression, hypotension, shivering
Fentanyl (Sublimaze)	Narcotic analgesic	Pain control; decreases surgical stress in lengthy procedures	Muscle rigidity, hypotension, Bradycardia, apnea/ respiratory depression, nausea/vomiting
Morphine	Narcotic analgesic	Decreases pain perception; sedation; aids in induction and maintenance of anesthesia	Same as sublimaze
Midazolium (Versed)	Neuroleptic/sedative	Produces sleep, amnesia or anesthesia, onset of anesthesia slow with use	Respiratory/cardiac depression
Diazepam (Valium)	Neuroleptic/sedative	Produces sleep, amnesia, or anesthsia	Respiratory/cardiac depression
Droperidol (Inapsine)	Neuroleptic/sedative	Maintains general anesthesia; decreases anxiety and pain	Hypotension, tachycardia
Ketamine (Ketalar)	Nonbarbiturate anesthetic	Used alone or a supplement to other agents; aids in induction	Tachycardia, hypertension, laryngospasm, respiratory depression, hallucinations, delusions
Pancuronium (Pavulon)	Nondepolarizing muscle relaxant	Neuromuscular blocker, induces skeletal muscle relaxation for intubation	Tachycardia, increased salivation

**TABLE 20-3. Common Anesthetic Agents
Used With Burn Patients (Continued)**

Medication	Classification	Usage	Adverse Actions
Vercuronium (Norcuron)	Nondepolarizing muscle relaxant	Same as pancuronium; short duration in low doses; has less cumulative effect and cardiovascular side effects; easily reversed when discontinued	Duration short
Atracurium (Tracrium)	Nondepolarizing muscle relaxant	Same as pancuronium	Release of histamine causes flushing and hypotension; bronchospasm

TABLE 20-4. Stages of Anesthesia

Stage I—Analgesia   Procedure
  Disorientation
  Muscle relaxation   Intubation
  Diminished gag reflex
Stage II—Excitement
  Loss of consciousness
  Delirium
  Increased reflexes
  Rapid eye movement
  Rhythmic respirations
Stage III—Surgical Anesthesia
  Plane 1   Rhythmic respirations
  Plane 2   Cessation of eye movement
            Fixed pupils
            Depressed ocular reflex
            Depression of skeletal muscle tone   Surgery performed
  Plane 3   Irregular, diaphragmatic respirations
            Complete relaxation of skeletal muscles   Ventilator dependent
            Respiratory muscle paresis
  Plane 4   Respiratory and involuntary muscle paresis
            All reflexes absent
Stage IV—Medullary Paralysis
  Apnea—no spontaneous respirations
  Cardiovascular collapse

Nursing Diagnosis: Breathing Pattern, Ineffective (*Continued*)

Interventions	Rationale
• Inspect finger and toes for capillary refill throughout surgery.	• Assessment for capillary refill is a quick way to determine tissue perfusion.

COLLABORATIVE

Interventions	Rationale
• Position patient so that the anesthesiologist will have complete access for respiratory interventions.	• Some surgical procedures require awkward positioning of the patient. The anesthesiologist must have access to the patient's respiratory system at all times throughout surgery.
• Maintain emergency equipment.	• Prevents delays in treatment if complications arise.
• Keep patient calm; explain all procedures step by step.	• Providing support to lessen fears and anxiety will facilitate a smooth induction and decrease the chance of complications secondary to laryngospasm.
• Maintain the operating room quiet and free of disturbances.	• Environmental disturbances can cause untoward effects (i.e., hallucinations and excitability) with some anesthetic agents during induction.

Nursing Diagnosis: Impaired Gas Exchange

May Be Related To:

- Airway deviation or obstruction
- Accumulated pulmonary secretions
- Aspiration of gastrointestinal contents secondary to vomiting

Possibly Evidenced By: Wheezing, stridor, coughing, rales, rhonchi, altered arterial blood gases, cyanosis, and vomiting.

Desired Patient Outcomes: Patient oxygenation will be maintained.

Interventions	Rationale
INDEPENDENT	
• Assess and record breath sounds preoperatively; review patient record for respiratory status.	• Baseline information is necessary to recognize deviations.
• Inspect fingers and toes for capillary refill throughout surgery.	• Assessment for capillary refill is a quick way to determine tissue perfusion.
• Maintain suction equipment and emergency equipment.	• Prevents delays in treatment if complications arise.

Intervention	Rationale
• Take measures to decrease the chance of hypothermia (refer to Hypothermia. Potential for, page 396).	• Hypothermia will increase oxygen consumption.
• Verify that patient is NPO. If a nasogastric tube is present, maintain its patency and proper function.	• Keeping the patient NPO reduces the risk of vomiting and aspiration. A properly functioning nasogastric tube will help decompress the stomach and reduce the risk of vomiting.

COLLABORATIVE

• Monitor oxygen saturation by use of oximeter or transcutaneous monitoring.	• Provides continuous feedback regarding oxygen saturation so that necessary changes can be made quickly.
• Monitor blood gases. Provide that there is no delay in transporting bloodwork to the laboratory or obtaining results. Notify the physician immediately of the results.	• Arterial blood gases are a tool for evaluating acid/base balance and oxygenation. Results should remain at patient's normal range; if not, treatment should be initiated immediately.
• Suction as necessary.	• Suctioning frees secretions and maintains a patent airway.

Nursing Diagnosis: Tissue Perfusion, Alteration In

May Be Related To:

- Trauma to blood vessels secondary to surgical debridement
- Excessive blood/fluid loss through burn wounds
- Anesthesia
- Edema formation

Possibly Evidenced By: Skin cool, pale and clammy; increased heart rate; diminished or absent peripheral pulses; decreased urine output; increasing respiratory rate; bleeding; decreased blood pressure

Desired Patient Outcomes: Patient will be hemodynamically stable throughout the surgical procedure. Vital signs will remain within the preoperative baseline range. Optimal tissue perfusion is maintained.

Interventions	Rationale
INDEPENDENT	
• Place patient on a cardiac monitor.	• Information will be utilized as a baseline throughout surgery.
• Assess and record vital signs and urine output prior to surgical procedures.	• Treatment measures can be initiated for critical deviations.

Nursing Diagnosis: Tissue Perfusion, Alteration In (*Continued*)

Interventions	Rationale
• Maintain readily available blood or intravenous fluids. Check blood products prior to surgery and note that there are at least two units of packed red blood cells available and in the operating room.	• Prevents delays in blood/fluid replacement. Viable bleeding tissue is a parameter used by the surgeons during debridement of a burn wound to determine depth of excision.
• Notify physician if hemoglobin is less than 10 and hematocrit is less than 30 prior to surgery. Infuse blood products as prescribed.	• Blood loss is common during wound debridement. A transfusion might be necessary before starting the surgical procedure.
• Secure an access for an intravenous line. Maintain an intravenous line no smaller than an 18- to 20-gauge needle.	• Manipulation of the line may cause dislodgement or infiltration causing a delay in fluid replacement. Blood products need to be infused via a large-bore catheter.
• Keep an accurate account of the patient's intake and output.	• Accurate intake and output is necessary for proper assessment of fluid therapy. A balanced intake and output is necessary for cardiovascular stability.
• Maintain an accurate sponge count before, during, and after the surgical procedure.	• An accurate sponge count will give approximate information regarding blood and fluid loss.

COLLABORATIVE

• Check blood and blood products prior to starting the procedure.	• Prevents delays in blood replacement after the procedure has begun.
• Keep the operating room quiet and free of distractions.	• To facilitate communication between physician and anesthesiologist regarding vital signs, fluid therapy, and other pertinent information.
• Secure an area for continuous monitoring of blood pressure.	• Deviations will be recognized quickly and emergency interventions can be initiated. Anesthesia can cause fluctuations in blood pressure as can large amounts of fluid or blood loss.
• Monitor blood studies and notify physician of abnormalities.	• Electrolyte imbalance will cause cardiovascular instability.

Nursing Diagnosis: Hypothermia/ Potential For

May Be Related To:

• Inability to regulate heat loss secondary to the burn wound	• Prolonged exposure during surgical procedure
• Circulatory impairment	

Possibly Evidenced By: Decrease in body temperature; poor capillary refill; decreased pulse; cool skin

Desired Patient Outcomes: Temperature of patient will remain no less than 96.8°F throughout the surgical procedure. Patient will remain hemodynamically stable.

Interventions	Rationale

INDEPENDENT

Assess patient record. Obtain temperature prior to anesthesia and throughout the procedure. Use a temperature probe for continuous temperature monitoring.
- Maintain room temperature no less than 76°F. Keep the flow of traffic in and out of the operative suite at a minimum.
- Cover patient with warm sterile blankets. Use sterile drapes that are plastic or paper.

- A baseline temperature is essential for determining any deviations throughout the procedure. Measures can be initiated for critical changes at any time.
- A warm room will lessen the chance of chilling and air flow around the patient.

- Maintains patient's warmth and reduces evaporative and conductive heat losses.

COLLABORATIVE

- Warm fluids prior to infusion. Warm inspired gases. Use overhead heat shields or warmers. Prepare operative sites with warm solutions. Place patient on a warming blanket upon arrival to the operating room.

- Reduces heat loss, keeps patient warm, and maintains body temperature greater than 96.8°F. Keeping the patient warm will lessen the effects of a depressed metabolic rate caused by anesthesia.

Nursing Diagnosis: Infection, Potential For

May Be Related To:

- Exposure of burn wound to contaminants
- Surgical incision
- Wound debridement with bacterial showering
- General anesthesia with intubation and suctioning
- Increased resistance to infection with frequent antibiotic use

Desired Patient Outcomes: During the operative procedure, the patient will be protected from infection and physiologic stability will be maintained. There will be no signs of infection postoperatively. Grafted areas will have 100 percent take.

Interventions	Rationale

INDEPENDENT

- Maintain sterile operative environment at all times. Take action at once to eliminate any breaks in sterile field.

- Contaminated operative fields are a risk to any surgical patient.

Nursing Diagnosis: Infection, Potential For (*Continued*)

Interventions

- Assess patient's record for documentation of active infection. Communicate information to surgical team.
- Prepare burn wound for surgery, inspect patient's chart for preoperative wound preparation.
- Wound preparation is best accomplished in the operating room after anesthesia is achieved.

- After removing old dressings and preparing the wound, clean the work area by mopping and drying the floor prior to set up of new sterile field. Use new dry sterile sheets around and under patient.
- Prepare donor site for surgery as ordered: Wash area with sterile cleansing agent and shave. If scalp is to be used, save hair for patient.
- Assess burn wound: Observe the color of the tissue bed, color of drainage and any odor from the wound. Note if the perimeter of the wound is red, edematous, warm, or hard. Notify physician of findings prior to surgery.

COLLABORATIVE

- Minimize interruptions and flow of traffic in the operating room. Keep doors closed at all times.

- Maintain sterility of intubation and suction equipment. Provide numerous sterile suction catheters available for use with sterile gloves.

Rationale

- Active wound infection will cause graft loss and showering of bacteria during surgery.
- Scrubbing and shaving the wound several hours prior to surgery may increase the risk for infection.
- Preparing the wound after the onset of anesthesia will lessen the pain of the patient and reduce the risk of preoperative infection.
- Maintains sterility of area and reduces risk of infection.

- Sterile preparation of the donor site reduces the risk of infection.

- Permits early detection and treatment of infection.

- Cross-contamination by airborn organism can occur secondary to high incidence of air flow. Frequent interruption or distraction can lead to a break in sterility.
- Since burn patients are so susceptible to infection, sterile technique must be enforced to ensure no contamination of the pulmonary system.

Nursing Diagnosis: Anxiety

May Be Related To:

- Unpreparedness
- Fear of the unknown
- Fear of general anesthesia
- Inadequate preoperative medication

Possibly Evidenced By: Nervousness, increase pulse, increase blood pressure, increase respiratory rate, difficult intubation, limited attention span, and pallor.

Desired Patient Outcomes: Patient's anxiety level will be reduced. Patient remains able to follow instructions. There will be no problems with intubation. Anesthesia induction will be smooth and safe. The patient will have an uneventful surgical course. The patient's recovery will be stable. Untoward effects of anesthesia will be none or kept to a minimum.

Interventions

INDEPENDENT

- Be calm. Reassure patient. Maintain close attention to patient at all times.
- Assess patient's level of understanding and orientation. Explain all procedures in a way the patient will understand.

- Assess for signs of physiologic instability. Monitor oxygen saturation frequently.
- Observe effects of drugs, especially preoperative medications and anesthetic agents.

COLLABORATIVE

- Assist patient to concentrate on relaxing. Instruct patient to take slow deep breaths during induction of anesthesia.
- Prevent distractions.

Rationale

- A calm supportive atmosphere will help minimize fears the patient will have.
- Clear explanations and a chance to ask questions will aid in minimizing fears and provide the patient with a better understanding of what is to be expected.
- Hypoxia will cause restlessness and increase anxiety.

- Drug effects may be causing anxiety rather than alleviating it.

- Helping the patient to relax will help reduce the risk of hyperventilation and enable induction to take place.
- Distractions and frequent interruptions can cause more anxiety, making it difficult to anesthetize the patient. Some anesthetic agents can cause nightmares if the period of induction is noisy and disorganized.

Nursing Diagnosis: Knowledge Defect Regarding Surgical Procedure

May Be Related To:

- Unfamiliarity with procedure
- No prior surgical experience

Possibly Evidenced By: Verbalizations, inability to answer questions regarding surgery.

Desired Patient Outcomes: Patient verbalizes understanding of the procedure.

Nursing Diagnosis: Knowledge Defect Regarding Surgical Procedure (*Continued*)

Interventions	Rationale
INDEPENDENT	
• Provide age-appropriate preoperative teaching regarding preoperative and postoperative procedures and restrictions, deep breathing, and other appropriate exercises (for example, appearance of graft/donor sites; areas of discomfort; where patient will be postoperatively; special devices such as splints; mobility level postoperatively; length of procedure).	• Providing accurate information decreases anxiety. Practicing before surgery encourages adherence to deep breathing and exercises afterward.
• Determine information given to patient by physician.	• Allows the nurse to build upon that knowledge and base teaching plan on needs.
• Provide an environment conducive to learning.	• Allows patient to be attentive. Patient will be free to express fears or concerns.
• Provide written instructions for patient to refer to as necessary.	• Provides reinforcement of information verbally presented.

Nursing Diagnosis: Fluid Volume Deficit

(Refer to Chapter 9, page 165, for etiology, manifestations, desired patient outcomes, and interventions.)

Nursing Diagnosis: Skin Integrity, Impairment Of

(Refer to Chapter 4, page 64, for etiology, manifestations, desired patient outcomes, and interventions.)

Nursing Diagnosis: Airway Clearance, Ineffective

(Refer to Chapter 9, page 162, for etiology, manifestations, desired patient outcomes, and interventions.)

Nursing Diagnosis: Pain

(Refer to Chapter 9, page 169, for etiology, manifestations, desired patient outcomes, and interventions.)

Nursing Diagnosis: Powerlessness

(Refer to Chapter 7, page 96, for etiology, manifestations, desired patient outcomes, and interventions.)

Nursing Diagnosis: Fear

(Refer to Chapter 7, page 175, for etiology, manifestations, desired patient outcomes, and interventions.)

Nursing Diagnosis: Anxiety

(Refer to Chapter 7, page 98, for etiology, manifestations, desired patient outcomes, and interventions.)

BIBLIOGRAPHY

Ando, M and Ando, Y: Anesthetics in Grafting of Burn Injuries on Children. Bull Clin Rev Burn Injuries 1:56, 1984.
Boswick, J: The Art and Science of Burn Care. Aspen Publications, Rockville, MD, 1987.
Campbell, C: Nursing Diagnosis and Intervention in Nursing Practice, ed 2. John Wiley & Sons, New York, 1984.
Churchill-Davidson, HC: A Practice of Anesthesia, ed 5. Year Book Medical, Chicago, 1984.
Crane, H and Miner, D: Thermo-resuscitation for post-operative hypothermia using reflective blankets. AORN 47:222, 1988.
Larson , S and Parks, D: Managing the difficult airway in patients with burns of the head and neck. Journal of Burn Care and Rehabilitation 9(1):1988.
Lee, K, Weedman, D, and Peters, W: Use of fiberoptic bronchoscope to change endotracheal tubes in patients with burned airways. Journal of Burn Care and Rehabilitation 7(4):1986.
Norwicki, C and Sprenger, C: Temporary skin substitutes for burn patients. JBCR 9(2):1988.
Prasaad, J, Feller, I, and Thomson, P: A prospective controlled trail of biobrane versus scarlet red on skin graft donor areas. Journal of Burn Care and Rehabilitation 8(5):1987.
Sendack, M: Getting the patient to surgery and back 11. Common recovery room problems. Emerg Med Nov 30:117, 1986.
Wiener, M, et al: Clinical Pharmacology and Therapeutics in Nursing. McGraw-Hill, New York, 1979.

Chapter 21

PATRICIA SMITH-REGOJO

CARE OF THE BURN PATIENT IN THE RECOVERY ROOM

When surgery for the burn patient is nearing an end, the recovery period commences. The operating room nurse has already notified the recovery room as to the approximate time the surgery will be over, the status of the patient intraoperatively, and what special equipment will be necessary for the recovery period.

Patients who are stable and require minimal respiratory care go directly to the recovery room. Patients who require intensive care nursing and/or further respiratory care and intubation return directly to the burn intensive care unit. It is imperative that the patient recovers without any untoward reactions. He or she will most likely be returning to surgery in the near future.

A quick and uneventful recovery will lessen the chance of complication. The recovery room nurse must be able to identify potential problems that can lead to unnecessary complications, maintain safety and stability of the patient, and promote wellness for the postsurgical burn patient.

COMMON POSTOPERATIVE PROBLEMS

Complications can happen at any time during the course of surgery and afterward. The most common complications the burn patient will face after surgery are bleeding, respiratory insufficiency, sepsis, gastrointestinal problems, and pain. A thorough patient assessment with continuous monitoring will alert the burn team of impending problems.

Bleeding

Burn surgery will cause a significant amount of blood loss. Particular areas of importance are those of wound debridement, especially with tangential incisions and donor sites (Color Plate 48). Bleeding is controlled in surgery but there are times when a continuous ooze from operative areas occurs. If a pressure dressing does not work, the physician is notified immediately, especially if a patient has a bleeding disorder. There have been occasions when the patient must be brought back to the operating room to control the bleeding. Monitoring postoperative hemoglobin and hematocrit is imperative.

Respiratory Insufficiency

Frequent, often lengthy, surgeries under general anesthesia compromise a patient's respiratory system. Without aggressive respiratory care including deep-breathing exercises and mobilization of excessive secretions, atelectasis can occur. The threat of a pulmonary embolus is real with the frequency of immobilization secondary to prolonged bedrest.

Sepsis

Often the patient who shows no sign of sepsis preoperatively demonstrates septic episodes postoperatively. This is due to the overwhelming showering of bacteria from an infected wound during the debridement procedure. The patient's vital signs change drastically. The temperature climbs suddenly, then drops to the point of hypothermia. The patient's blood pressure sometimes falls below his or her normal range. Bowel sounds once present may disappear. Confusion and disorientation in subtle undertones are generally picked up by the nurse. Not able to pinpoint the problem, the nurse is nevertheless aware that something is not right with the patient as manifested by inappropriate verbal responses or actions. The effects of sepsis on the patient's hemodynamic status must be monitored very closely.

Gastrointestinal (GI) Complications

It is possible the patient's bowel sounds will be diminished or absent secondary to the effects of anesthesia. As the anesthesia wears off, however, bowel sounds should reappear. Frequent monitoring of the GI tract will alert the practitioner to changes. If tube feedings were used preoperatively they are restarted as soon as the bowel sounds return, checking every 2 hours for any residuals. Patients who have the ability to eat can be started with sips of water or ice chips and advanced to diet as tolerated, as long as there is no vomiting postoperatively. Vomiting is another effect of anesthesia that can lead to aspiration. Vomiting also results from the onset of an ileus which in turn can be an early sign of sepsis, or is an early complication of burn shock.

Pain

The majority of patients complain about the pain from their donor sites postoperatively rather than from the burn wounds themselves. Along with pain comes stiffness and muscle soreness after lengthy positioning in the operating room. Postoperative positioning and splint application will also add to the patient's discomfort. The nurse evaluates the patient's pain and need for medication; but, most important, the nurse must evaluate the effectiveness of the prescribed treatment. Postoperative pain might be the worst complication for the patient. Patients in pain cannot eat properly and will not want to cough and deep-breathe, turn, or position themselves, which can lead to many other complications if not monitored carefully. This is the time the nurse pulls all his or her resources together to give the needed comfort to the patient.

TRANSPORTING THE PATIENT TO THE RECOVERY ROOM

The surgery is over and it is time for the patient to recover quickly, completely, and without any complications. The operating room nurse, anesthesiologist, and surgeon accompany the patient to the recovery room or ICU.

Care must be taken when moving the patient from a stretcher to a bed. Areas of new graft are not to be manipulated so as to avoid graft dislodgement. If this happens the physician is notified immediately.

The patient is lifted completely clear of the mattress to prevent shearing of the graft, donor site, and other wounds. Donor site pain is the most common complaint of the postoperative burn patient. Any type of movement will aggravate that pain.

Once in the recovery room, a total assessment of the patient is performed. The anesthesiologist will notify the nurse as to what type of respiratory care (including ventilator setting) should be initiated. The surgeon will give information regarding wound care.

The nurse is responsible for monitoring the patient until recovery is achieved and the patient can safely be transported to his or her original room or the patient is completely reversed and vital signs are stable. Parameters for vital signs are listed in the Nursing Assessment section of this chapter, which follows.

NURSING ASSESSMENT

Because the patient has been placed in a drug-induced coma, maintaining a functioning airway and obtaining a set of vital signs are the first priority of the recovery room nurse. Additional priorities of the recovery room nurse are to minimize pain and promote comfort in the postoperative burn patient, and to prevent or minimize postoperative complications. It is the responsibility of the nurse to obtain a full report on the status of the patient including the type of anesthesia used before initiating any treatment. A thorough assessment must be performed quickly and accurately in order to maintain the safety and stability of the postsurgical burn patient and to promote a complete recovery.

Neurologic System

The nurse identifies the responsiveness of the patient. Has the anesthesia been reversed? Is the patient awake and moving the extremities? Can the patient follow commands? Do the pupils react to light? What is the pupil size and reaction time? If the anesthesiologist elects not to reverse the anesthesia but to let the patient awaken spontaneously, then it is important to note the time the patient begins to wake and move. It is common for the burn patient to be excited and disoriented in the recovery room. Neurologic checks are performed every 30 minutes for 1 hour, then every hour until the patient is completely recovered. Frequent orientation and reassurance are offered to the patient. If family members are allowed to visit, the patient's neurologic status and physical appearance are explained to them.

Cardiovascular System

The patient is attached to a cardiac monitor and a set of vital signs are obtained and communicated to the anesthesiologist before he or she leaves the patient. The heart rate and rhythm and the blood pressure are compared to the preoperative and intraoperative record, and any deviations noted. Vital signs, including temperature, respirations, pulse, and blood pressure, are monitored and recorded: every 15 minutes for the first hour; every 30 minutes for the next 2 hours; every hour for the following 4 hours, and as long as the patient is stable, every 4 hours unless otherwise noted. All additional hemodynamic monitoring are re-established as soon as possible including Swan Ganz lines, arterial lines, and other necessary continuous drips to stabilize the patient. Parameters for hemodynamic monitoring will be set by the anesthesiologist or surgeon. The patient is kept warm and the temperature is evaluated as soon as possible. Since postsurgical burn patients are usually hypothermic, it is important to have extra warm blankets or warming devices readily available.

The operative site is assessed for bleeding. A report is obtained on blood loss and fluid replacement from anesthesia. Intravenous sites are assessed. Intravenous fluids and or blood products are maintained in the recovery room for necessary administration. Postoperative laboratory studies are obtained as needed, especially hemoglobin, hematocrit, and electrolytes.

Respiratory System

The lungs are auscultated to determine if the patient has a clear airway and spontaneous respirations. All findings are documented. If the patient is intubated or to remain intubated; the endotracheal tube is inspected for size and location. The anesthesiologist will determine the proper ventilator settings for the patient. An arterial blood gas value is obtained after 20 minutes on the ventilator. Suction equipment is available at all times so that the patient can be suctioned whenever necessary. If the patient is to be extubated, a high-humidity oxygen mask is readily available.

Gastrointestinal System

The patient's bowel sounds are auscultated, remembering that bowel sounds may take a few hours to return postoperatively depending on the length of the procedure. Frequent inspection of the abdomen is necessary to determine bowel function, distention, or the onset of an ileus (common in postoperative burn patients). If a nasogastric tube or feeding tube is present, its position and patency is ensured. Antacid therapy is administered, if indicated.

Genitourinary System

Information is obtained regarding the patient's intake and output during surgery. Urine output is recorded every hour if the patient has a Foley catheter. If the patient has no Foley catheter, the time of the last void is verified. The color of urine is assessed and the specific gravity is recorded every 4 to 6 hours.

Musculoskeletal System

Any splinted areas are inspected for proper alignment and pressure points (Fig. 21–1). Identify how the patient can move and what areas need to be immobilized. The patient is positioned as prescribed, maintaining comfort as much as possible. Extremities are kept elevated and joints extended or abducted as ordered using extra pillows for support.

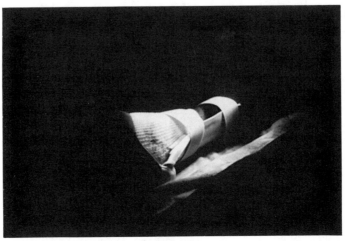

FIGURE 21-1. Splinted areas need to be inspected for pressure points and proper alignment. (Photo courtesy of D. Hensell, St. Agnes Medical Center Burn Treatment Center, Philadelphia, PA.)

Integumentary System

Donor sites must be inspected for excessive bleeding. Grafted areas are freed from pressure points and shearing due to movements across a bed. The use of a bed cradle will relieve added discomfort from heavy blankets. Other areas of the body are assessed for excessive pressure during the surgery. Proper positioning is very important.

Psychosocial Considerations

The patient is safeguarded, reassured, and oriented to time and place, as he or she might be confused or delerious. Medicate for pain as ordered. The charge nurse is notified on the patient's floor as soon as the patient has arrived in the recovery room and is stable. The floor nurse will keep the patient's family or significant other(s) informed of the patient's progress and condition. If the patient has returned to the intensive care unit (ICU), the nurse caring for the patient will inform the family of the patient's condition as soon as possible. The patient is kept informed of his or her own progress, the time sequence in the recovery room, and what to expect in the next few hours.

DISCHARGE FROM THE RECOVERY ROOM

Once the patient is fully awake and vital signs are stable, the anesthesiologist will determine if the patient is ready to be discharged from the recovery room. A full report will be called to the floor nurse taking care of the patient. The report should include the type of surgery performed, the status of the patient during surgery and immediately postoperatively, and any complications experienced. Fluid and/or blood therapy and medication administration should also be reported to the nurse.

NURSING CARE PLAN: CARE OF THE BURN PATIENT IN THE RECOVERY ROOM

Nursing Priorities

1. Maintain patent airway.
2. Maintain hemodynamic stability.
3. Prevent trauma to wounds and operative sites.
4. Prevent hypothermia.
5. Minimize pain and discomfort.
6. Maintain holistic approach in meeting psychosocial needs of patient and significant others.

Nursing Diagnosis: Gas Exchange, Impaired

May Be Related To:

- Obstructed airway
- Increased secretions
- Hypothermia
- Hypotension
- Decreased cardiac output

Possibly Evidenced By: Confusion, restlessness, irritability, hypoxia, inability to move secretions, cyanosis, dyspnea, and tachycardia.

Desired Patient Outcomes: Patient will demonstrate improved ventilation and adequate oxygenation demonstrated by arterial blood gases (ABGs) within patient's normal ranges and be free of symptoms.

Interventions	Rationale
INDEPENDENT	
• Upon arrival of the patient from surgery obtain report from the anesthesiologist regarding brief preoperative history, type of anesthetic used, fluid therapy, and perioperative vital signs.	• Existing and potential problems can be discussed. Plan of care can be formulated and immediate treatment initiated.
• Auscultate for breath sounds. Note if the patient has been reversed from anesthesia.	• Those patients not reversed will have a longer recovery time. Brain concentration of anesthesia is proportionate to alveolar concentration. The longer the patient is under anesthesia, the longer it will take to eliminate it.
• Provide oxygen that is warm and humidified as ordered.	• Humidity will facilitate alveolar oxygenation and ventilation. Warm oxygen will help to warm the patient.
• Suction the patient for secretions.	• Removing secretions will facilitate oxygenation.

Nursing Diagnosis: Gas Exchange, Impaired (*Continued*)

Interventions	Rationale
• Have the patient take slow deep breaths and cough as ordered.	• Coughing and deep-breathing will help eliminate secretions and anesthetic agents and lessen the chance of atelectasis.
• Keep the patient warm (refer to Nursing Diagnosis: Hypothermia, page 396. If the patient is hypothermic, obtain ABGs to assess pO_2 and pCO_2.	• Hypothermic patients will have a decreased pO_2 and pCO_2.
• Connect the patient to a cardiac monitor. Obtain vital signs every 15 minutes until the patient is fully recovered.	• Continual assessment of the postoperative patient's vital signs is imperative so that any potential problems will be quickly recognized and treated.
• Obtain ABGs 20 minutes after the patient has been placed on the ventilator without any interruptions. Notify the anesthesiologist of the results.	• An uninterrupted time span will give the patient the best opportunity for adequate measurement of oxygenation capabilities. Changes can be initiated if necessary.

COLLABORATIVE

• Warm the patient slowly but steadily. Determine that anesthesia has been completely reversed before extubation. Have emergency equipment readily available.	• Patients sometimes become reanesthetized after warming and may need reintubation.
• If used, make sure an oral airway device has been placed correctly and that an esophageal stethoscope has been removed. Maintain the patient's head tilted back and chin up.	• Obstruction can be caused by a misplaced oral airway device or esophageal stethoscope. Proper positioning is necessary to open up the patient's airway and promote ventilation.
• Know the current anesthetic agents used and their side effects. Review the patients record for administration of medication that can potentiate the effects of anesthesia (Table 21–1).	• Certain medications will prolong anesthesia. The longer the patient is under anesthesia, the longer it will take to eliminate it.

TABLE 21–1. Common Drugs Used With Burn Patients That Can Potentiate Anesthesia

Clindamycin	Tetracycline
Gentamicin	Quinidine
Neomycin	Narcotics

Nursing Diagnosis: Tissue Perfusion, Alteration In

May Be Related To:

- Blood loss
- Hypovolemia
- Cardiac ischemia

Possibly Evidenced By: Postoperative hypotension or hypertension, changes in skin color (pale blue) and temperature (cold extremities), and weak peripheral pulses.

Desired Patient Outcomes: The patient will be hemodynamically stable upon discharge from the recovery room or within 3 hours after surgery.

Interventions	Rationale
INDEPENDENT	
• Obtain report from the anesthesiologist. Assess the patient record for preoperative and perioperative vital signs. Monitor vital signs every 15 minutes until patient is fully recovered.	• Documents the physiologic status of the patient including any problems that occurred during surgery. Knowing the vital signs prior to and during surgery will give the nurse baseline information to use for comparison. Deviations from the baseline will be easily recognized and treated.
• Assess the patient closely for rise or fall in blood pressure, especially if the patient is hypothermic (refer to Nursing Diagnosis: Hypothermia, page 396). Notify the physician if the blood pressure is ±20 mmHg from baseline. A cause must be determined and the condition treated promptly.	• Hypothermia will cause a rise in blood pressure secondary to systemic vascular resistance. Pain will also cause the blood pressure to rise. Rewarming will decrease the blood pressure, as will hypovolemia.
• Auscultate heart sounds. Maintain patient on cardiac monitor to assess heart rate and rhythm and signs of instability or changing status.	• Anesthesia can affect cardiac contractility. Hypothermia can cause cardiac ischemia. Hypovolemia will increase the pulse, as will pain.
• Check capillary refill. Make sure pulses are palpable, especially in the extremity that was operated on. Use a Doppler device if pulse is not palpable. Notify physician immediately if pulses are lost.	• Loss of weakened pulses result from increased interstitial edema secondary to third spacing of fluid and diminished blood volume caused by surgery. Constrictive wound dressings will compromise pulses.
• Observe operative sites for bleeding. Reinforce dressings of debrided wounds. Notify the physician if bleeding increases or does not cease. Assess vital signs.	• Viable bleeding tissue is a parameter used for wound debridement. Blood loss is common in the surgical burn patient. Hypertension can cause bleeding at the operative sight.
• Monitor intake and output (I & O) carefully. Assess urine output for more than 30 ml/hour in the adult and more than 0.5–1.0 ml/kg per hour in the child.	• Destruction of tissue (due to burn injury and surgery) and release of myoglobin into the circulation will cause kidneys to clog and urine output to diminish. Hy-

Nursing Diagnosis: Tissue Perfusion, Alteration In (Continued)

Interventions	Rationale
Notify physician immediately for inadequate urine output. Verify that Foley catheter is draining properly. Obtain order from physician to insert Foley catheter if patient is unstable.	povolemia will cause a decrease in urine output. Urine output is a critical parameter used in burn patient assessment.

COLLABORATIVE

Interventions	Rationale
• Monitor intravenous (IV) fluid therapy carefully. Be prepared to increase fluids as ordered, as patient rewarms.	• The dilated vascular system will require more fluid to decrease the chance of hypotension. It is common to replace blood loss with added IV fluids or with packed red blood cells.
• Monitor hemoglobin and hematocrit closely.	• Hemoconcentration is a sign of hypovolemia or excessive blood replacement. Low values of hemoglobin and hematocrit may be a sign of excessive blood loss, acute bleeding, or fluid overload.
• Observe for side effects of anesthetic agents that cause hypotension and cardiac complications (refer to Chapter 20, Table 20–3).	• Knowledge of the anesthetic agents used will prepare the practitioner for potential problems.
• Use caution when administering narcotics for pain control or other medications that can potentiate the effects of anesthesia (refer to Table 21–1).	• Certain medications can prolong the effects of anesthesia.
• Monitor electrolytes closely. Notify the physician of changes that affect the patient's status.	• Electrolyte imbalance will cause cardiac instability.

Nursing Diagnosis: Hypothermia

May Be Related To:

- Extended exposure to air during the operative procedure
- Decrease skin barrier to cold, secondary to injury
- Creation of a donor site

Possibly Evidenced By: Decrease in body temperature, poor capillary refill, decrease pulse, and cold skin.

Desired Patient Outcomes: Patient's temperature will be within baseline range within 1 hour after surgery.

Interventions	Rationale
INDEPENDENT	
• Monitor vital signs every 15 minutes until fully recovered. Assess temperature fluctuations. Be prepared to take	• Continual assessment of vital signs will keep the nurse informed of the patient's changing needs. Anesthesia has a longer

Intervention	**Rationale**

appropriate action against any change in patient status.

- Monitor blood pressure closely as temperature increases. Verify that IV fluids are infusing properly.

- Maintain patient on a cardiac monitor. Note any changes in the ST segment.

- Cover patient with warmed blankets. Use a reflective blanket over the warm blanket. Tuck all blankets in at the side and around the shoulders.

COLLABORATIVE

- Assess temperature in patients who are shivering. If the temperature is stable but the shivering persists, obtain an order from the physician for meperidine 25 mg IV (adult dose).
- Utilize heat shields or warming blankets to warm patient. Administer IV fluids through warmers.
- Provide oxygen that is warmed and humidified. Monitor pO_2 and pCO_2 closely.

- Maintain recovery room temperature at no less than 75°F.

duration in hypothermic patients. The longer the patient is anesthetized the longer it will take the patient to recover and eliminate the anesthetic agent.
- A rise in temperature will cause vasodilation, resulting in decreased blood pressure and need for additional fluid to compensate the larger vascular system.
- Hypothermia can cause myocardial ischemia in patients, particularly those with coronary artery disease and the elderly.
- A warm blanket will help control shivering and conductive heat loss and create a heat source. The metallic blanket will direct heat toward the patient and reduce heat loss.

- Shivering can be caused by hypothermia or by the anesthetic agent fentanyl. Meperidine helps to eliminate shivering secondary to anesthesia.

- Actions are taken to provide patients with an added heat source.

- Low pO_2 and pCO_2 result from increased solubility of gases secondary to hypothermia. Physiologic response to hypoxia and hypercapnia are dulled secondary to hypothermia. Rewarming increases oxygen consumption.
- Action is taken to reduce chilling from circulating air.

Nursing Diagnosis: Pain

May Be Related To:

- Incisional or excisional sites
- Immobilization
- Burn injury
- Bladder distention
- Hypothermia

Possibly Evidenced By: Moaning, thrashing, restlessness, increased pulse

and blood pressure, increase respiratory rate, agitation, grimacing, or withdrawal.

Desired Patient Outcomes: The patient will express comfort. Postoperative pain will be minimized.

Nursing Diagnosis: Pain
(*Continued*)

Interventions	Rationale

INDEPENDENT

- Assess patient carefully. Determine what is altering vital signs.

- Assess location and cause of pain.

- Assess patient's response to pain medication.

- Pain can alter vital signs (e.g., it can increase pulse, blood pressure, and respiratory rate), as can other physiologic conditions.
- Postoperative pain can be from debridement, donor sites, surgical incisions, other burn injury, or other physiologic problems.
- Accurate assessment of patient response can determine a need for adjusting the medication dose.

COLLABORATIVE

- Carefully reposition patient every 2 to 4 hours as ordered. Support with pillows. Keep blankets snug but not too constricting.

- Use the same methods for assessing relief of discomfort (i.e., pain rating scales). Keep a consistent record.

- Check dressings. Determine that they are not too tight. Assess pulses on extremities. Note for sutures pulling excessively.

- Monitor urine output closely. Assess intake of fluids during surgery and postoperatively. If the patient has not voided for at least 8 hours and the bladder is distended, obtain an order for catheterization.
- If Foley catheter is present, monitor urine output hourly. Maintain Foley catheter patency. Note specific gravity and color of urine. Obtain an order from the physician to irrigate Foley catheter if necessary. Assess the need for low-dose dopamine infusion.

- Immobilization secondary to splinting and bulky dressings will cause added discomfort. Patients may be afraid to move on their own because of fear of causing more pain or injury.
- Consistent methods for evaluating pain will give the practitioner adequate information needed to assess effectiveness of treatment.
- Dressings that are too tight will be uncomfortable. Positioning the patient properly can relieve some tension on the sutures. Dressings that are too constricting will restrict blood flow to the area, causing more discomfort and swelling.
- Bladder distention will cause pain and discomfort.

- Muscle destruction secondary to surgery or injury will cause myoglobin to clog the urinary tract, decreasing urine output, and increasing bladder distention causing much discomfort. Urine will appear bloody and concentrated. Renal dose dopamine will increase urine output by dilating renal vasculature and increasing renal blood flow, which in turn will increase urine output.

Nursing Diagnosis: Anxiety

May Be Related To:

- Unfamiliarity with surgery
- Unknown factor of anesthesia
- Unpreparedness
- Preoperative stress
- Unpredictability of pain

Possibly Evidenced By: Apprehension, overexcitement, restlessness, inability to follow instructions, confusion, and agitation.

Desired Patient Outcomes: The patient will experience an uneventful emergence from anesthesia.

Interventions

INDEPENDENT

- Assess patient carefully for hypoxia, hypercarbia, and cerebral ischemia that will cause restlessness, confusion, and overexcitement that in turn will increase anxiety.
- Determine the effects of the anesthetic agents used.
- Allow patient to awaken in a quiet area of the recovery room. Subdue room by dimming the lights and pulling curtains closed. Slightly lower the volume on cardiac monitors, while making sure the monitor can still be heard.
- Give constant reassurance. Stay close to patient at all times. Orient patient when needed. Give instructions in simple but direct terms.

Rationale

- Determination for the cause of symptoms must be considered before treatment is initiated.

- Some anesthetic agents can cause confusion and hallucinations.
- A quiet environment will help keep patient calm and relaxed.

- Patients recovering from surgery need to feel safe and secure in the unfamiliar environment of the recovery room. Preoperative stress can cause confusion postoperatively.

COLLABORATIVE

- If patient is delirious and combative, obtain an order from the physician to restrain. Keep siderails up at all times.
- Medicate for pain appropriately. Keep patient comfortable.

- If possible, visit the patient before surgery. Get to know the patient and his or her feelings regarding the surgery. Offer support if needed at the time.

- Restraints will help prevent patient from harming self and others. Siderails help to prevent falls.
- Pain and discomfort can contribute to untoward effects from anesthesia emergence.
- Patients will be less disoriented postoperatively if they are familiar with their surroundings and caregiver. Patients who experience great emotional stress prior to surgery are prone to confusion and delirium postoperatively.

Nursing Diagnosis: Fear

(Refer to Chapter 9, page 175, for etiology, manifestations, desired patient outcomes, and interventions.)

Nursing Diagnosis: Powerlessness

(Refer to Chapter 7, page 96, for etiology, manifestations, desired patient outcomes, and interventions.)

Nursing Diagnosis: Coping, Possible Ineffective

(Refer to Chapter 7, page 92, for etiology, manifestations, desired patient outcomes, and interventions.)

Nursing Diagnosis: Fluid Volume Deficit

(Refer to Chapter 8, page 165, for etiology, manifestations, desired patient outcomes, and interventions.)

Nursing Diagnosis: Skin Integrity, Impairment Of

(Refer to Chapter 4, page 64, for etiology, manifestations, desired patient outcomes, and interventions.)

Nursing Diagnosis: Airway Clearance, Ineffective

(Refer to Chapter 9, page 162, for etiology, manifestations, desired patient outcomes, and interventions.)

BIBLIOGRAPHY

Boswick, J: The Art and Science of Burn Care. Aspen Publications, Rockville, MD, 1987

Campbell, C: Nursing Diagnosis and Intervention in Nursing Practice, ed 2. John Wiley & Sons, New York, 1984.

Harrison, M and Cotanch, P: Pain: Advances and issues in critical care. Nurs Clin North Am 22:691, 1987.

Crane, H and Miner, D: Thermo-resuscitation for post-operative hypothermia using reflective blankets. AORN 47:222, 1988.

Fraulini, K and Gorski, D: Don't let peri-operative medications put you in a spin. Nursing '83 13(12): 1983.

Sendack, M: Getting the patient to surgery and back 11. Common recovery room problems. Emerg Med 18(20):117, 1986.

Wiener, MY, et al: Clinical Pharmacology and Therapeutics in Nursing. McGraw-Hill, New York, 1979.

PROFESSIONAL ISSUES IN BURN CARE

Chapter 22

MARY M. WAGNER

NURSING EDUCATION

Giving nursing care to persons who have sustained a catastrophic injury is one of the most challenging, rewarding, and frustrating experiences a nurse can enjoy. In the early 1950s, there were no burn units or nurses specifically educated in the care of burn patients. Many patients were placed on surgical units. The state of the art left much to be desired. People interested in the care of burn patients had to meet at other professional meetings to share information; information was also disseminated in professional journals. With the advent of the American Burn Association (ABA) in 1967, the thrust for care, teaching, and research was begun. A few years later prevention was added to the mission statement of the ABA.

The purpose of this chapter is to assist others who have the responsibility for education of students, orientation of new employees, and continued competence of the burn unit staff.

ORIENTATION OF NEW PERSONNEL

To achieve a smooth transition from new employee to confident practitioner requires an organized program. This section contains preceptorships, general guidelines, and curricular content.

Preceptorship

For nurses who are newly employed in the burn unit and have not worked with or been exposed to burned persons, the initial experience can be overwhelming. It is of the utmost importance that new burn unit nurses be allowed to spend time coming to grips with their emotional shock. It is less traumatic if, at the outset, they are provided with a preceptor who will be working and teaching them throughout the orientation and probationary period. A preceptor or mentor is an experienced nurse who is an able teacher and with whom the new nurse can develop a trusting relationship.

To quote a former student and later colleague,

Watching someone else demonstrate the art of assembling an arterial flush system looks easy. For a novice the same tubing becomes coils of serpentine plastic with every portion defying union with another. Squawky ventilators need not precipitate inner panic once one learns to do a rapid check of probable causes.[1]

The selection of preceptors is vitally important because the new nurse is using the preceptor as the role model in adapting to burn care. In selecting the preceptor, the following factors should be considered:

- Professional and emotional maturity
- Knowledge of burn nursing standards[2]
- Skill as practitioner
- Participation in continuing education programs
- Good communication and organizational skills
- Willingness to participate

Preceptors are not automatically endowed with these qualities and should receive an orientation to the role. This role may be part of a clinical ladder program. The preceptor must know what is involved in terms of time and evaluation procedures. The program of study and schedule of activities of the new employee should be planned with the preceptor. At the beginning of the preceptorship, the time schedules of the two should coincide in order to develop a good working relationship. Later, as the new employee gains confidence, the time schedules do not need to mesh, as the gradual emergence from learner to colleague occurs. Optimally, the relationship is of a caring and nurturing nature, which leads to independence of practice.

It is important to develop staff to accept and perform the role of preceptor in order to prevent overuse of one person. Preceptorship can be used as a recognition of quality contributions and achievement. Acting as a preceptor presents the person with an opportunity to review and evaluate one's own practice as well as to teach. Teaching is a means of enhancing personal learning because questions raised by new learners often initiate a re-examination of current practice. Commitment to sound practice and care is transmitted to new persons when there is a pervasive team spirit within the unit. Philosophic unity provides the base for peer support and respect and can only contribute positively to staff morale and retention.

General Orientation Guidelines

A record of skills and procedures is maintained that demonstrates the progression toward competency. A skills checklist can be designed that incorporates the principles of competency-based learning. Practice of skills should be concurrent with didactic material. In determining what is to be taught with skills, priority is given to that which is of critical importance for patient care. Early participation in care, although limited by inexperience, provides the new staff member with a feeling of contribution and belonging. For further detail, a review of the articles by Bayley and Raverly[3] and Manning[4] is recommended.

The development of competency based skill requires the delineation of all steps. Questions to be answered are

- What are the steps?
- Are they absolutely essential or may some be omitted in a critical situation?
- Must the steps be done in a specific sequence?
- How often must the skill be performed?
- What is the level of importance?

As the procedures and skills are developed using this approach, the burn unit staff should review them for completeness and applicability. The use of competency-based tools provides the preceptor with a concrete and objective measure for evaluation of the new employee. The learner also knows what is expected and can achieve the desired outcome. Table 22–1 is an example of a sample tool.

Cost-effective orientation and course offerings have to be carefully planned in this age of economic constraints. The following factors need to be considered when developing a program:

- Numbers and mix of personnel
- Frequency of offerings
- Availability of lecturers and clinical preceptors
- Clinical facilities for demonstration and practice
- Evaluation of learning

The employment of new graduates in the hospital is a predictable factor, but not so with other personnel (e.g., technicians and nurses who have recently moved to the area). Scheduling of programs is easy with the influx of relatively large numbers of new graduate nurses, while the "out-of-season" employee presents a problem. It is not good for the morale of the latter to have to wait to receive the instruction necessary to give quality care. However, a course cannot be offered for one or two persons, even though this might be eminently desirable. The solution would be to design a course of study that is modular and self-paced. The didactic content can be videotaped, which also allows for updating knowledge with a study guide developed to assist the learner. Computer-assisted instruction (CAI) may be used for didactic content as well as patient-simulated learning.

The modules can be designed to meet learning needs in other critical care units since there is a core of content that is essential for all nurses working in these units. The content that is unique to each specialty area can be prepared as adjunctive modules. For example, the respiratory core module would contain

- Anatomy and physiology
- Pathologies
- Clinical assessment
- Ventilatory support
- Nursing interventions

TABLE 22–1: PERFORMANCE CHECKLIST:
Administration of IV Push Medications

Actions*	Yes	No	Comments
1. Obtains current medication			
2. Checks does and amount			
3. Knows speed at which medication may be safely administered.			
4. Checks patient identification			
5. Flushes IV line or heparin lock			
6. Administers medication			
7. Flushes IV line or heparin lock			
8. Records medication and patient's immediate response			
9. Returns at specified time to verify patient response			

*Steps cannot be omitted; must be done in sequence.

The specialty content in burn care would include

- Mechanisms of inhalation injuries
- Impaired ventilation due to circumferential injury
- Nursing assessment and interventions

Examples of Curricula

This section will present two excerpts from published curricula. These are the ABA Core Curriculum, based on the work done by Dr. Tarcinale at the University of Rochester, and the Core Curriculum for Critical Care Nursing, developed by the Association of Critical Care Nurses.

A CURRICULUM FOR BASIC BURN NURSING PRACTICE

Table of Contents
Developing and Maintaining Competency in Burn Nursing
A Curriculum Overview

Unit I	The burned person: biopsychosocial factors
Unit II	Initial assessment and care
Unit III	Systemic problems in burn care
Unit IV	Management of wound care and infection
Unit V	Nutrition
Unit VI	Psychosocial aspects of burn care
Unit VII	Surgical procedures: grafting and reconstruction
Unit VIII	Special age-related needs
Unit IX	Rehabilitation of the burned person
Unit X	Discharge planning and home care

Evaluation

Each unit is accompanied by learning objectives and an extensive bibliography.

EIGHT MAJOR SECTIONS FOR CRITICAL CARE NURSING

The Core Curriculum for Critical Care Nursing has eight major sections:

- Pulmonary System
- Cardiovascular System
- Neurologic System
- Renal System
- Endocrine System
- Hematologic System
- Gastrointestinal System
- Psychosocial Implications

The content just described can be found in greater detail in the core curricula of the ABA and of the American Association of Critical Care Nurses.[5,6]

Testing and evaluation of learning can be achieved by paper and pencil tests or through CAI.

STAFF RECRUITMENT AND RETENTION

Many gimmicks have been used to recruit nurses, including bonuses for coming to work at "our place." The best and most economic recruitment method is to have a sound retention program. There is no magic solution to the problem of maintaining experienced staff. The bottom line is that the employer and employee must develop a mutually beneficial relationship.

Review of the literature reveals some suggestions that may be incorporated into a unit's retention program. For example, an incentive program as described by Newman[7] recognizes staff achievement and contributions and plans rewards based on a point system. A sample reward is an all-expense-paid trip to a continuing education offering such as an ABA national meeting. Other incentives need to be designed to fit the individual situation.

Nurturance of staff is an essential aspect of retention. Working with the burn-injured person requires a great deal of physical and mental energy. Staff meetings should provide not only content related to the functioning of the unit but also built-in interventions that decrease staff grief. Recognition of the emotional trauma that accompanies a long siege of high patient census and high levels of acute care must be recognized as a potentially explosive situation. In this period of time, one spark can trigger a rash of absenteeism or resignations, or both. Crisis intervention techniques are useful in defusing the "bomb." The intervention at this time needs to be done by an individual who is familiar with the phenomenon of staff grief and has had personal experience going through a similar crisis. The individual referred to previously may be the clinical nurse specialist for the unit, the psychiatric liaison nurse with whom the staff has developed rapport and trust, or both.

Staff members may be so caught up in their personal conflict that they may not recognize that they are grieving. Focusing on the problems by having staff identify the sources of their pain is one method of helping staff recognize their grief. After a catharsis session about their irritations with themselves, patients, patient's families, and other members of the burn team, priorities can be assigned to the worst problems; that is, the ones the staff perceive as the greatest barrier to effective unit functioning.

At the initial catharsis session, only the burn unit nurses should be involved. (This is not to say that other members of the burn team do not have problems, but they are not involved with total patient care on a continuous basis. Some of the conflicts may arise from this very fact.) The staff may perceive that they are being "dumped on" when they have to work on weekends, do shift work, and get stuck with left over tasks. This type of negative thinking and attitude—that things are beyond the individual's control—is what precipitates a major eruption in the unit. The group leader may want to have the staff look at their perception of control. A simple test of locus of control may be a pivotal stimulus to direct thinking toward a more positive outlook. The administrator in charge of the unit should be on the alert that there is a potential for explosion when patient census and acute care cases are on the rise.

The other potential time for major upheaval is when patient census is low and staff members are transferred to other areas. Again, the administrator needs to look carefully at the reasons for transfer. Are the nurses being transferred because of numbers of patients and a real need on other units? If there is not a valid reason, then this is an ideal time for continuing education, vacations, and bonus days off, which are a recognition of dedication during the high patient census time. Bonus days off will not cost a hospital more money. This is based on an experience at the University of Iowa when bonus checks were received by those who did not use sick time. In fact when census is low and staff are pulled, sick calls may increase; this not only costs the hospital just as much in money but also may erode staff morale. A sick call to avoid being unnecessarily transferred puts a burden of guilt on the individual, which requires some form of rationalization for the behavior. This leads to an erosion of character that can be tolerated only for so long, whereupon the person feels lack of self-worth and is forced to look elsewhere for personal satisfaction.

Personal satisfaction and recognition of achievement are the keys to retention. Respect from other members of the burn team for the nursing required by burn-injured patients is paramount. If an occupational or physical therapist is lost from the unit, care will still go on because the nurse can do the exercises and improvise splinting. If a nurse is lost, the other nurses can work overtime until one or more of them get discouraged and leave. If too many nurses leave, beds must be closed and care is denied to those who might otherwise survive in terms of life and quality of life. When beds are closed, the hospital loses money. Does monetary loss become the bottom line? Why spend thousands of dollars on recruitment and pennies on retention? The retention program must be given priority and must be geared toward maintaining the dignity of the nurses' contributions to care.

Within the retention program, some suggestions for recognition include

- Participation in outreach programs structured to improve the transfer of patients to the burn unit[8]
- Participation and cooperation with others in the community in burn prevention programs
- Involvement in unit management
- Development of a clinical ladder that rewards direct patient care
- Tuition reimbursement for higher education
- Yearly recognition dinner for all outstanding employees with the awarding of plaques or certificates of achievement
- Yearly picnic reuniting patients and staff as a means of reaffirming success in caring

None of these ideas are new but rather reaffirm that in order to keep valued persons, the persons must realize that they are valued. The retention of staff is only as good as the effort that is put into a comprehensive, well-thought-out program.

One of the most effective methods of recruitment seems to be the extern program, which is structured to allow students to practice in selected areas and to develop relationships with their colleagues and with other professionals. The extern gets to see "real nursing" and experiences the frustrations and joys of working with patients. According to Jonason and McCue, the extern program continues to be the best in terms of recruitment and retention.[9] This program has been in existence for over 15 years at the Medical University of South Carolina. From 1985 through 1987, the recruitment rate from the general extern program was 40 to 60 percent; while in 1985 and 1986, it was 100 percent for the burn unit.

Another method of recruitment is closely tied to educational experiences. Providing clinical facilities for students allows them to see realities of care. Optimally, faculty members who teach in these specialty areas should be certified as clinical nurse specialists (CNS) and hold a joint appointment with college and hospital. The joint appointment of a CNS with an academic rank enhances the prestige of burn nursing and boosts unit morale. Allowing access for graduate and undergraduate students fosters a climate of enthusiasm for scholarship and research.

An enthusiastic, happy employee is a very good advertisement; therefore, sending staff members to meetings such as the student nurses' conventions can generate interest within the unit. The staff member also feels valued to be selected. Attendance of a staff member along with a recruiter at career days at nursing schools is another means of visibility. Displays and giveaways may be used to attract people to a booth but there needs to be something that will hold the individual's interest long enough for a "sales pitch." Selection of meetings for recruiting is important so that the recruiter does not wind up trying to recruit other recruiters, which is a waste of money.

BURN CARE IN NURSING CURRICULA

The amount of time allotted to burn unit nursing is minimal in most undergraduate programs. Two to three class hours may be devoted to an overview of the problem. When it comes to clinical practice, there may be no place available for the student to work with a burned person. Often nursing schools are too far away from a burn care facility.

The student may also be able to take an independent elective course in critical care and focus on burn patients if the school is located near a burn unit. If the curriculum is designed so that a student can take an off-campus elective course at a different school, the student can be advised to do so near a burn unit. If the recruiter is familiar with schools that have this option, a program of study can be offered. Another suggestion is to have a staff member from a regional burn unit come as a guest lecturer. It also may be feasible to arrange a lecture in conjunction with a tour of the burn unit facilities.

Video tapes and films can also be used to help the student gain some understanding of the problem. A listing of available teaching aids and location of burn units may be obtained from the ABA.

The content of an undergraduate program should be as follows:

• Pathophysiology of the injury
• Nursing care and treatment during the emergent and acute phases of the injury
• Psychosocial aspects
• Prevention and rehabilitation

To present all of this content in three class hours is an arduous task.

Graduate programs in burn nursing are usually found as an emphasis track within the critical care elective or major. The curriculum is variable and dependent upon the college of nursing in which it is housed. In the United States, there are a few programs that are specifically devoted to burn nursing. For further information concerning graduate education programs, contact the National League for Nursing.

SUMMARY

It is beyond the scope of this book to present all of the information that is necessary for burn nursing education. However, some of the ideas and suggestions, although not new or original, may be helpful in planning one's own program. If expertise is needed, assistance is available from the ABA and the contributing authors of this text.

REFERENCES

1. Heffley, DL: Burn care—A nursing perspective. In Wagner, MM: Care of the Burn Injured Patient. PSG Publishing, Littleton, MA, 1981, pp 235–236.
2. American Burn Association: Guidelines for Burn Nursing Practice, 1980.
3. Bayley, EW and Raverly, AN: Development of a competency based orientation for burn nursing. Journal of Burn Care and Rehabilitation 4(6):36, 1983.

4. Manning, S: Characteristics of a burn orientation program. Journal of Burn Care and Rehabilitation 4:49, 1983.
5. American Burn Association: A Curriculum for Basic Burn Nursing Practice, ed 4. University of Texas, Galveston, 1985.
6. Alspach, JG and Williams, SM: Core Curriculum for Critical Care Nursing, ed 3. WB Saunders, Philadelphia, 1985.
7. Newman, NL: A nursing incentive program. Journal of Burn Care and Rehabilitation 4(56): 1983.
8. Hallberg, PW: Developing outreach programs in community hospitals. Journal of Burn Care and Rehabilitation 4:41, 1983.
9. Jonason, AM and McCue, P: Personal communication. Feb 1988.

BIBLIOGRAPHY

American Journal of Nursing News: No head nurse need apply. AJN 87:862, 1987.
Bayley, EW: Nursing education in a burn unit. Critical Care Quarterly 7:67, 1984.
Brack, G, et al: A survey of attitudes of burn nurses. Journal of Burn Care and Rehabilitation 8:299, 1987.
Bruce, GL and Ingersoll, GL: Critical care orientation of the burn nurse. CCQ 7:79, 1984.
Bunker, BJ and Carnes, RW: Burn unit experience for nursing students. DCCN 5:363, 1986.
Dixon, MJ, et al: Vocational interest as a predicator of tenure in the burn unit. Journal of Burn Care and Rehabilitation 8:327, 1987.
Gonzales, EL: Burn clinical nursing specialist/nurse clinician roles and role development. Journal of Burn Care and Rehabilitation 8:25, 1987.
Kenner, CV, et al: Guidelines for burn nursing practice: Discussion. Journal of Burn Care and Rehabilitation 4:59, 1983.
Kibbee, E, et al: Borrowed burn nurses. Journal of Burn Care and Rehabilitation 8:220, 1987.
Scherer, P: Hospitals that keep and attract nurses. AJN 88:43, 1988.
Rotter, JB: Generalized expectancies for internal vs external control of reinforcements. Psychol Monog, 80, 1966.
Sovie, MD: The primary nurse system. Journal of Burn Care and Rehabilitation 4:43, 1983.

Chapter 23

PATRICIA M. ORR

BURN PREVENTION

Burn injury causes medical, social, environmental, and financial problems that have grown to epidemic proportions in the United States. Approximately 2 million burn injuries occur per year with 20,000 victims needing hospitalization and 9000 deaths.[1] The advent of major burn centers using a multidisciplinary approach to burn care has contributed to a decrease in mortality and morbidity from this type of injury. The gradual evolution of these burn care facilities with specialized staff—along with supportive burn foundations, firefighters, industrial safety inspectors, and community groups—has developed an increasing awareness of the burn injury problem. Prevention programs have been developed by these groups, in the belief that prevention of a burn injury is the best cure of the problem.

To develop an effective prevention program, research into causative factors has led to target population groups. Data collection by interested prevention groups has demonstrated the following facts. Scalds are the major cause of burns in children. Approximately 17 percent of all hospitalized children are scalded, often the victims of child abuse. The other population at risk from scald burns is the elderly (age 65 or older), and sometimes they are victims of abuse by caregivers. Flame injuries, although not as numerous as scalds, are the more serious injury. Flame-injured victims comprise 70 percent of the burn population who are hospitalized. Chemical injuries, industrial in nature, usually affect young men aged 21 to 50. These injuries comprise about 3 percent of the burn population. Electrical injuries constitute about 8 percent of the burn population and are catastrophic in nature. This trauma occurs also in young men aged 20 to 50.[2]

Where the burn occurs is important in prevention project development. Eighty percent of burn injuries occur in the home. Flame injuries occur most frequently in kitchens from cooking accidents, and in bedrooms from smoking in bed. Scald injuries occur most frequently in bathrooms from excessive hot water temperatures in the bath or shower and in the kitchen from spills of boiling water. Chemical and electrical injuries occur most often in an industrial setting.

Prevention efforts have also focused on appliances that decrease burn injury such as the smoke detector in the home. Development of fire drills in the home with the use of escape routes and fire ladders is also targeted by prevention groups. Campaigns by prevention groups have proved effective by decreasing the incidence of scald injuries and increasing public awareness of the dangers of excessively high hot water temperature settings. Enforcement of safety rules and regulations and the use of newer or well-repaired equipment around hazardous materials are the prevention efforts of safety engineers.

In Philadelphia, the Nurse Advisory Council of the Burn Foundation developed a data collection system to develop effective burn prevention projects in the region. The 1987 data from the five participating hospitals reviewed the cases of 714 patients treated in the burn centers. Thirty-three percent of the patients were flame injured, and 20 percent had experienced flame and inhalation injury. The majority of flame injuries were caused by cigarettes, followed in order of frequency by matches, stoves, and electricity. The scald-injured represented 24 percent of the patients. This type of burn injury most frequently resulted from stove-heated water, followed by tap wataer and other beverage scalds. Injuries in the work place occurred in 18 percent of the burn population, the majority of which were flame injuries, followed by electrical and contact burns. The statistics also demonstrated that very young children (birth to age 3) requiring burn center care were most often victims of scald or contact burns. The elderly were more likely to require hospitalization for flame and inhalation injuries. Electrical and chemical burns requiring burn center care were most common in the 21- to 45-year age group.[3]

AGE-RELATED INJURIES

Infants and Toddlers

Curious and energetic infants or toddlers, constituting the majority of victims of scald injury in the home, are burned by hot liquids or hot grease in the kitchen, hot tub water in the bathroom, and hot surfaces such as irons or alternate heating methods. Children in this age group are also prone to electrical injury by chewing on electrical wires left within easy reach. These injuries frequently occur due to inadequate supervision in the home. When the parent or responsible caregiver is most distracted or busy, such as at mealtimes or holidays, the unattended toddler is burned. In the kitchen the toddler will bump into someone carrying hot water or reach for a pot or cup containing hot liquids. Investigative children of this age group will often lean on or pull over hot objects. Increasingly, scald burns in this age group are due to heating babies' bottles in microwave ovens; hot milk sprays the infant's face as the bottle is inverted for feeding.

Accidents in this age group could be prevented with adequate supervision. Educational efforts of prevention groups are aimed at new mothers and other caregivers targeted adequate supervision, especially in the bath, and the development of a safe play area in the home to decrease the incidence of injury. At times of stress or hurriedness, it is important to keep toddlers out of the kitchen, or to place them in a safe area such as a high chair. Items such as hot liquids on tables should be placed out of reach. Tablecloths should be removed to prevent a child from pulling a hot object over by tugging on the tablecloth. Bottles should not be heated in microwave ovens. All electrical cords that are within reach of the child should be removed. Hot water temperature in the home can be controlled through the use of preset thermostats on hot water heaters. Children should wear fire-retardant clothing.

Preschoolers

In the 3- to 8-year age group, children begin learning what is dangerous. They also begin to imitate adult behavior and want to help the parent. Risk-taking behavior increases, and the child begins reaching and climbing. Burn injury is caused by scalding as the child reaches for hot liquids usually on the stove. Ingestible chemicals stored in reachable cabinets are also hazardous. The child in this age group begins playing with matches or lighters, creating fire hazards in the home. Usually, after a fire is started, the child hides from it, thereby leading to a greater loss of life or property. Hot water placed on top of kerosene heaters has created a new hazard for this age group, as they frequently bump into objects while running or playing. Children left home alone are at risk of burning in house fires due to faulty wiring or heating by alternate methods such as wood-burning stoves.

Preventive efforts of burn injury in this age group are aimed at parental education. Matches, lighters, and chemical agents should be kept out of the reach of children. No food should be stored above the stove, in order to prevent a child from climbing or reaching, risking injury. Responsible caregivers should be employed, never leaving young children home unattended. Fire-retardant clothing should be used. Encourage children not to use the kitchen as a play area, especially during meal preparation times.

Educational efforts begin with the very young by drills on fire safety and what to do during a house fire. "Stop, drop, roll, and cool" to extinguish a fire should be practiced, as should fire drills in the home. Materials such as coloring books (Fig. 23–1), readily available from some fire departments and burn foundations, educate children about fire, burn hazards, and prevention behaviors.

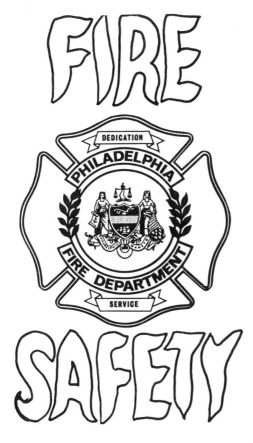

COLORING
BOOK

FIGURE 23–1. Fire safety coloring book. (Courtesy of the Philadelphia Fire Department, Philadelphia, PA.)

AIRPORT CRASH TRUCK

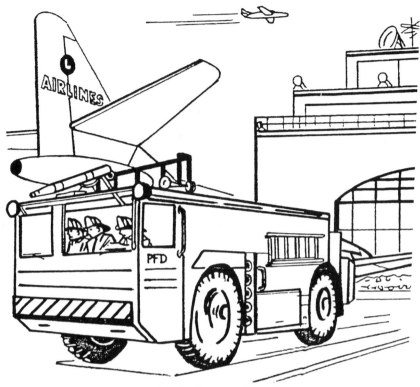

FIGURE 23-1. *Continued.*

Adolescents

Older children develop more risk-taking behaviors, especially under peer pressure. They require less supervision and increasingly attempt to perform adult tasks. Burns occur through the use of flammable materials when attempting to perform tasks such as starting a lawnmower (gasoline) or an outdoor barbecue (lighter fluid). Children in this age group may play with flammable substances or climb an electrical power station fence to retrieve a ball, risking burn injury.

Education through the school system has been a very effective method in preventing these types of injuries. High-tension electrical injury prevention programs are provided through the electric companies. Fire departments provide demonstrations in schools and shopping malls of the "stop, drop, roll, and cool" method of smothering flames. Adult supervision is recommended when children are using volatile substances, no matter what the child's age.

Teenagers, who are generally of the opinion that "it won't happen to me," present a special educational task. This group is often looking for something to do out of boredom. Burn injuries may result from experimentation with drugs or working with automobiles. Image, also of concern in this age group, can lead to extended exposure from sun or sunlamps, resulting in extensive, painful burn injury. Individuals in this age group may seek part-time employment as cooks in fast food restaurants and pumping gasoline in gas stations, which frequently results in burns occurring due to lack of education regarding hazardous substances.

MATCHES & CARELESS SMOKING HAZARDS   YES   NO

    Do you keep matches away from sources of heat such
as stoves or heaters?   ___   ___
    Do you make sure matches and smoking materials are
out before disposing of them?   ___   ___
    Do you have plenty of large, non-combustible ash
trays in every room?   ___   ___

ELECTRICAL HAZARDS
    Are there enough electrical outlets in every room
to avoid the need for multiple attachment plugs and
long extension cords?   ___   ___
    Are all extension cords in the open - not run under
rugs, over hooks or through partitions or door openings? ___   ___

HOUSEKEEPING HAZARDS
    Do you keep your basement storage area and closets
cleaned of old rags, papers, mattresses, broken
furniture and other combustible odds and ends?   ___   ___
    After using oily polishing rags or waste, do you
destroy them or place them in covered metal cans?   ___   ___
    If you store paint, varnish, etc., do you keep the
containers tightly closed?   ___   ___
    Has everyone in your family been warned never to use
gasoline, benzine or other flammable fluids for cleaning
clothes, furnishings or floors?   ___   ___

SPECIAL FOR PARENTS
    Do you keep matches out of the reach of children?   ___   ___
    Do you leave a responsible person with your children
when you go out, even for a little while?   ___   ___
    When you employ baby-sitters, do you instruct them
carefully on what to do in case of fire?   ___   ___
    IMPORTANT: A child learns by example as well as by
instruction. In regard to fire safety, do you always
set a good example?   ___   ___

HEATING AND COOKING HAZARDS
    Is your stove, including oven and broiler, kept clean
of grease?   ___   ___
    Are curtains near stoves and heating equipment
arranged so as not to blow over them?   ___   ___
    Are all heaters set level, and placed out of the way
of traffic?   ___   ___
    Since gas and oil heaters use up oxygen as they burn,
do you always keep a door or window slightly open in any
room where such a heater is being used?   ___   ___

FIGURE 23-1. *Continued.*

    Prevention efforts are aimed at educating the teenager in safety factors when exposed to thermal agents. Safe exposure time in the sun or under a sunlamp should be emphasized. Many of the dangers associated with cars—such as hot radiators, hot mufflers, battery acid, and gasoline fumes—need to be part of a prevention program. Fire safety with "stop, drop, roll, and cool" to prevent extensive flame injury should be part of the fire department education program in the school system. Electrical safety aimed at this age group can be provided by the electric company and by television public service announcements.

Adults

For adults, prevention efforts are aimed at home and work place safety standards. Injuries in this age group are related to house fires, alcohol or drug abuse, smoking in bed, faulty electrical wiring, or alternate heating methods such as kerosene heaters. Contact injuries, caused by tar or molten metals, occur in the workplace, usually when persons are not wearing protective gear. Burns due to carelessness or lack of education occur as gasoline is poured into hot radiators of cars or kerosene heaters. Unextinguished cigarettes create a major hazard, as the cigarette will smolder for a few hours prior to igniting.

Preventive efforts are aimed to heighten adult awareness of the hazards in everyday living. Home fire drills are mandatory. The use of smoke detectors has effectively decreased the number of fire-related deaths. Smoking areas should be designated in the home, and one should *never* smoke in bed. Labels on flammable liquids should be read prior to use and stored in their appropriate container outside the home.

In the work setting, protective gear should be worn as recommended by safety inspectors. There should always be an awareness of electrical safety when working around high-tension wires. Workers need to be alert and aware of any heat source and the dangers that might exist in relation to the heat. They should not work in these areas when stressed, overworked, or overtired. All workers should be cognizant of the regular safety inspections utilizing a fire prevention checklist following guidelines of the National Fire Code (Fig. 23–2).

The elderly, age 60 and older, need special prevention education. Mostly through senior citizen groups, fire prevention, emphasizes avoiding hazards. The decreased motor responses, neuropathies, handicaps, and sensory deficits of elderly persons cause serious injuries to occur from hot water spills, hot tub or shower water temperature, and the inability to exit the home quickly when a fire starts. Prevention aspects focuses on fire drills, fire extinguishers, and smoke detectors in the home. Presetting hot water temperatures and testing bath or shower water temperature before getting in prevents serious injury. Regarding cooking, emphasis must be on the state of health of the cook (history of fainting, frequent dizzy spells, uncontrolled seizures, or other disabilities that create a hazard when cooking) and the type of clothing being worn when cooking (loose flowing sleeves). Elderly individuals, due to the aging process, have a difficult time surviving burn injury.

COMMUNITY PROJECTS

A number of communities and organizations across the United States develop projects for burn prevention. The Fire and Burn Safety Alliance is an organization of groups interested in fire safety and burn prevention. Developed in 1984, this alliance set its goals as follows:

To promote a spirit of cooperation among burn organizations
To disseminate current information
To involve community and national organizations.[4]

FIRE PREVENTION CHECK LIST

ELECTRICAL EQUIPMENT

- ☐ No makeshift wiring
- ☐ Extension cords serviceable
- ☐ Motors and tools free of dirt and grease
- ☐ Lights clear of combustible materials
- ☐ Safest cleaning solvents used

- ☐ Fuse and control boxes clean and closed
- ☐ Circuits properly fused
- ☐ Equipment approved for use in hazardous areas (if required)
- ☐ Ground connections clean and tight

FRICTION

- ☐ Machinery properly lubricated
- ☐ Machinery properly adjusted and/or aligned

SPECIAL FIRE-HAZARD MATERIALS

- ☐ Storage of special flammables isolated
- ☐ Nonmetal stock free of tramp metal

WELDING AND CUTTING

- ☐ Area surveyed for fire safety
- ☐ Combustibles removed or covered
- ☐ Permit issued

OPEN FLAMES

- ☐ Kept away from spray rooms and booths
- ☐ Portable torches clear of flammable surfaces
- ☐ No gas leaks

PORTABLE HEATERS

- ☐ Set up with ample horizontal and overhead clearances
- ☐ Secured against tipping or upset

- ☐ Safely mounted on noncombustible surface
- ☐ Not used as rubbish burners
- ☐ Combustibles removed or covered

HOT SURFACES

- ☐ Hot pipes clear of combustible materials
- ☐ Ample clearance around boilers and furnaces

- ☐ Soldering irons kept off combustible surfaces
- ☐ Ashes in metal containers

SMOKING AND MATCHES

- ☐ "No smoking" and "smoking" areas clearly marked
- ☐ Butt containers available and serviceable

- ☐ No discarded smoking materials in prohibited areas

SPONTANEOUS IGNITION

- ☐ Flammable waste material in closed, metal containers
- ☐ Flammable waste material containers emptied frequently

- ☐ Piled material cool, dry, and well ventilated
- ☐ Trash receptacles emptied daily

STATIC ELECTRICITY

- ☐ Flammable liquid dispensing vessels grounded or bonded
- ☐ Moving machinery grounded

- ☐ Proper humidity maintained

HOUSEKEEPING

- ☐ No accumulations of rubbish
- ☐ Safe storage of flammables
- ☐ Passageways clear of obstacles
- ☐ Fire doors unblocked and operating freely with fusible links intact

- ☐ Premises free of unnecessary combustible materials
- ☐ No leaks or drippings of flammables and floor free of spills

EXTINGUISHING EQUIPMENT

- ☐ Proper type
- ☐ In proper location
- ☐ Unobstructed
- ☐ Clearly marked

- ☐ In working order
- ☐ Service date current
- ☐ Personnel trained in use of equipment

FIGURE 23–2. Fire prevention check list. (Courtesy of the National Safety Council, Chicago, IL.)

This alliance was developed to provide a communication network for all groups interested in burn safety and prevention. It can also provide a unified group to address public policy on today's issues regarding burn safety.

Many groups individually have addressed fire safety, such as fire departments, burn foundations, former burn victims, and burn centers staffs. Education based on data collection most commonly addresses scald burns and their causes, burn prevention and fire safety behaviors, and burn prevention in the young, elderly, and handicapped. Individuals also begin campaigns against a specific unsafe product because of an increased incidence in burns related to the product (i.e., kerosene heaters in the home).

Scald Burns

Burn injury due to scalds has been addressed by many organizations interested in burn prevention. Prevention efforts have been aimed at two groups—the very young, under age 5, and the elderly, over 65. Seventeen percent of childhood burn injuries are attributable to hot tap water. Six percent of scald victims are admitted to hospitals, with 112,000 individuals treated in emergency departments annually.[5]

The time-temperature relationship from Moritz and Henrique's study have implications for prevention efforts (refer to Chapter 3, Fig. 3–1). Heightened awareness of hot water temperatures in the home is the goal of these prevention groups. In the public sector, efforts have been made to have hot water heater temperatures preset at factories no higher than 130°F. In response to this recommendation of the Consumer Product Safety Commission (CPSC) and the National Safety Council, the American National Standards Committee revised standards to 130°F (54°C) as the maximum setting for new gas hot water heaters, with guidelines recommending standard temperature setting on all hot water heaters.

The use of tempering valves to prevent scald injury is also recommended by safety groups. These valves are useful in buildings in which hot water temperatures are greater than 130°F by necessity such as high-rise apartment buildings. These tempering valves can lower the in-line temperature of the water at the use site, thus reducing the risk of scald injury.

Lastly, control of the hot water handles is emphasized by prevention groups. Making the handles more difficult to turn on or removing the handles completely can decrease the risk of scald injury in the home.

Education efforts by prevention groups must be aimed at changing behaviors of the child or elderly person. Testing water temperature prior to bathing is emphasized. Temperature testing devices are available on the market for consumers. Prevention activities are mostly directed at caregivers. Instructions on scald prevention emphasize supervision of any activities in the bathroom and/or kitchen.

The American Burn Association (ABA) emphasizes two major points in the education of the parent or caregiver regarding scald prevention:

1. Constant supervision . . .
2. Run cold water . . . and test water temperature.[6]

Burn Prevention and Fire Safety Behaviors

Community educational efforts are aimed at instructing groups on how to create a fire-safe home and on what actions should be taken if one is involved in a fire. Items on the market to prevent home fires include smoke and fire detectors, fire extinguishers, electric charcoal starters, and long-handled barbecue tools. Educational materials for fire safety in the home are available through burn foundations, burn centers, and local fire departments.

One major area of concern of fire prevention groups is safe smoking habits. Common ignition sources in home fires are cigarettes, cigars, pipes, and lighters, with cigarettes being the most common. Many prevention campaigns have been aimed at producing a fire-safe cigarette. Although a technical study group mandated by the Cigarette Safety Act of 1984 reported the feasibility of developing a cigarette that has a reduced capacity to ignite furniture, fire-safe cigarettes are not yet mandated by federal law.[7] Developing safe smoking habits and designating specific smoking areas in the home constitute subjects of educational efforts by prevention groups.

Another major area of interest for burn prevention groups is electrical safety. As reported by the CPSC, 192,500 home fires each year are electrical in origin. One thousand deaths are attributed to these fires annually, with 100,000 people being injured.[8] Second in frequency only to cigarette smoking, this cause of fires is attributed to arching and overloading electrical equipment. Some goals of the educational groups are to increase knowledge of wattage and to use extension cords, electrical appliances, electrical space heaters, and electrical circuits. All appliances must also meet the minimum safety standards marketed by Underwriters Laboratories or other recognized testing facilities.

Preventive education on "what to do in case of a fire" emphasizes the use of a home fire drill (e.g., EDITH, Exit Drills In The Home). Exit drills in the home teach families how to exit from each area in case of fire, and designate a meeting area outside the home to ensure the safe exit of all family members from a fire scene. Fire departments, burn center personnel, and other interested community members should make sure neighborhood malls, schools, and fire stations display the "stop, drop, roll, and cool" method of extinguishing fires. People of all ages must be taught this behavior, along with how to exit a fire area to avoid burns and smoke inhalation. Heightened public awareness occurs during Fire Prevention Month as many communities have parades and displays of fire-fighting equipment and home safety devices.

Public education on the use of smoke detectors, kerosene heaters, wood-burning stoves, and other heating appliances is available through pamphlets found at the fire department, television public service announcements, or newspaper articles.

The Learn Not to Burn Foundation was established by the National Fire Protection Association in December 1986 to reduce fire-related deaths, injuries, and property loss. Educational activities of this group include television public service announcements, "Learn Not to Burn" curricula for elementary students, "Firesafety for the Rest of Your Life" curricula for high school students, and regional representatives for implementation of prevention projects. This group also sponsors the annual national fire safety poster contest.

Prevention in Young, Elderly, and Handicapped

Successful burn and fire safety programs for the young include puppet shows such as "Kids Around the Block" or the Sesame Street program. School programs are developed by concerned burn centers staffs and fire departments. Coloring books demonstrating fire-safe behavior instruct children as they play (Fig. 23–3). Many prevention programs, through continuing research to determine causes of burn injuries, are aimed at a burn-prone population. Other programs are developed for juvenile fire-setters. Dade county firefighters and nurses from the University of Miami/Jackson Memorial Burn Center utilize a computerized robot named "Snuffy" in a program aimed at elementary school children. Prevention programs have also been developed for use in maternity units to educate new mothers in safety hazards for infants and toddlers.

Prevention programs for the elderly are presented at community and senior citizen centers. Programs developed by fire departments or burn center staff are usually taught by a group of instructors from within the community. Identifying the elderly as being most at risk for burn injury, fire prevention efforts adapt their teaching to the potential hazards and safety needs of this community. Fabric ignition relating to fabric flammability spurred the federal government to pass the Flammable Fabrics Act.

Handicapped individuals are especially prone to major injury during a fire. Attention to fire safety programs for the disabled and use of smoke detectors or sprinkler

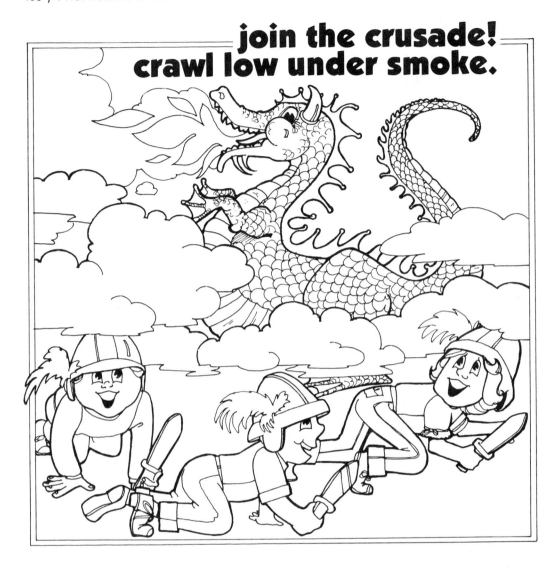

MESSAGE TO ADULTS: Sit down with your family today and make a step-by-step plan for an emergency fire escape.

FIGURE 23-3. Learn About Burns coloring book. (Courtesy of the Burn Foundation, Philadelphia, PA.)

systems in their living quarters increases their chances for survival. Disabled persons should be included in fire drills, fire training, and fire planning exercises. In 1978 a task force on "Life Safety and the Handicapped" assembled to discuss specific problems of disabled persons with respect to fire safety. The proceedings of this and further conferences held in 1980 and 1981 are available from the United States Government Printing Office as a reference when planning an educational curriculum for this group. Another publication, "Wheeling to Fire Safety," was developed by the Eastern Paralyzed Veterans Association and is available not only to the handicapped but also to fire departments, senior citizen groups, and fire-safety organizations. Fire safety for the hearing impaired has led to the development of flashing-light alarms and/or flashing exit signs to help them survive in a fire emergency.

cool a burn

Unscramble the words to find these places to cool a burn.
Write the words in the spaces.

KNSI

— — — —

ERRVI

— — — — —

SHOE

— — — —

WREHOS

— — — — — —

MESSAGE TO ADULTS: No matter how a burn happens, immediately apply cool water or cool compresses to stop the burning process. Call the doctor or emergency number for anything but a slight burn. Don't use ice, butter, or ointments.

FIGURE 23-3. *Continued.*

Many other groups develop fire-safety programs for communities. One very effective group consists of recovered burn patients. A recovered burn patient group in St. Louis developed the "Alarms for Life" prevention campaign, aimed at installation of smoke detectors within the community. Insurance companies, businesses, and foundations are also interested in burn prevention activities and will frequently provide support for fire-safety programs in industry as well as the community.

An example of a special campaign for a fire-safe product was printed in *The Courier-*

Journal in Louisville and *The Philadelphia Inquirer* in Philadelphia to heighten awareness of the dangers of disposable cigarette lighters. The crusade was started in order to develop stricter regulations on the design and manufacture of these lighters. Since 1979, 10 deaths have been attributed to the use of disposable lighters. The CPSC has received complaints about this type of lighter since 1974 and is the agency responsible for warning the public about safety issues with the use of this product. Due to public response shown by this campaign, companies have begun to correct the defective mechanism in the lighters and to create a more fire-safe lighter.

Fire safety and prevention is a responsibility of all members of society. The public consistently need to be made aware of burn hazards in order to decrease the number of annual burn-related injuries and preventable fire-related deaths. Again, *prevention of a burn injury is the best cure for this problem.*

REFERENCES

1. Fisher, SV and Helm, PA: Comprehensive Rehabilitation of Burns. Williams & Wilkins, Baltimore, 1984, p 7.
2. Artz, CP, Moncrief, JA, and Pruitt, BA: Burns: A Team Approach. WB Saunders, Philadelphia, 1979.
3. 1987 Burn Center Admission Data: Burn Causes and Treatment Costs. Burn Foundation, Philadelphia, 1988, p 1.
4. Mieszala, P: The fire and burn safety alliance. Journal of Burn Care and Rehabilitation 8:427, 1987.
5. Maley, MP and Achauer, BM: Prevention of tap water scald burns. Journal of Burn Care and Rehabilitation 8:62, 1987.
6. American Burn Association: Scald Burn Prevention. Burn Prevention Committee. p 2.
7. McGuire, A: The role of the American Burn Association on the campaign for firesafe cigarette: A ten-year progress report. Presented at an American Burn Association Meeting. Unpublished Material, 1989.
8. Horan, M: Electrical wires and electrical fires. Journal of Family Safety and Health 45:28–30, 1986.

BIBLIOGRAPHY

Burke, R: Ten deaths, hundreds of injuries tied to Bic lighters. *The Philadelphia Inquirer*, Philadelphia, April 12, 1987.
Cohen, H: Firesafety for the hearing impaired. Fire Journal Jan, 1982.
How to spot fire hazards. National Safety and Health News 133, 1988.
Kaplan, J: Hot tap water can cause fatal burns. Medical World News 18(10):20, 1977.
Katcher, MI: Scald burns from hot tap water. JAMA 246:1219, 1981.
Levin, BM and Nelson, H: Firesafety and Disabled Persons. Fire Journal Sept, 1981.
Maley, MP and Achauer, B: Prevention of tap water scalds. Journal of Burn Care and Rehabilitation 8:62–65, 1987.
McCraven, M: Nurse leads charge against lighter brigade. Courier-Journal, Louisville, May 9, 1986.
Meiszala, P: The fire and burn safety alliance. Journal of Burn Care and Rehabilitation 8:427–428, 1987.
Meiszala, P and Williams, JS: Project L.I.F.E.: Local Involvement in Fire Education. Journal of Burn Care and Rehabilitation 8:561–565, 1987.
Morrison, MIS, Horath, K, and Chase, C: Puppets for prevention: Playing safe is playing smart. Journal of Burn Care and Rehabilitation 9:650–651, 1988.
Off-The-Job: Can your family escape a fire. National Safety and Health News 133, 1986.
Powell, PA: Learn Not to Burn Foundation. Fire Journal 80(4):12, 1986.
Schmeer, S, Stern, N, and Monafo, WW: An effective burn prevention program initiated by a recovered burn group. Journal of Burn Care and Rehabilitation 7:535–536, 1986.
Tideiksaar, R: Environmental dangers to the elderly. Am, J Public Health 70:1218–1219, 1980.
Williams, RA: Keep 'em rolling. Firehouse Oct, 1982.

Chapter 24

JANET A. MARVIN

FUTURE OF BURN CARE AND BURN NURSING

HISTORY OF BURN CARE AND BURN NURSING

To be a prognosticator of the future, one must be an avid student of history. We can guess what the future holds only when we know what our past has been. Burn care today (i.e., the burn unit concept) began just over 50 years ago with the development of the first burn unit in Dzhandelidze, Russia, in 1938. The purpose for a burn unit was to place all burn patients on the same ward to facilitate the complex nursing management of these patients. Soon after World War II a number of burn units (both military and civilian) were formed in the United States and abroad. Today there are more than 200 such units in the United States and Canada.

In the mid 1960s two organizations were developed to promote the care of the burn-injured patient. The International Society for Burn Injuries had its inaugural meeting in 1965 in Edinburgh. The stated objectives of that association are

1. Dissemination of information about the current state of the science and prophylaxis of burns
2. Initiation and promotion of scientific, therapeutic, and sociological research on burns
3. Education in the treatment of all stages of burns, including first aid
4. Elaboration and improvement of methods that give higher percentage of cures in burn cases
5. Cooperation of surgeons and *nurses* in all countries with the problem of burn treatment[1]

In a similar fashion the American Burn Association (ABA) was founded in 1967 and emphasized the team approach to burn care, focusing on the areas of patient care, teaching, and research. Prevention was added as a specific area of interest in 1972.[2] The ABA adopted the "Specific Optimal Criteria for Hospital Resources for Care of Patients with Burn Injuries,"[3] in April 1976. These criteria were adopted also by the American College of Surgeons in 1977[4] and have served as the basis for many documents outlining the guidelines for burn care. Over the years, nurses, as well as other members of the burn team, have enriched the organization with their contributions. A joint committee of the ABA and the American Nurses Association (ANA) developed "Guidelines for Burn Nursing Practice"[5] based on the "Specific Optimal Criteria for Hospital Resources for Care of Patients with Burn Injury;"[3] the 1974 ANA "Standards of Medical Surgical Nursing Practice;"[6] the 1974 ANA "A Statement of the Scope of Medical Surgical Nursing Practice;"[7] and the 1980 ANA's "Nursing: A Social Policy Statement."[8] These guidelines were developed to provide a definition of burn nursing practice, to describe the professionals who function therein, delineate the dimensions of the practice, and describe the factors that influence it.

As defined in the "Guidelines for Burn Nursing Practice," burn nursing is defined as

> . . . the nursing care of adults and children with known or predicted physiologic, psychologic and social alterations related to burn injury and associated trauma. Nursing practice includes the care and treatment necessary to provide comfort; to prevent, detect, and treat illness; to promote restoration to the highest possible productive capacities; to assist individuals in the promotion and maintenance of health; and when necessary, to assist with a dignified death. Burn nursing practice encompasses patient assessment, planning, intervention, and evaluation. It takes into account the interrelatedness of physiologic, psychologic, and social components of the patient's response or adjustment to the burn injury.[5]

Within this document the dimension of practice is described according to three broad areas: patient care, research, and prevention of burn injury. The factors that influence practice are described as the patient's physiologic and psychologic alterations, administrative support, interdisciplinary practice arrangements, and professional autonomy in the practice setting. Crucial to these guidelines was the definition of the levels of nursing practice. It is recognized that nurses caring for burn patients may range from generalists, or nurses who are novices in burn care, to nurses with advanced education and experience in burn nursing. Through formal and informal training programs and experience, a nurse can become an expert clinician in the delivery of burn care. As Benner has so aptly described the levels of the learner in "From Novice to Expert,"[9] there are several levels of advancement to becoming an expert. In burn nursing these levels of clinical expertise are often described in the clinical ladders used in many institutional settings.[10]

CLINICAL NURSE SPECIALISTS

The most advanced level described in the guidelines is that of the clinical nurse specialist (CNS), a nurse having a master's degree in nursing. This nurse is considered to be the clinical expert and is expected to provide and manage the nursing care of the burn patient with highly complex or unusual nursing problems, to provide education, to develop standards of care and evaluate the quality of patient care, to participate in research, and to promote interdisciplinary collaboration in patient care problems. The CNS has been considered the key to improvement in the quality of nursing care delivered to burn patients.

Special education programs for the training of CNS in burn care began in 1972 at Texas Woman's University as a program developed jointly by Texas Woman's University and the University of Texas Southwestern Medical School through a grant from the Division of Nursing of the Department of Social and Health Services. Similar programs have since begun at the University of Cincinnati (1975), University of Washington (1976), and Widener College, Pennsylvania (1978). In addition to these special programs, many graduate programs in medical, surgical, physiologic, or critical care nursing offer the student the opportunity for advanced study in burn care.

History and Role Development of the CNS

Although the role of the CNS was first described by Reiter,[11] it actually had its genesis in the late-1940s and 1950s. Soon after World War II several factors favored advanced specialization:[12]

1. Depletion of experienced nurses on the homefront
2. Nurses returning from overseas being forced to enter clinical areas such as tuberculosis or psychiatric nursing for which they had no formal preparation
3. Funds available to veterans for postgraduate education
4. Other forces that included the rapid increase in knowledge, development of new technology, and increased complexity of the health care system.

A major problem facing nursing then, as now, is how to enable nurses to "really practice nursing." Because the more lucrative areas of nursing practice were in administration and education, more and more nurses were leaving the bedside. This left the inexperienced, task-oriented nurse at the bedside with little help in learning to make appropriate clinical decisions based on scientific knowledge, principles, and experience.

Although the concept of the clinical specialist role was envisioned as early as the 1940s, programs to prepare nurses to function in these roles were not developed until the 1950s. This was followed in the late-1950s by the implementation of these roles in various health care settings. Even by 1970, Edith Lewis introduced her book on the CNS with the statement: "No one is yet quite sure of exactly *who* the CNS is; *how* she should be prepared; or *what* and *how* she fits into the institutional and agency structure."[13] In 1973, Kinsella[13a] noted that the public was dissatisfied with the technical approach to illness care and predicted that if nurses did not seize the opportunity to improve health care, society would mandate new functionaries to replace them. By 1981, 81 programs in the United States offered clinical specialty preparation.[14]

As with any new role, the development of that role requires a period of adjustment, before the role becomes well defined. According to Montemuro, a survey of nursing literature from 1965 to 1980 described the CNS as having 17 different functions or responsibilities.[12] More recently the functions of the CNS are more consistently defined as expert practitioner, consultant, educator, and researcher. Although the role of expert practitioner is the backbone of clinical specialization, CNSs are finding that their role continues to evolve in this area so that they are becoming case managers for a number of complex patients instead of providing direct care to a few patients. In this way the CNS can guide the care of several nurses in providing a higher quality of care. What with the growing nursing shortage of the 1980s, the lack of qualified nurses at the bedside is rapidly reaching catastrophic proportions. The US Department of Health and Human Services (DHHS) predicts a 50 percent undersupply of BSN-prepared nurses by 1990 and a 65 percent oversupply of associate degree– and diploma-prepared nurses.[15] Additionally, the DHHS projects a demand for 500,000 master's degree–prepared nurses by the year 2000, whereas the current supply is about 170,000.[16] What does this mean to nursing and especially to burn nursing? Fraliac suggests that the paramount question is "how to provide high-quality nursing care with fewer available RNs?" She further suggests that, "If we do not design those systems, others will design them for us."[17] Thus, if we are to provide high-quality burn care, what will be the role of the CNS, and how will this role be integrated into a system of care? The CNS in the role of case manager allows the CNS to use his or her expertise and knowledge to direct the care given by others through consultation, collaboration, teaching, and research. This model has the potential to give close clinical supervision to the less experienced nurse and allow the registered nurse to gain the needed level of expertise over time. Holt noted that "Nurses are bombarded with expectations to be super humans."[18] She suggests that

TABLE 24–1. Developmental Stages of Clinical Nurse Specialist Role

Stages and Timeframe	Direct Caregiver	Teacher	Consultant	Researcher	Change Agent	Primary Focus of Development	Sphere of Influence
Stage I Pre-CNS BSN graduate (1–2 yr)	Staff nurse-generalist All conditions ages, stages, settings	Teach individual patient and family		Read regularly to keep current in practice Read research reports critically	Active membership in professional organizations ANA, NLN, and so on	Develop skill and confidence in direct patient care Integration of theory and practice	Individual patient and families Own case load
Stage II BSN (3–4 yr) Study for MS	Leadership role in patient care (e.g., primary nurse, team leader)	Group teaching Develop teaching materials for patients	Participate in research directed by others	Use research findings in own practice Identify clinical problems needing research	Present papers or publish on patient care (e.g., case study)	Focus on still developing skill as direct caregiver	Local service unit Local chapter of professional organization
Stage III MSN graduate CNS (1–2 yr)	Beginning CNS Direct care to individual patients Develop own conceptual framework for care of specialty patients	Role-model direct patient care Teach patient and families individually or group	Assist individual nursing staff in giving care to specialty patients Develop role informally	Use research findings in own practice Identify clinical problems needing research	Read comprehensively and regularly in specialty area Attend meetings, workshops, and the like Communicate new knowledge and others' research findings to colleagues	Focus on improving care of individual patients Has knowledge and clinical competence in specialty Develop confidence and expertise in clinical area	Stay visible in service agency and professional organization Local service unit Local chapter professional organization

| Stage IV 3–4 yr post-MS | Planning/giving/evaluating care of groups of specialty patients Test out own conceptual framework of care on groups of patients | Systematically plan/teach care of patients within specialty area Use conceptual framework as basis for teaching | Serve as resource to nurses and other disciplines on specialty patients | Set up small research studies to address clinical nursing problems. | Keep self and others current on all aspects of care to specialty patients Communicate results of own studies to colleagues Publish, give papers locally and regionally on nursing care of specialty patients Work as participant in change | Focus on improving care to groups of specialty patients via teacher and researcher role while maintaining skill as individual patient care giver | Expand contact areas to state and regional Other CNSs in specialty area Keep active in nursing community Develop contacts in interdisciplinary arena |

Reprinted with permission from Holt, FM: Executive Practice Role Editorial. Clinical Nurse Specialist 1(3):117–118, 1987. Copyright by Williams & Wilkins, 1987.

TABLE 24-2. US Burn Care Facilities for Clinical Nurse Specialists

	Facilities		No. of CNSs Needed
143	facilities with <20 beds	=	143
24	facilities with >20 beds	=	48
33	facilities with no specific burn unit of which 17 had 6 or more beds	=	17
	Total		208

it takes time for the CNS to evolve into the role and that this can best be conceptualized in six stages (Table 24-1).[18] As noted, the first two stages are pre-master's degree and are necessary for the nurse to move from the novice or generalist to a leadership role in which an area of expertise has begun to be defined. This pre-master's degree experience is invaluable to preparation of the graduate-level CNS. Likewise, the post-master's degree experience must be viewed as a stepwise progression to attaining a high level of expertise in the role. This model fits well with the levels of nursing practice as defined in the "Guidelines for Burn Nursing Practice" of 1982.

Upon reflecting on the predictions of the DHHS, one might ask how burn nursing is doing in the development of nurses at this advanced level. A review of the nursing membership of the ABA in 1986 shows that there were 64 nurses with master's and doctorate degrees. Although not all of these nurses function as a CNS, many are continuing to provide nursing leadership through administration and educational activities. If one asked how many CNSs are needed to provide quality burn care, one only has to look at the number of burn units and the number of beds within those units. Based on a ratio of one CNS to 10 to 15 patients in a case manager type of role, all burn units with less than 20 beds would need at least one CNS and those with more than 20 beds (assuming at least an 80 percent occupancy rate) would need more than one CNS (Table 24-2). Thus, by comparing the number of nurses with advanced preparation in the field of burn care (as evidenced by ABA membership) and the number of positions required to meet the 1 to 10 or 1 to 15 ratio, we can see that more than 200 CNSs are currently needed.

NURSING RESEARCH

One of the prescribed roles of the nurse with an advanced degree is that of researcher. Research is the backbone of any body of knowledge and serves as a framework for our professional practice. As Bunge stated in 1958, "Research is every professional nurse's business."[19] In looking to the future of research in burn nursing, it might be asked, "Where have we been and where are we going?" It is difficult to look back at our research record before the inception of the ABA because whatever nursing research was done in burn care was published in a variety of journals. Since the inception of the ABA in 1967, a review of the programs at the annual meetings may serve as a record of reported research. Between the years 1967 and 1980 there were less than 100 papers presented by nurses, most of which were not data based. Table 24-3 depicts the number of papers presented at the ABA annual from 1980-1988. During those years almost 200 papers have been presented by nurses. As noted in the table, about 15 percent of all papers presented over the last nine years have been by nurses. If one looks at the number of papers presented by nurses for the years 1980 through 1983, the number of papers actually reporting research findings averaged 52 percent. More re-

TABLE 24-3. ABA Papers Presented 1980-1988

Year	Total	No. Nursing	Percent Nursing†	No. With Data	Percent With Data
1980	106	15	14	10	66
1981	116	21	18	11	52
1982	105	15	14	8	53
1983	139	23	17	9	39
1984	165	27	16	19	70
1985	168	15	9	13	86
1986	170	21	12	17	81
1987	179	28	16	22	78
1988	184	31	17	23	74

*Nurse as first author.
†Percent of total papers presented by nurses.

cently (1984 to 1988) this number has increased to 78 percent. Likewise, the average number of papers presented in the two time periods has increased from a mean of 18 to a mean of 24 annually. This would suggest that, as a professional group, burn nurses are engaged in or at least reporting the results of more research studies.

Another important question to ask about burn nursing research is, "in what areas are nurses doing research?" Table 24-4 lists the number of papers in several major areas by year. It is of interest to note that the areas of the most papers presented are physiologic response of the patient and prevention. Germane to the area of direct patient care are the first four categories listed in the table. Approximately 50 percent of the papers relate directly to patient care; another 20 percent concern prevention, which leaves about 30 percent of the articles to deal with the nurse, nursing education, and administrative issues.

In what other way can we measure our progress in burn nursing research? In 1983 the American Association of Critical Care Nurses (AACN) published the results of their Delphi study.[20] In this study 67 topics were identified as areas in which further research is needed within critical care nursing. Table 24-5 lists the top 20 priorities for critical care nursing research and the number of papers presented by nurses at ABA meetings

TABLE 24-4. Areas of Nursing Papers Presented

Area	1980	1981	1982	1983	1984	1985	1986	1987	1988	Total
Patient (Psych, Rehab, Educ)	1	6	4	5	2	1	0	2	5	26
Patient (Pain)	3	2	2	4	3	0	4	3	1	22
Patient (Physio, Nutrition)	5	4	3	2	6	3	5	6	10	44
Infection Control	1	0	0	1	1	1	1	3	2	10
Audit/Classification/ Cost	0	2	0	1	2	2	4	4	0	15
Nurse Education	3	1	0	3	1	2	1	0	0	11
Nurse Staffing/Stress	0	2	3	1	5	0	1	0	3	15
Prevention	0	3	2	4	7	6	4	9	7	42
Miscellaneous	2	1	1	2	0	0	1	1	3	11
Totals	15	21	15	23	27	15	21	28	31	206

TABLE 24-5. Influence of AACN Study Priorities in Critical Care Research

Top Priorities	1980-1983	1984-1988
1. Sleep/rest	0	2
2. "Burnout"	0	0
3. Cost-effective orientation	4	2
4. Increased ICP	0	0
5. Ventilator weaning	0	0
6. Patient classification	0	4
7. Incentive/clinical ladder	1	0
8. Decreased nurse stress	1	3
9. Impaired communication	1	0
10. Position/CV and pulmonary function	0	0
11. Staffing patterns	5	4
12. Prevention of infection/invasive lines	1	4
13. PEEP/suctioning	1	0
14. Incorporation of research findings into nurse practice	0	0
15. Pain relief	11	11
16. Staff development/competence retention	0	4
17. Quality of care/LPNs and technicians	0	1
18. Impact of CNS on quality of care	0	0
19. Decreasing patient stress	0	6
20. Visiting policy on patient and family stress	1	1
Total Studies (percent of all nursing papers presented)	26(35)	42(34)

since 1980 on these topics. The papers presented are categorized as before 1983 and after 1983 to see if this list of priorities may have influenced burn nursing research. As noted on the table, the actual number of papers presented in these 20 priority areas divided by the total number of papers presented shows that the percentage of papers addressing these priority areas has not changed. One might then ask: "Are the priorities for burn nursing research the same as for critical care?" Yet when one looks at the categories chosen for research, nurses have chosen to present papers in 14 of the 20 top priority categories. Perhaps burn nurses need to do a similar Delphi study to assess the priorities within burn care.

Future of Burn Nursing Research

Facilitation of research in burn nursing is the key to our future. We need to have a plan, to decide what needs to be researched, to develop resources for doing research, and to encourage collaborative efforts to accomplish our research goals. When we ask what needs to be researched or what our priorities are, the world is our oyster. As noted in the AACN Delphi study there are still many unanswered questions that apply to burn nursing (Table 24-6). These 32 areas chosen from the 69 priorities of the AACN study is at least a starting place for burn nursing research. These include both areas related to direct patient care and studies that deal with the administrative or educational aspects of the delivery of care.

For another organizing framework for burn nursing research, one might look to relevant nursing diagnoses. Table 24-7 lists a number of nursing diagnoses pertinent to the patient with a burn injury. By using these diagnoses as the organizing framework we can pose many questions at varying levels of knowledge generation. For example, we might ask the simple question: How frequently are any one of these diagnoses pertinent to the burn patients? Or we may wish to go further and ask questions about nursing

TABLE 24-6. 32 Areas of Research from AACN Study With Particular Relevance to Burn Nursing

1. What are the most effective ways of promoting optimum sleep-rest and preventing sleep deprivation?
2. What measures can be taken to prevent or lessen burnout?
3. What type of orientation program is most effective in terms of cost, safety, and retention?
4. What classification systems are most valid, reliable, and sensitive in determining staff ratios?
5. What incentives will retain "burn" nurses?
6. What are effective ways to reduce staff stress?
7. What are the most effective staffing patterns?
8. What measures are most effective in preventing infections in invasive lines?
9. What are the most effective measures in relieving pain in critically ill patients?
10. What is the relationship between staff development and competency or retention?
11. What methods for developing and implementing interdisciplinary teams are most effective in reducing conflict and developing mutual respect and support?
12. What is the impact of increased technology on the reactions of patients and families and on the roles and philosophy of care of the staff?
13. How can nurses utilize families and/or significant others of critically ill patients to reduce stress (of nurses, families, and the patients) and benefits the patient?
14. What techniques are most effective in preventing infections in monitoring lines with stopcocks?
15. What is the effect of early initiation of selected nursing measures (e.g., passive range of motion, body positioning, sleep/rest periods) on successful rehabilitation of trauma patients?
16. What is the effect of primary nursing on the anxiety levels of critically ill patients and their families and on ultimate patient recovery?
17. What are the effects of various methods of administration of nutritional alimentation (e.g., route, rate, temperature) on absorption, gastrointestinal motility, patient comfort, and prevention of complications?
18. What nursing interventions are effecting in helping patients maintain basic stress reduction techniques?
19. Does implementing primary nursing in a critical care setting increase nurses' job satisfaction and decrease burnout?
20. What are the most effective methods (e.g., exercises, TED stockings) of preventing circulatory complications in patients?
21. What are effective methods of maintaining good lip and mucosal integrity in patients with prolonged tubation?
22. Which nursing interventions are most effective in increasing a sense of and control in the critically ill patient?
23. What are some of the clinical indices differentiating pain and anxiety in various types of critically ill patients?
24. Which indicators most accurately reflect the nutritional status of the critically patient?
25. What nursing interventions are most effective in assisting the patient with a long-term disfiguring injury to adjust to his or her altered self-image
26. What position(s) is (are) most effective in preventing aspiration in patients with feeding tubes?
27. What criteria are most effective in identifying patients at risk for developing psychosis in critical care areas?
28. What combination of content and teaching method is most effective in preparing a severely burned patient to return to the community?
29. How do the lay public, hospital administrators, physicians, and other nursing disciplines view the critical care nurse?
30. What factors are associated with attracting nurses to critical care?
31. What are the most effective methods of managing critically ill patients with diarrhea?
32. What personality characteristics are associated with success in critical care nursing?

therapies used to treat these patient problems: Do the therapies work? What are the advantages or disadvantages of one therapy versus another? How can we prevent a specific potential problem? Thus, using nursing diagnoses as the framework for research allows one to direct research more specifically to patient care. This is not to say that research in education or administration is not important; quite the contrary is true, we

TABLE 24-7. Areas of Future Research by Nursing Diagnosis

Actual or potential fluid volume deficit
Potential for relative fluid volume excess
Potential fluid and electrolyte imbalance
    Hyponatremia
    Hypernatremia
    Hyperkalemia
    Hypokalemia
Potential for impaired gas exchange
Potential for infection
Potential alteration in tissue perfusion
Deficit in nutrition related to hypermetabolism
Alterations in comfort (pain)
Decreased mobility and potential joint contraction
Actual or potential alterations in sensory perception or disturbances in sleep patterns
Potential self-care deficits related to cognitive impairment, lack of motivation, or physical limitations
Fear, anticipatory grieving, depression, and social isolation
Decreased activity tolerance
Potential impaired skin integrity (post-healing)
Potential noncompliance/potential sexual dysfunction

still need research in these areas as well. Without knowing what causes or reduces stress for the caregiver, how many nurses we need or do not need, or how best to provide the nurse with the knowledge necessary to deliver quality care, it will be difficult to define the therapeutic value of nursing to patient care. One area of nursing that has generally escaped in-depth study is the therapeutic use of "the nurse" or "therapeutic use of self." It is not uncommon to hear patients, colleagues, and even other nurses comment that when Nurse X is here, "everything will go well." What does this nurse do that is different from the others? How does this nurse structure patient-staff interactions to improve the perceived quality of care? Is this "therapeutic use of self?"

A second step in a plan for burn nursing research is the development of resources or at least to seek out existing resources. Depending on the scope of the specific research project, there are many avenues open to the nurse researcher. Certainly on the national level, the Center for Nursing Research at the National Institutes of Health, the American Nurses Foundation, Sigma Theta Tau, AACN, and private organizations such as the Robert Wood Johnson foundation exemplify sources of financial support for major research projects. Even within the ABA the International Association of Fire Fighters Burn Foundation is a potential source of money. Other regional and local foundations should also be considered. In addition to monetary resources needed to accomplish a research project, help with study design, statistical consulting, and computer access are also important—hence the need for collaboration.

Collaboration with other professionals, nursing or non-nursing, is another step in a research plan. This is especially true for the nondoctorally prepared researcher. Establishing the appropriate collaborative arrangements early with other nurses, statisticians, computer analysts, physicians, and others can be invaluable in developing an appropriate study design and to gain access to patients, computers, and laboratory space to carry out a research project.

So where do we go from here? As stated by Ada M. Lindsey in 1984, "Nursing practice must be influenced and directed by empirical findings rather than by practice, beliefs and intuitions."[21] Herein lies the importance of nursing research to our future and a challenge to nurses involved in burn care. Only through research in patient care issues and the delivery of quality of care will we see further improvements in burn care.

REFERENCES

1. International Society for Burn Injuries: Constitution. Edinburgh, adopted Sept 1982, Rev Feb 1986.
2. MacMillan, BG: The development of burn care facilities. In Boswick, JA (ed): The Art and Science of Burn Care. Aspen Publications, Rockville, MD, 1987, p 19.
3. American Burn Association: Specific Optional Criteria for Hospital Resources for Care of Patients with Burn Injuries. April 1976.
4. Total care for burn patients. Bull Am Coll Surg 62:6, 1977.
5. American Burn Association: Guidelines for burn nursing practice. Boston, Mass, May 1982.
6. American Nurses Association, Division of Medical Surgical Nursing Practice: Standards of medical surgical nursing practice. ANA, Kansas City, MO, 1974.
7. American Nurses Association, Division of Medical Surgical Nursing Practice: A statement of the scope of medical surgical nursing practice. ANA, Kansas City, MO, 1974.
8. American Nurses Association: Nursing: A social policy statement. ANA, Kansas City, MO 1980.
9. Benner, P: From Novice to Expert: Power and Excellence in Clinical Nursing Practice. Addison Wesley, Menlo Park, CA, 1984.
10. Kravitz, M, Workman, J, and Warden, GD: Planning and implementation of career ladder for burn nurses. Presented at the 11th Annual Meeting of the American Burn Association, New Orleans, March 15–17, 1979.
11. Reiter, F: The nurse clinician. Am J Nurs 66:274, 1966.
12. Montemuro, MA: The evolution of the clinical nurse specialist: Response to the challenge of professional nursing practice. Clinical Nurse Specialist 1(3):106, 1987.
13. Lewis, EP (ed): The clinical nurse specialist. American Journal of Nursing, Educational Services Division, New York, 1970.
13a. Kinsella, CR: Who is the clinical nurse specialist? Hospitals 47:72–80, 1973.
14. Feild, L: Current trends in education and implications for the future. In Hamric, A and Spross, J (eds): The Clinical Nurse Specialist in Theory and Practice. Grune and Stratton, New York: 1983, p 237.
15. The new nursing shortage: Is it here to stay? California Nurse 00:8, 1987.
16. Testimony presented on appropriations for nursing education and research (1987). Capital Update 5:5, 1987.
17. Fraliac, MF: Again so soon? Thoughts on the nurse shortage. Nursing and Health Care 8:209, 1987.
18. Holt, FM: Executive practices. Clinical Nurse Specialist 1(3):116, 1987.
19. Bunge, HL: Research is every professional nurse's business. Am J Nurs 58:816, 1958.
20. Lewandowski, LA and Kositsky, AM: Research priorities for critical care nursing: A study by the American Association of Critical Care Nurses. Heart Lung 12(1):35, 1983.
21. Lindsey, AM: Research for clinical practice: Physiological phenomena. Heart Lung 13(5):496, 1984.

INDEX

A page # followed by an "F" indicates a figure; A "T" following a page # indicates a table